Drug Calculations for Nurses

A step-by-step approach

SECOND EDITION

Robert Lapham BPharm Clin Dip Pharm MRPharmS

Clinical Pharmacist, Sunderland Royal Hospital, City Hospitals
Sunderland NHS Trust, UK

Heather Agar RGN BSc (Hons)

Rheumatology Specialist Nurse, Northumbria Healthcare
NHS Trust, UK.

Hodder Arnold

A MEMBER OF THE HODDER HEADLINE GROUP

First published in Great Britain in 2003 by
Hodder Arnold, a member of the Hodder Headline Group,
338 Euston Road, London NW1 3BH

http://www.hoddereducation.co.uk

Distributed in the United States of America by
Oxford University Press Inc.,
198 Madison Avenue, New York, NY10016
Oxford is a registered trademark of Oxford University Press

Whilst the advice and information in this book are believed to be true and
accurate at the date of going to press, neither the author[s] nor the publisher can
accept any legal responsibility or liability for any errors or omissions that may be
made. In particular (but without limiting the generality of the preceding
disclaimer) every effort has been made to check drug dosages; however it is still
possible that errors have been missed. Furthermore, dosage schedules are
constantly being revised and new side-effects recognized. For these reasons the
reader is strongly urged to consult the drug companies' printed instructions
before administering any of the drugs recommended in this book.

British Library Cataloguing in Publication Data
A catalogue record for this book is available from the British Library

Library of Congress Cataloging-in-Publication Data
A catalog record for this book is available from the Library of Congress

ISBN-10   0 340 81028 9
ISBN-13   978 0 340 81028 6

5 6 7 8 9 10

Commissioning Editor: Georgina Bentliff
Development Editor: Heather Smith
Project Editor: Anke Ueberberg
Production Controller: Lindsay Smith
Cover Design: Amina Dudhia

Typeset in 9.5/11 Minion by Tech-Set Ltd, Gateshead
Printed and bound in Spain

Hodder Headline's policy is to use papers that are natural, renewable and
recyclable products and made from wood grown in sustainable forests. The
logging and manufacturing processes are expected to conform to the
environmental regulations of the country of origin.

What do you think about this book? Or any other Hodder Arnold title?
Please send your comments to **www.hoddereducation.co.uk**

Contents

Preface

Drug treatments given to patients in hospital are becoming increasingly complex. Sometimes, these treatment regimes involve potent and, at times, new and novel drugs. Many of these drugs are toxic, possibly even fatal if administered incorrectly or in overdose. It is therefore very important to be able to carry out drug calculations correctly to avoid putting the patient at risk.

In current nursing practice, the need to calculate drug dosages is not uncommon. These calculations have to be performed competently and accurately, so the nurse is not put at risk, and, more importantly, to protect the patient. This book aims to provide an aid to the basics of mathematics and drug calculations. It is intended to be of use to all nurses of all grades and specialities, and to be a handy reference for use on the ward.

The concept of this book arose from nurses themselves; a frequently asked question was: 'Can you help me with drug calculations?' Consequently, we wrote a small booklet to help nurses with their drug calculations, particularly those studying for their IV certificate. This was very well received, and copies were being produced from original copies, indicating the need for such help and a book like this. The contents of the book were determined by means of a questionnaire sent to nurses, asking them what they would like to see featured in a drug calculations book. As a result, this book was written and, hopefully, covers the topics that nurses would like to see.

Although, this book was primarily written with nurses in mind, others who use drug calculations in their work may also use it. Some topics have been dealt with in greater detail for this reason, e.g. moles and millimoles. So this book can be used by anyone who wishes to improve their skills in drug calculations, or to use it as a refresher course.

How to use this book

This book is designed to be used for self-study.

Before you start, you should attempt the pre-test to assess your current ability in carrying out drug calculations. After completing the book, repeat the same test and compare the two scores to see if you have made any improvement.

To attain maximum benefit from the book, start at the beginning and work through one chapter at a time, as subsequent chapters increase in difficulty. For each chapter attempted, make sure you understand it fully and can answer the problems confidently before moving on to the next chapter.

Alternatively, if you wish to skip quickly through any chapter, you can refer to the 'Key points' at the end of each chapter.

MINIMIZING ERRORS

- Write out the calculation clearly. It is all too easy to end up reading from the wrong line.
- If you are copying formulas from a reference source, double-check what you have written down.
- Write down every step.
- Do not take short cuts; you are more likely to make a mistake.
- Try not to be totally dependent on your calculator. Have an approximate idea of what the answer should be. Then, if you happen to hit the wrong button on the calculator you are more likely to be aware that an error has been made.
- Finally, always double-check your calculation. There is frequently more than one way of doing a calculation, so if you get the same answer by two different methods the chances are that your answer will be correct. Alternatively, try working it in reverse and see if you get the numbers you started with.

> **Remember**
> **If you are in any doubt about a calculation you are asked to do on the ward, stop and get help.**

Drug names

In the past, the British Approved Name (BAN) was used for drugs in the UK. A European Directive (92/27/ECC) now requires the use of the Recommended International Non-proprietary Name (rINN) for medicinal substances. In most cases, the BAN and the rINN are identical. Where the two differ, the BAN has been modified to the new rINN; for example, amoxicillin instead of amoxycillin.

In cases where a change of name is considered to pose a high potential risk to patients, both names will be required to appear on labels and leaflets in the UK for a transitional period of 5 years.

For a full list of all the name changes, see the current edition of the *British National Formulary* (BNF). Affected drugs are referred to in this book by their new name (rINN) followed by their old name (BAN) in brackets:

New name (rINN)	Old name (BAN)
aciclovir	acyclovir
epinephrine	adrenaline*
amoxicillin	amoxycillin
furosemide	frusemide
lidocaine	lignocaine
levothyroxine	thyroxine

* In this case the old BAN will continue be used with the new rINN in brackets, i.e. adrenaline (epinephrine).

Pre-test

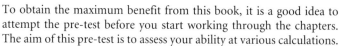

To obtain the maximum benefit from this book, it is a good idea to attempt the pre-test before you start working through the chapters. The aim of this pre-test is to assess your ability at various calculations.

The pre-test is divided into several sections that correspond to each chapter in the book, and the questions try to reflect the topics covered by each chapter. You don't have to attempt every section, only the ones that you feel are relevant to you. Answering the questions will help you identify particular calculations you have difficulty with.

You can use calculators or anything else you find useful to answer the questions, but it is best to complete the pre-test on your own, as it is **your** ability that is being assessed and not someone else's.

Don't worry if you can't answer all of the questions. As stated before, the aim is to help you to identify areas of weakness. Once again, you don't have to complete every section of the pre-test, just the ones you want to test your ability on.

Once you have completed the pre-test and checked your answers, you can start using the book. Concentrate particularly on the areas you are weak on and, if necessary, miss out the chapters you are confident with.

It is up to you as how you use this book, but hopefully the pre-test will help you to identify areas you need to concentrate on if you wish.

BASICS

The aim of this section is to test your ability on basic principles such as fractions, decimals, powers and using calculators before you start any drug calculations.

FRACTIONS

Solve the following, leaving your answer as a fraction:

1 $\dfrac{5}{9} \times \dfrac{3}{7}$

2 $\dfrac{3}{4} \div \dfrac{9}{16}$

Convert to a decimal:

3 $\dfrac{2}{5}$

DECIMALS

Solve the following:

4 0.25×0.45 **5** $3.5 \div 0.2$

6 1.38×100 **7** $25.64 \div 1,000$

Convert the following to a fraction:

8 1.2

ROMAN NUMERALS

Write the following as ordinary (Arabic) numbers:

9 VII   **10** IX

POWERS

Convert the following to a proper number:

11 3×10^5

Convert the following number to a power of 10:

12 $5,000,000$

UNITS AND EQUIVALENCES

This section is designed to test your knowledge on units normally used in clinical medicine, and how to convert from one unit to another. It is important that you can convert units easily, as this is the basis for most drug calculations.

Convert the following:

UNITS OF WEIGHT

1 0.0625 milligrams (mg) to micrograms (mcg)

2 600 grams (g) to kilograms (kg)

3 50 nanograms (ng) to micrograms (mcg)

UNITS OF VOLUME

4 0.15 litres (L) to millilitres (mL)

UNITS OF AMOUNT OF SUBSTANCE

Usually describes the amount of electrolytes, as in an infusion (see Chapter 5, Moles and millimoles, for a full explanation).

5 0.36 moles (mol) to millimoles (mmol)

DOSAGE CALCULATIONS

These are the type of calculations you will be doing every day on the ward.

CALCULATING THE NUMBER OF TABLETS OR CAPSULES REQUIRED

The strength of the tablets or capsules you have available does not always correspond to the dose required. Therefore you have to calculate the number of tablets or capsules needed.

1 The dose prescribed is furosemide (frusemide) 120 mg. You have 40 mg tablets available. How many tablets do you need?

DRUG DOSAGE

Sometimes the dose is given on a body weight basis, or in terms of body surface area. The following tests your ability at calculating doses on these parameters.

Work out the dose required for the following:

2 Dose = 0.5 mg/kg   Weight = 64 kg
3 Dose = 3 micrograms/kg/min   Weight = 73 kg
4 Dose = 1.5 mg/m^2 surface area = 1.55 m^2

CALCULATING DOSAGES

Calculate how much you need for the following dosages:

5 You have aminophylline injection 250 mg in 10 mL

  Amount required = 350 mg

6 You have digoxin injection 500 micrograms/2 mL

  Amount required = 0.75 mg

7 You have morphine sulphate elixir 10 mg in 5 mL

  Amount required = 15 mg

8 You have gentamicin injection 40 mg/mL, 2 mL ampoules

  Amount required = 4 mg/kg for a 74kg patient.

How many ampoules?

PERCENT AND PERCENTAGES

This section is designed to see if you understand the concept of percent and percentages.

1 How much is 28% of 250 g?
2 What percentage is 160 g of 400 g?

MOLES AND MILLIMOLES

This section is designed to see if you understand the concept of millimoles. Millimoles are used to describe the 'amount of substance', and are usually the units for body electrolytes, (e.g. sodium 138 mmol/L).

1 Approximately how many millimoles of sodium are there in a 10 mL ampoule of sodium chloride 30% injection? (Molecular weight of sodium chloride = 58.5.)

DRUG STRENGTHS OR CONCENTRATIONS

This section is designed to see if you understand the various ways in which drug strengths can be expressed.

PERCENTAGE CONCENTRATION

1 How much sodium (in grams) is there in a 500 mL infusion of sodium chloride 0.9%?
2 You need to add 2 g of potassium chloride to 1 litre of sodium chloride 0.9% infusion. You have 10 mL ampoules of 20% potassium chloride. What volume of potassium chloride do you need to draw up?

CONCENTRATIONS IN MG/ML

3 What is the concentration (in mg/mL) of an 8.4% sodium bicarbonate infusion?

CONCENTRATIONS OR RATIO STRENGTHS – '1 IN … '

4 You have a 10 mL ampoule of adrenaline (epinephrine) 1 in 10,000. How much adrenaline (epinephrine) – in milligrams – does the ampoule contain?

DRUGS EXPRESSED IN UNITS

5 You need to give an infusion of heparin containing 29,000 units over 24 hours. You have ampoules of heparin containing 25,000 units/mL and 5000 units/mL. How much of each ampoule do you need to draw up?

MOLARITY

6 How many grams of sodium chloride is required to make 200 mL of an 0.5 M solution? (Molecular weight of sodium chloride = 58.5.)

INFUSION RATE CALCULATIONS

This section tests your knowledge of various infusion rate calculations. It is designed to see if you know the different drop factors for different giving sets and fluids, as well as being able to convert volumes to drops and vice versa.

CALCULATION OF DRIP RATES

1 What is the rate required to give 500 mL of sodium chloride 0.9% infusion over 6 hours using a standard giving set?

2 What is the rate required to give 1 unit of blood (500 mL) over 8 hours using a standard giving set?

3 You are asked to give a 250 mL infusion to a child over 8 hours. What rate should the infusion run using a microdrop (paediatric) giving set?

CONVERSION OF INFUSION RATES (ML/HOUR) TO DROPS/MIN

Sometimes, in order to give an infusion, you may need to convert the rate from mL/hour to drops/min.

4 You are asked to give a 1 litre infusion of sodium chloride 0.9% at a rate of 125 mL/hour using a standard giving set. What is the rate in drops/min?

CONVERSION OF DOSAGES TO ML/HOUR

Sometimes it may be necessary to convert a dose (mg/min) to an infusion rate (mL/hour).

5 You are asked to give 500 mL of doxapram 0.2% infusion at a rate of 3 mg/min using an infusion pump. What is the rate in mL/hour?

CONVERSION OF ML/HOUR TO MICROGRAMS/KG/MINUTE OR MG/MIN

With infusion pumps, it may be necessary to convert from mL/hour to micrograms/kg/minute or mg/min in order to check the rate at which the pump is set.

6 An infusion pump containing 50 mg of sodium nitroprusside in 50 mL is running at a rate of 13 mL/hour. The dose wanted is 3 micrograms/kg/minute and the patient's weight is 72 kg. Is the pump rate correct?

CALCULATION OF LENGTH OF TIME OF INFUSIONS

Sometimes it may be necessary to calculate the number of hours an infusion should run at a specified rate, e.g. to check the drip rates.

7 You have a 250 mL infusion at a rate of 21 drops/min using a standard giving set. Approximately how long will the infusion run?

PAEDIATRIC CALCULATIONS

The principles covered by the other sections apply to paediatric calculations. However, doses are usually based on a 'mg/kg' basis, so it is important that you can calculate doses on this basis.

Other factors to take into account are displacement volumes for antibiotic injections, body surface area nomograms, and how to interpret paediatric dosage books. See Chapter 9, Paediatric dosage calculations, for a fuller explanation.

1 You need to give trimethoprim to a 7-year-old child weighing 23 kg at a dose of 4 mg/kg twice a day. Trimethoprim suspension comes as a 50 mg in 5 mL suspension. How much do you need for each dose?

2 You need to give benzylpenicillin at a dose of 25 mg/kg four times a day to a 6-month-old baby weighing 8 kg. How much do you need to draw up for each dose assuming each 600 mg vial is to be reconstituted to 5 mL?

ANSWERS

BASICS

Fractions

1 $\dfrac{5}{21}$ **2** $\dfrac{4}{3}$ **3** 0.4

Decimals

4 0.1125   **5** 17.5   **6** 138

7 0.02564   **8** $\dfrac{6}{5}$

Roman numerals

9 7   **10** 9

Powers

11 300,000   **12** 5×10^6

UNITS AND EQUIVALENCES

Units of weight

1 62.5 micrograms   **2** 0.6 kilograms (kg)
3 0.05 micrograms

Units of volume

4 150 millilitres (mL)

Units of amount of substance

5 360 millimoles

DOSAGE CALCULATIONS

Calculating the number of tablets or capsules required

1 Three furosemide (frusemide) 40 mg tablets

Drug dosage

2 32 mg   **3** 219 micrograms/min
4 2.325 mg

Calculating dosages

5 14 mL   **6** 3 mL
7 7.5 mL   **8** 4 ampoules

PERCENT AND PERCENTAGES

1 70 g   **2** 40%

MOLES AND MILLIMOLES

1 51.3 mmol (rounded to 51 mmol)

Sometimes it is necessary to adjust the dose by rounding like this for
ease of calculation and administration, as long as the adjustment is not
so much that it makes a large difference in the dose.

DRUG STRENGTHS OR CONCENTRATIONS

Percentage concentration

1 4.5 g   **2** 10 mL

Concentrations in mg/mL

3 84 mg/mL

Concentrations or ratio strengths ('1 in . . . ')

4 1 mg

Drugs expressed in units

5 $1 \times 25,000$ units/mL ampoule **and** 0.8 mL of a 5,000 units/mL ampoule

Molarity

6 5.85 g sodium chloride

INFUSION RATE CALCULATIONS

Calculation of drip rates

1 27.7 drops/min (rounded to 28 drops/min)
2 16.625 drops/min (rounded to 17 drops/min)
3 31.3 drops/min (rounded to 31 drops/min)

Conversion of infusion rates (mL/hour) to drops/min

4 41.67 drops/min (rounded to 42 drops/min)

Conversion of dosages to mL/hour

5 90 mL/hour

Conversion of mL/hour to micrograms/kg/min or mg/min

6 Dose = 3 micrograms/kg/min, so the pump rate is correct

Calculation of length of time of infusions

7 238 min = 3 hours 58 min (approximately 4 hours)

PAEDIATRIC CALCULATIONS

1 9 mL   **2** 1.67 mL

Basics

OBJECTIVES

At the end of this chapter, you should be familiar with the following:

- Arithmetic symbols
- Fractions and decimals
- Powers or exponentials
- Estimating answers
- Rules of arithmetic
- Roman numerals
- Using a calculator
- Measuring liquids

Before dealing with any drug calculations, we will briefly go over a few basic mathematical concepts that may be helpful in some calculations.

This chapter is designed for those who might want to refresh their memories, particularly those that are returning to healthcare after a long absence. You can simply skip some parts of this chapter, or all of it. Alternatively, you can refer back to any part of this chapter as you are working through the rest of the book.

ARITHMETIC SYMBOLS

The following is a table of mathematical symbols generally used in textbooks. The list is not exhaustive, but only covers common symbols you may come across.

Table 1 Arithmetic symbols

Symbol	Meaning	Symbol	Meaning
+	plus **or** positive; add in calculations	≠	not equal to
		≡	identically equal to
−	minus **or** negative; subtract in calculations	>	greater than
		<	less than
±	plus or minus; positive or negative	≤	equal to or less than
		≥	equal to or greater than
×	multiply by	%	percent
/ or \	divide by	Σ	sum of
=	equal to	≯	not greater than
≈	approximately equal to	≮	not less than

RULES OF ARITHMETIC

Consider the following sum: $3 + 4 \times 6$

- Do we add 3 and 4 together, and then multiply by 6, to give 42? **or**
- Do we multiply 4 by 6, and then add 3, to give 27?

There are two possible answers, depending on how you would solve the above sum – which one is right?

The correct answer is 27.

RULES FOR THE ORDER OF OPERATIONS

Adding $(+)$, subtracting $(-)$, multiplying $(\times)$ and dividing $(/$ or $\div)$ numbers are known as **operations**. When you have complicated sums to do, you have to follow simple rules known as the **order of operations**. Initially (a long time ago) people agreed on an order in which mathematical operations should be performed, and this has been universally adopted.

The acronym or word BEDMAS is used to remember the correct order of operations: Each letter stands for a common mathematical operation; the order of the letter matches the order of doing the mathematical operations.

Brackets	e.g.	$(3 + 4)$
Exponentiation	e.g.	2^3
Division	e.g.	$6 \div 3$
Multiplication	e.g.	3×4
Addition	e.g.	$3 + 4$
Subtraction	e.g.	$4 - 3$

The basic rule is to work from **left to right**.

B   Calculations in brackets are done first. When you have more than one set of brackets, do the inner brackets first.

E   Next, any exponentiation (or powers) must be done – see later for a fuller explanation of exponentiation or powers.

D and **M**   Do the division and multiplication in order from left to right.

A and **S**   Do the addition and subtraction in order from left to right.

To help you to remember the rules, you can remember the acronym **BEDMAS** or the phrase **Big Elephants Destroy Mice And Snails**. You can even make up your own phrase to remember the correct order of operations.

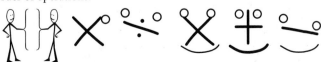

Get us in the right order

WORKED EXAMPLE 1

Work out the sum:

$20 \div (12 - 2) \times 3^2 - 2$

First of all – everything in the brackets is done first:

$(12 - 2) = 10$

So the sum becomes:

$20 \div 10 \times 3^2 - 2$

Next, calculate the exponential:

$3^2 = 3 \times 3 = 9$

So the sum becomes:

$20 \div 10 \times 9 - 2$

Next multiply and divide as they appear:

$20 \div 10 = 2$

then multiply:

$2 \times 9 = 18$

So the sum becomes:

$18 - 2$

Finally, add or subtract as they appear:

$18 - 2 = 16$

Answer: 16

WORKED EXAMPLE 2

If we look at the example on page **219** (calculating creatinine clearance), we can see that it is quite a complicated sum:

$$\text{CrCl (mL/min)} = \frac{1.23 \times (140 - 67) \times 72}{125} = 51.7$$

In the top line, the sum within the brackets is done first, i.e. $(140 - 67)$, then multiply by 1.23 and then by 72.

Thus, $(140 - 67) = 73$, so the sum is $1.23 \times 73 \times 72 = 6464.88$
Then divide by 125 to give the answer of 51.7

> **Tip** If there is a 'line', work out the top, then the bottom, and finally divide.

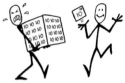

Use a power to make cumbersome numbers more manageable

FRACTIONS AND DECIMALS

A basic knowledge of fractions and decimals is helpful since they are involved in most calculations. It is important to know how to multiply and divide fractions and decimals, as well as to be able to convert from a fraction to a decimal and vice versa.

FRACTIONS

Before we look at fractions, a few points need to be defined to make explanations easier.

Definition of a fraction

A fraction is part of a whole number or one number divided by another. For example:

$$\frac{2}{5}$$

is a fraction and means 2 parts of 5 (where 5 is the whole).

- The number above the 'line' is called the **numerator**. It indicates the number of parts of the whole number that are being used (i.e. 2 in the above example).
- The number below the 'line' is called the **denominator**, and it indicates the number of parts into which the whole is divided (i.e. 5 in the above example).

Thus in the above example, the whole has been divided into 5 equal parts and you are dealing with 2 parts.

$$\frac{2}{5} \quad \begin{array}{l} \text{numerator} \\ \text{denominator} \end{array}$$

Simplifying (reducing) fractions

When you haven't a calculator handy, it is often easier to work with fractions that have been 'simplified' or reduced to their lowest terms.

To reduce a fraction, choose any number that divides exactly into the numerator (number on the top) and the denominator (number on the bottom).

A fraction is said to have been reduced to its lowest terms when it is no longer possible to divide the numerator and denominator by the same number. This process of converting or reducing fractions to its simplest form is called **cancellation**. It is often referred to as: 'whatever you do to the top line, you must do to the bottom line'.

Remember – reducing or simplifying a fraction to its lowest terms does not change the value of the fraction.

Examples

1) $\dfrac{\cancel{15}^{3}}{\cancel{25}_{5}} = \dfrac{3}{5}$

2) $\dfrac{\cancel{\cancel{135}^{27}}^{3}}{\cancel{\cancel{315}_{63}}_{7}} = \dfrac{3}{7}$

Remember:

- any number that ends in 0 or 5 is divisible by 5
- any even number is divisible by 2
- there can be more than one step (see Example 2 above).

If you have a calculator, then there is no need to reduce a fraction to its lowest terms: the calculator does all the hard work for you!

Equivalent fractions

Consider the following fractions:

$$\frac{1}{2} \qquad \frac{3}{6} \qquad \frac{4}{8} \qquad \frac{12}{24}$$

Each of the above fractions has the same value: they are called **equivalent fractions**. If you reduce them to their simplest form, you will notice that each is exactly a half ($\frac{1}{2}$).

Now consider the following fractions:

$$\frac{1}{3} \qquad \frac{1}{4} \qquad \frac{1}{6}$$

If you want to convert them to equivalent fractions with the **same** denominator, you have to find a common number that is divisible by all the individual denominators. This number is known as the **lowest common denominator**. For example, in the above case, multiply each denominator by 2, 3, 4, etc. until the smallest common number is found, as illustrated in the following table:

	3	**4**	**6**
× 2	6	8	**12**
× 3	9	**12**	18
× 4	**12**	16	24

In this case, the common denominator is 12. For each fraction, multiply the number above the line the same number of times as the number below the line. So for the first fraction, multiply the numbers above and below the line by 4; for the second, multiply them by 3; and for the third, multiply them by 2. So the fractions become:

$$\frac{1 \times 4}{3 \times 4} = \frac{4}{12} \text{ and } \frac{1 \times 3}{4 \times 3} = \frac{3}{12} \text{ and } \frac{1 \times 2}{6 \times 2} = \frac{2}{12}$$

Thus:

$$\frac{1}{3} \; \frac{1}{4} \; \frac{1}{6} \quad \text{equals} \quad \frac{4}{12} \; \frac{3}{12} \; \frac{2}{12}$$

Adding and subtracting fractions

To add (or subtract) fractions with the **same** denominator, add (or subtract) the numerators and place the result over the common denominator, i.e.

$$\frac{14}{32} + \frac{6}{32} - \frac{4}{32} = \frac{14 + 6 - 4}{32} = \frac{16}{32}$$

To add (or subtract) fractions with **different** denominators, first convert them to equivalent fractions with the same denominator, then add (or subtract) the numerators and place the result over the common denominator as before, i.e.

$$\frac{1}{4} - \frac{1}{6} + \frac{1}{3} = \frac{3}{12} - \frac{2}{12} + \frac{4}{12} = \frac{3 - 2 + 4}{12} = \frac{5}{12}$$

Multiplying fractions

It is quite easy to multiply fractions. You simply multiply all the numbers above the line (the **numerators**) and the numbers below the line (the **denominators**).

For example:

$$\frac{2}{5} \times \frac{3}{7} = \frac{2 \times 3}{5 \times 7} = \frac{6}{35}$$

However, it may be possible to simplify the fraction before multiplying, i.e.

$$\frac{\overset{3}{\cancel{9}}}{\underset{5}{\cancel{15}}} \times \frac{2}{5} = \frac{3 \times 2}{5 \times 5} = \frac{6}{25}$$

In this case, the first fraction has been reduced to its lowest terms by dividing both the numerator and denominator by 3.

You can also 'reduce' both fractions by dividing diagonally by a common number, i.e.

$$\frac{\overset{2}{\cancel{6}}}{7} \times \frac{5}{\underset{3}{\cancel{9}}} = \frac{2 \times 5}{7 \times 3} = \frac{10}{21}$$

In this case, each fraction contains a number that is divisible by 3 (6 and 9).

Dividing fractions

Sometimes you may have to divide fractions expressed or written like this:

$$\frac{\frac{2}{5}}{\frac{3}{7}} \quad \text{OR} \quad \frac{2}{5} \div \frac{3}{7}$$

In this case, you simply invert the second fraction (or the bottom one) and multiply, i.e.

$$\frac{2}{5} \times \frac{7}{3} = \frac{2 \times 7}{5 \times 3} = \frac{14}{15}$$

If, after inverting, you see that reduction or cancellation is possible, you can do this before multiplying. For example,

$$\frac{5}{2} \div \frac{25}{8}$$

becomes:

$$\frac{\overset{1}{\cancel{5}}}{\underset{1}{\cancel{2}}} \times \frac{\overset{4}{\cancel{8}}}{\underset{5}{\cancel{25}}} = \frac{1 \times 4}{1 \times 5} = \frac{4}{5}$$

Converting fractions to decimals

This is quite easy to do. You simply divide the top number (**numerator**) by the bottom number (**denominator**).

If we use our original example:

$$\frac{2}{5} = 2 \div 5$$

$$\begin{array}{r} 0.40 = 0.4 \\ 5\overline{)2.00} \\ \underline{2.0} \\ 0 \end{array}$$

It's important to place the decimal point in the correct position, usually after the number that is being divided (in this case it is 2).

> **Tip** Simplifying fractions will always make calculations easier to do.

DECIMALS

Decimals describe 'tenths' of a number, i.e. in terms of 10. A decimal number consists of a decimal point and numbers both to the left and right of that decimal point. Just as whole numbers have positions for units, tens, hundreds etc., so do decimal numbers, but on both sides of the decimal point, i.e.

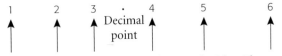

1	2	3	.	4	5	6

Hundreds   Tens   Units   Tenths   Hundredths   Thousandths

- Numbers to the **left** of the decimal point are **greater** than 1.
- Numbers to the **right** of the decimal point are **less** than 1.

Thus:

- 0.25 is a **fraction** of 1.
- 1.25 is **1 plus a fraction** of 1.

Multiplying decimals

Decimals are multiplied in the same way as whole numbers except there is a decimal point to worry about.

    If you are not using a calculator, remember to put the decimal point in the correct place in the answer.

    Consider the sum:

$$
\begin{array}{r}
0.65 \\
\times\ 0.75 \\
\hline
325 \\
4550 \\
\hline
4875 \\
\end{array}
$$

0.65 × 0.75

You may use another method, but the answer should be the same. The decimal point is placed as many places to the **left** as there are numbers after it in the sum. In this case there are four, two in each of the number to be multiplied.

$$0.6\,5 \times 0.7\,5$$
$$1\,23\,4 = 4$$

Therefore the decimal point has to be moved four places to the **left**:

$$.4\ 8\ 7\ 5\ = 0.4875$$

Multiplying by multiples of 10

To multiply a decimal by a multiple of 10 (100, 1000, etc.) you simply move the decimal point the same number of places to the **right** as there are zeros in the number you are multiplying by.

For example:

Number to multiply by	Number of zeros	Move the decimal point to the right
10	1	1 place
100	2	2 places
1,000	3	3 places
10,000	4	4 places

and so on.

Dividing decimals

Division of decimals is quite simple, but once again it's important to get the decimal point in the right place.

To make it easier to explain, the following terms are used:

$$\frac{\text{dividend}}{\text{divisor}} = \text{quotient (answer) or}$$

$$\text{divisor } \overline{)\text{dividend}}^{\text{quotient (answer)}}$$

Consider:

$\frac{34.8}{4}$ which can be rewritten as $34.8 \div 4$

The decimal point in the answer (quotient) is placed directly above the decimal point in the dividend:

$$\begin{array}{r} 8.7 \\ 4\overline{)34.8} \\ \underline{32} \\ 28 \end{array}$$

Dividing a decimal by another decimal

This involves an extra step. Consider:

$$\frac{1.55}{0.2}$$

which could also be written as:

$1.55 \div 0.2$

- First, make the divisor equal to a **whole number**, i.e. in this case, move the decimal point one place to the right.

- Then, move the decimal point in the dividend the **same number** of places to the right.

In this case:

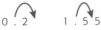

$$0 \,.\, 2 \qquad 1 \,.\, 5\,5$$

which equals:

$$2\overline{)15.5}$$

Then the decimal point in the answer (quotient) is placed directly above the decimal point in the dividend as before.

```
      7.75
   2)15.5
      14 ·
      15
      14
       10
```

Dividing by multiples of 10

To divide a decimal by a multiple of 10, you simply move the decimal point the same number of places to the **left** as there are number of zeros or zeros in the number you are dividing by.

Number to divide by	Number of zeros	Move the decimal point (to the left)
10	1	1 place
100	2	2 places
1,000	3	3 places
10,000	4	4 places

and so on.

For example:

$$\frac{546}{1000}$$

Move the decimal point three places to the left (because there are three zeros in the bottom number):

$$0 \,.\, 5 \;\; 4 \;\; 6$$

Rounding of decimal numbers

Sometimes it is necessary to 'round up' or 'round down' a decimal number to a whole number.

This is particularly true in infusion rate calculations, as it is impossible to give a part of a drop or a millilitre (mL) when setting an infusion rate.

- If the number after the decimal point is 4 or less, then ignore it, i.e. **round down**.
  For example: 31.35
  The number after the decimal point is 4 or less, so it becomes 31.
- If the number after the decimal point is 5 or more, then add 1 to the whole number, i.e. **round up**.
  For example: 41.67
  The number after the decimal point is 5 or more, so it becomes 42.

Converting decimals to fractions

It is unlikely that you would want to convert a decimal to a fraction, but this is included here just in case.

- First, you have to make the decimal a whole number by moving the decimal point to the **right**, i.e.

  0. 7 5

  becomes 75 (the **numerator** in the fraction)
- Next, divide by a multiple of 10 (the **denominator**) to make a fraction.

The value of this multiple of 10 is determined by how many places to the **right** the decimal point has moved, i.e.

  1 place = a denominator of 10
  2 places = a denominator of 100
  3 places = a denominator of 1,000

Thus in our example, 0.75 becomes 75, i.e. the decimal point has moved two places to the right, so the denominator is 100:

$$\frac{75}{100}$$

To simplify, divide the numerator and denominator by 25:

$$\frac{3}{4}$$

ROMAN NUMERALS

Although it is not recommended as best practice, roman numerals are still commonly used when writing prescriptions. With roman numerals, letters are used to designate numbers.

The following table explains the roman numerals most commonly seen on prescriptions.

Table 2 Roman numerals

Roman numeral	Ordinary number
I (or i)	1
II (or ii)	2
III (or iii)	3
IV (or iv)	4
V (or v)	5
VI or (vi)	6
VII or (vii)	7
VIII or (viii)	8
IX or (ix)	9
X (or x)	10
L (or l)	50
C (or c)	100
D (or d)	500
M (or m)	1,000

RULES FOR READING ROMAN NUMERALS

There are some simple rules for roman numerals. It doesn't matter whether they are capital letters or small letters, the value is the same. The position of one letter relative to another is very important, and determines the value of the numeral.

Rule 1   Repeating a roman numeral twice doubles its value; repeating it three times triples its value.

Examples II = 1 + 1 = 2   III = 1 + 1 + 1 = 3

Rule 2   The letter I can usually be repeated up to three times; the letter V is written once only.

Example   III = 3 is correct; IIII = 4 is not correct

Rule 3   When a smaller roman numeral is placed **after** a larger one, add the two together.

Example   VI = 5 + 1 = 6

Rule 4　When a smaller roman numeral is placed **before** a larger one, subtract the smaller numeral from the larger one.

　　　Example　$IV = 5 - 1 = 4$

Rule 5　When a Roman numeral of a smaller value comes **between** two of larger values, first apply the subtraction rule, then add.

　　　Example　$XIV = 10 + (5 - 1) = 10 + 4 = 14$

POWERS OR EXPONENTIALS

Powers or exponentials are a convenient way of writing very large or very small numbers. Powers of 10 are often used in scientific calculations.

Consider the following:

$10 \times 10 \times 10 \times 10 \times 10$

Here you are multiplying by 10, five times. Instead of all these 10s, you can write:

10^5

We say this as '10 to the power of 5' or just '10 to the 5'. The small raised number 5 next to the 10 is known as the **power** or **exponent** – it tells you how many times the same number is being multiplied together.

$10^5 \longleftarrow$ power or exponent

Now consider this:

$$\frac{1}{10} \times \frac{1}{10} \times \frac{1}{10} \times \frac{1}{10} \times \frac{1}{10} = \frac{1}{10 \times 10 \times 10 \times 10 \times 10}.$$

Here we are repeatedly dividing by 10. For short, you can write:

10^{-5}

instead of:

$$\frac{1}{10 \times 10 \times 10 \times 10 \times 10}$$

In this case, there is a minus sign next to the power or exponent.

10^{-5}　minus power or exponent

This is a **negative power** or **exponent**, and is usually called '10 to the power of -5' or minus 5.

In conclusion:

- A positive power or exponent means **multiply** by the number of times of the power or exponent.
- A negative power or exponent means **divide** by the number of times of the power or exponent.

You will probably come across powers used as in the following:

3×10^3 or 5×10^{-2}

This is known as the **standard index form**. It is a combination of a power of 10 and a number with just one unit in front of a decimal point, i.e.

$5 \times 10^6 \quad (5.0 \times 10^6)$

1.2×10^3

4.5×10^{-2}

$3 \times 10^{-6} \quad (3.0 \times 10^{-6})$

The number in front of the decimal point can be anything from 0 to 9. This type of notation is the type seen on a scientific calculator when you are working with very large or very small numbers. It is a common and convenient way of describing numbers without having to write a lot of zeros.

Here are some more examples:

$3 \times 10^5 = 3 \times 100,000$

$1.4 \times 10^3 = 1.4 \times 1,000$

$4 \times 10^{-2} = 4 \div 100$

$2.25 \times 10^{-3} = 2.25 \div 1,000$

Because you are dealing in 10s, you will notice that the number of zeros you multiply or divide by is equal to the power.

EXAMPLE 1

3×10^5

You move the decimal point five places to the right (positive power of 5). So it becomes:

$3 \times 10^5 = \underbrace{3\,0\,0\,0\,0\,0}_{\text{5 zeros}}. = 300,000$

EXAMPLE 2

4×10^{-2}

You move the decimal point two places to the left (negative power of 2). So it becomes

$4 \times 10^{-2} = \underbrace{0.04}_{\text{2 zeros}} = 0.04$

Table 3 Powers of ten

Power of 10	Written out in full	Power of 10	Written out in full
10^9	1,000,000,000	10^{-1}	0.1
10^8	100,000,000	10^{-2}	0.01
10^7	10,000,000	10^{-3}	0.001
10^6	1,000,000	10^{-4}	0.0001
10^5	100,000	10^{-5}	0.00001
10^4	10,000	10^{-6}	0.000001
10^3	1,000	10^{-7}	0.0000001
10^2	100	10^{-8}	0.00000001
10^1	10	10^{-9}	0.000000001
10^0	1		

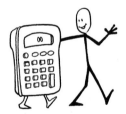

Get to know your calculator

USING A CALCULATOR

Numbers should be entered in a certain way when using a calculator, and you need to know how to read the display. The manual or instructions that came with your calculator will tell you how to do this.

This section explains how to use your calculator correctly.

Consider the following calculation:

$\frac{2}{500} \times 140$

There are two ways of entering this into your calculator:

METHOD 1

Enter [2]	DISPLAY = 2
Enter [×]	DISPLAY = 2
Enter [1][4][0]	DISPLAY = 140

You are doing the sum:

2×140

Enter [÷]	DISPLAY = 280
Enter [5][0][0]	DISPLAY = 500

You are doing the sum:

$$\frac{2 \times 140}{500}$$

Enter [=]	DISPLAY = 0.56 (answer)

METHOD 2

Enter [2]	DISPLAY = 2
Enter [÷]	DISPLAY = 2
Enter [5][0][0]	DISPLAY = 500

You are doing the sum:

$$\frac{2}{500}$$

Enter [×]	DISPLAY = 4^{-3} or 0.004

This is the way a scientific calculator shows small numbers. (See 'Powers or exponentials').

Enter [1][4][0]	DISPLAY = 140

You are doing the sum:

$$\frac{2}{500} \times 140$$

Enter [=]	DISPLAY = 0.56 (answer)

Now consider the following calculation:

$$\frac{20}{60} \times \frac{1,000}{8}$$

Again, there are two possible ways of doing this.

METHOD 1

Enter [2][0]   DISPLAY = 20
Enter [÷]   DISPLAY = 20
Enter [6][0]   DISPLAY = 60

You are doing the sum:

$$\frac{20}{60}$$

Enter [×]   DISPLAY = 0.3333333
Enter [1][0][0][0] DISPLAY = 1000

You are doing the sum:

$$\frac{20}{60} \times 1,000$$

Enter [÷]   DISPLAY = 333.33333
Enter [8]   DISPLAY = 8

You are doing the sum:

$$\frac{20}{60} \times \frac{1,000}{8}$$

Enter [=]   DISPLAY = 41.66667 (answer)

METHOD 2

Enter [2][0]   DISPLAY = 20
Enter [×]   DISPLAY = 20
Enter [1][0][0][0] DISPLAY = 1000

You are doing the sum:

$$20 \times 1,000$$

Enter [÷]   DISPLAY = 20000
Enter [6][0]   DISPLAY = 60

You are doing the sum:

$$\frac{20 \times 1,000}{60}$$

Enter [÷]   DISPLAY = 333.33333
Enter [8]   DISPLAY = 8

You are doing the sum:

$$\frac{20 \times 1,000}{60 \times 8}$$

Enter [=]   DISPLAY = 41.66667 (answer)

Whatever method you use, the answer is the same. However, it may be easier to split the sum into two parts:

1) $20 \times 1,000$ 2) 60×8

then dividing (1) by (2), i.e.

$$\frac{20}{60} \times \frac{1,000}{8} = \frac{20,000}{480} = 41.66667$$

Now consider a sum written as:

$$\frac{6}{4 \times 5}$$

You could simplify the sum first, i.e.

$$\frac{6}{20}$$

then divide 6 by 20 = 0.3 (answer).
   Alternatively, you could enter the following on your calculator:

Enter [6]	DISPLAY = 6
Enter [÷]	DISPLAY = 6
Enter [4]	DISPLAY = 4

You are doing the sum:

$$\frac{6}{4} = 1.5$$

Enter [÷]	DISPLAY = 1.5
Enter [5]	DISPLAY = 5

You are doing the sum:

$$\frac{\frac{6}{4}}{5} \text{ i.e. } \frac{1.5}{5}$$

Enter [=]	DISPLAY = 0.3 (answer)

Again, you can use either method, but it may be easier to simplify the top line and the bottom line before dividing the two.
   See the section on 'Powers and calculators' for an explanation of how your calculator displays very large and small numbers.

Tip   Get to know how to use your calculator – read the manual! If you don't know how to use your calculator properly, then there is always potential for errors. You won't know if the answer you've got is correct or not.

POWERS AND CALCULATORS

The display on a normal calculator is usually eight numbers:

1 2 3 4 5 6 7 8.

The maximum number that can be displayed in this way is:

99 999 999

and the smallest number that can be displayed is:

0.0000001

On a scientific calculator, if an answer is either larger or smaller than this, the answer will be shown as a power or exponential of 10, i.e.

4.0^9 or $7.^{-09}$

As mentioned earlier (p. 22), this is known as **standard index form**.

$5.^{06} = 5 \times 10^6 = 5 \times 1,000,000 = 5,000,000$

$3.^{-06} = 3 \times 10^{-6} = \dfrac{3}{1,000,000} = 0.000003$

So if the answer is displayed like this on your calculator and you want to convert to an ordinary number, you simply move the decimal point the number of places as indicated by the power and to the left or to the right depending on whether it is a negative or positive power.

$5.^{06} = 5 \times 10^6 = \underbrace{5\,0\,0\,0\,0\,0\,0.}_{6 \text{ zeros}} = 5,000,000$

$3.^{-06} = 3 \times 10^{-6} = \underbrace{0.0\,0\,0\,0\,0\,3}_{6 \text{ zeros}} = 0.000003$

ESTIMATING ANSWERS

It's often useful to be able to estimate the answer for a calculation. The estimating process is basically simple: numbers are rounded either up or down, in terms of tens, hundreds or thousands to give numbers that can be calculated easily.

For example, 41 would be rounded down to 40; 23.5 to 20; and 58.75 rounded up to 60. Single-digit numbers (less than 10) should be left as they are (although 8 and 9 could be rounded up to 10).

Once numbers have been rounded up or down, it's possible to do a simple calculation, and the result is close enough to act as an estimate.

No set rules for estimating can be given to cover all the possibilities that may be encountered. The following examples should illustrate the principles involved.

EXAMPLE 1

Add the following numbers:

3,459 + 11,723 + 7,895 + 789

There are several methods for estimating the answer: pick the method most suited to you.

Method 1

- Change the numbers so that they can be easily added up in your head. Look at the numbers. Three are numbers in the thousands and one in the hundreds. For now, ignore the number in the hundreds.
- First, add the thousands column (the number which is to the left of the comma), i.e.

3 + 11 + 7 = 21

Then add the three zeros (to convert back to a number in the thousands):

21,000

- Second, look at the hundreds column (the number just to the right of the comma). Add those numbers:

3,459 + 11,723 + 7,895 + 789
   4   +   7   +   8   + 7   = 26

Then add the two zeros (to convert back to a number in the hundreds)

2800 (2,800)

Round up or down to a number in the thousands (i.e. 3,000) and add to the 21,000:

21,000 + 3,000 = 24,000   estimated answer
3,459 + 11,723 + 7,895 + 789 = 23,866   actual answer

Method 2

Round the numbers up or down to numbers that can be added up easily. Therefore in this case:

original number		number after rounding up or down	
3,459		3,400	
11,723		11,700	
7,895		7,900	
789		800	
23,866	actual answer	23,800	estimated answer

EXAMPLE 2

Multiply 3018 by 489

Step 1

Round the numbers up or down in terms of hundreds, i.e.

3018 = 3000 and 489 = 500

You are now considering the sum:

3000 × 500

Step 2

For now, ignore the zeros in the sum, so consider the sum as:

3 × 5 = 15

Step 3

Now bring back the zeros to ensure that the answer is of the right magnitude. In this case five zeros were ignored, so add them to the end of the answer from Step 2:

15 00000 = 1,500,000

The estimated answer is:

1,500,000

The actual answer is:

3018 × 489 = 1,475,802

EXAMPLE 3

Multiply 28.67 by 67.66.

Step 1

Round up or down the numbers in terms of tens, i.e.

28.67 = 30 and 67.66 = 70

You are now considering the sum:

30 × 70

Step 2

For now, ignore the zeros in the sum, so consider the sum as

$3 \times 7 = 21$

Step 3

Now bring back the zeros to ensure that the answer is of the right magnitude. In this case 2 zeros were ignored, so add them to the end of the answer from Step 2:

21 00 = 2,100

The estimated answer is:

2,100

The actual answer of the sum 28.85 by 67.25 is:

1,940.1625

Don't forget – the answer is only an estimate.

- If you **round up** numbers, the estimated answer will be **more** than the actual answer.
- If you **round down** numbers, the estimated answer will be **less** than the actual answer.

EXAMPLE 4

Divide 36,042 by 48.

Step 1

Round the numbers up or down in terms of thousands and hundreds, i.e.

36,042 = 36,000 and 48 = 50

You are now considering the sum:

$36,000 \div 50$

Step 2

In division, more care is needed with the zeros. If there is a zero in the divisor (the number you are dividing by), then this must be cancelled out with a zero from the dividend (the number you are dividing). This may, at first, appear confusing, but the following example may make it clearer:

3 6 0 0∅ ÷ 5∅

Cancel out 1 zero from each side of the division sign (÷) to give:

$3,600 \div 5$

If there were two zeros in the divisor, then you would have to cancel two zeros from the dividend, i.e.

3 6 0 0̸0̸ ÷ 50̸0̸

Cancel out two zeros from each side of the division sign (÷) to give:

360 ÷ 5

Step 3

The zeros in the sum can be ignored, so consider the sum as:

36 ÷ 5 = 7.2 (rounded down to 7)

Step 4

Now bring back the zeros, to ensure that the answer is of the right magnitude. In this case 2 zeros were ignored, so add them to the end of the answer from Step 3:

7 00 = 700

The estimated answer is 700.
The actual answer is:

36,042 ÷ 48 = 750.875

Don't forget – the answer is only an estimate.

- If you **round up** numbers, the estimated answer will be **more** than the actual answer.
- If you **round down** numbers, the estimated answer will be **less** than the actual answer.

NUMBERS LESS THAN 1

What happens if there is a number less than 1? You obviously cannot round down to zero, as this would not give a proper answer – multiplying anything by zero gives an answer of zero. You simply convert the number to a fraction (see 'Converting decimals to fractions', p. 19). If there is more than one number after the decimal point, then round up or down to one decimal place.

For example:

0.28 becomes 0.3

Then convert to a fraction:

0.3 equals $\dfrac{3}{10}$

Tip In this case, to convert to a fraction, **always** divide by 10.

Once the decimal has been converted to a fraction, then calculate the sum as if you are multiplying or dividing by fractions (see 'Multiplying and dividing fractions', pp. 14–15).

For example:

27 × 0.28 would become $30 \times \dfrac{3}{10}$ (27 rounded up to 30)

$\overset{3}{\cancel{30}} \times \dfrac{3}{\cancel{10}}$ would become 3 × 3 = 9 (estimated answer)

27 × 0.28 = 7.56 (actual answer)

MEASURING LIQUIDS

The proper way to measure large volumes of liquid is to use a specific measure. However, it is unlikely that you will find a proper measure on the ward; liquids are usually measured with medicine pots and syringes (especially liquids or medicines to be administered to patients). All three methods of measuring liquids will be covered here.

CYLINDRICAL AND CONICAL MEASURES

These measures are mainly used for liquids that are for oral or external use. They range in size from 1 mL to 1,000 mL (1 litre).

Cylindrical measures are more accurate and are mainly used in chemical laboratories; conical flasks or measures are mainly found in dispensaries. Each measure must bear the stamp of a Weights and Measures Inspector.

When liquid is poured into a measure, the liquid 'clings' to the sides, creating a curved level that is known as the meniscus. This is due to the surface tension of the liquid.

When measuring, the top of the graduation line must be aligned with the true meniscus, i.e. the lowest part of the liquid (see Figure 2.1).

It is important that the measure should be on a flat surface, or held as level as possible. The graduation mark to which you are measuring

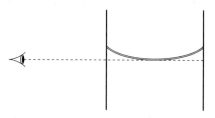

Fig. 2.1 Meniscus

should be at eye level. If viewed from above, the level may appear higher than it really is; if viewed from below, it appears lower. There are usually guidelines at the back of the measure to help align the meniscus properly, preventing these eye-level errors.

It is good practice to choose the most appropriate measure. If possible, do not split the volume between two measures because this increases errors, i.e. you are measuring 300 mL, it would be better to use a 500 mL measure than to measure out 100 mL and 200 mL.

When pouring, carefully pour the liquid into the centre of the measure; any that falls on to the sides above the relevant graduation mark has to be allowed to drain down before adjusting to the final volume.

MEASURING POTS

These are used on the ward to measure individual patient doses. They measure volumes ranging from 5 mL to 30 mL, and are not meant to be accurate. However, the same principles apply as when using cylindrical measures: measure at eye level.

SYRINGES

When measuring a volumes with a syringe, it is important to expel all the air first before adjusting to the final volume. The volume is measured from the bottom of the plunger.

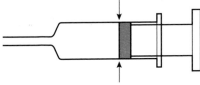

Fig. 2.2 Measure volume from the bottom of the plunger

The small amount of liquid that is left in the nozzle of the syringe after administering the drug has already been taken into account by the manufacturer when calibrating the syringe: it is known as 'dead space' or 'dead volume'. You shouldn't try to administer this small volume.

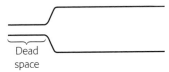

Dead
space

Fig. 2.3 'Dead space' in the nozzle of a syringe

Once again, you should use the most appropriate syringe for your dose.

Syringe calibrations

Table 4 Syringe calibrations

Syringe size (mL)	Division (mL)	Sub-division (mL)
1	0.1	0.01
2	0.5	0.1
5	1	0.5
10	1	0.5
20	5	1
50	10	1

It is important that injection doses are measured correctly. An overdose can be dangerous; too low a measure may result in an ineffective dose.

When calculating doses for injections, the number of decimal places in the answer should match the graduations on the syringe being used. For example, if you were going to use a 2 mL syringe with 0.1 mL graduations, you would calculate and round up your answer to **one** decimal place, i.e.

- If your calculated dose is 1.63 mL, you would draw up 1.6 mL.
- If your calculated dose is 1.68 mL, you would draw up 1.7 mL.

Accuracy of syringe calculations

Table 5 Accuracy of syringe calculations

Syringe size (mL)	Graduations (mL)	Answer (mL)
1	0.01	TWO decimal places
2	0.1	One decimal place
5	0.5	One decimal place
10	0.5	One decimal place

KEY POINTS

Basic arithmetic rules

Simple basic rules exist when adding (+), subtracting (−), multiplying (×) and dividing (/ or ÷) numbers – these are known as **operations**.

The acronym **BEDMAS** can be used to remember the correct **order of operations**:

B Do calculations in **brackets** first. When you have more than one set of brackets, do the inner brackets first.

E Next, do any **exponentiation** (powers).

D and **M** Do the **division** and **multiplication** in order from left to right.

A and **S** Do the **addition** and **subtraction** in order from left to right.

Fractions

● A fraction consists of a numerator and a denominator:

$\dfrac{2}{5}$ numerator
denominator

● With calculations, it is best to try and simplify or reduce fractions to their lowest terms.

● **Equivalent fractions** are those with the same value, e.g.

$$\frac{1}{2} \qquad \frac{3}{6} \qquad \frac{4}{8} \qquad \frac{12}{24}$$

If you reduce these to their simplest form, you will notice that each is exactly a half.

● If you want to convert fractions to equivalent fractions with the same denominator, you have to find a common number that is divisible by all the individual denominators.

Operations with fractions

● To add (or subtract) fractions with the same denominator, add (or subtract) the numerators and place the result over the common denominator.

● To add (or subtract) fractions with the different denominators, first convert them to equivalent fractions with the same denominator, then add (or subtract) the numerators and place the result over the common denominator as before.

● To multiply fractions, multiply the numerators and the denominators.

● To divide fractions, invert the second fraction and multiply (as above).

● To convert a fraction to a decimal, divide the numerator by the denominator.

Decimals

● When multiplying or dividing decimals, ensure that the decimal point is placed in the correct place.

Rounding up or down

● If the number after the decimal point is 4 or less, then ignore it, i.e. **round down**.

● If the number after the decimal point is 5 or more, then add 1 to the whole number, i.e. **round up**.

Roman numerals

In Roman numerals, letters are used to designate numbers.

Powers or exponentials

- Powers or exponentials are a convenient way of writing large or small numbers.
- A **positive** power or exponent (e.g. 10^5) means **multiply** by the number of times of the power or exponent.
- A **negative** power or exponent (e.g. 10^{-5}) means **divide** by the number of times of the power or exponent.

Measuring liquids

- Use the most appropriate measure for the volume you are measuring.
- When using cylindrical or conical measures and measuring pots, try to measure at eye level to prevent meniscus errors.

Units and equivalences

OBJECTIVES

At the end of this chapter, you should be familiar with the following:

- SI units and prefixes
- Equivalences of weight, volume and amount of substance
- Converting from one unit to another
- How to write units

Many different units of measurement are used in medicine. For example:

- drug strengths, e.g. digoxin injection 500 micrograms in 1 mL
- dosages, e.g. dobutamine 3 micrograms/kg/min
- patient electrolyte levels, e.g. sodium 137 mmol/L

and many more.

It's important to have a basic knowledge of the units used in medicine and how they are derived. It's particularly important to have an understanding of the units in which drugs can be prescribed, and how to convert from one unit to another – this last part is vital, as it forms the basis of all drug calculations.

SI UNITS

SI stands for Système Internationale, and is another name for the metric system of measurement. The aim of metrication is to make calculations easier than it was with the imperial system (ounces, pounds, stones, inches, pints, etc.). SI units are generally accepted in the United Kingdom and many other countries for use in medical practice and pharmacy. They were introduced to the NHS in 1975.

SI BASE UNITS

The main units are those used to measure weight, volume and amount of substance:

- weight: kilogram (kg)
- volume: litre (L or l)
- amount of substance: mole (mol).

SI PREFIXES

When an SI unit is inconveniently large or small, prefixes are used to denote multiples or sub-multiples. It is preferable to use multiples of a thousand, e.g.

- gram
- milligram (one thousandth, 1/1,000th of a gram)
- microgram (one millionth, 1/1,000,000th of a gram)
- nanogram (one thousand millionth, 1/1,000,000,000th of a gram).

For example, one millionth of a gram could be written as 0.000001 g or as 1 microgram. The second version is easier to read than the first, and easier to work with once you understand how to use units and prefixes. It is also less likely to lead to errors, especially when administering drug doses.

Prefixes used in clinical practice

Table 6 SI prefixes

Prefix	Symbol	Division/multiple	Factor
Mega	M	×1,000,000	10^6
Kilo	K	×1,000	10^3
Deci	d	÷10	10^{-1}
Centi	c	÷100	10^{-2}
Milli	m	÷1,000	10^{-3}
Micro	μ	÷1,000,000	10^{-6}
Nano	n	÷1,000,000,000	10^{-9}

The main prefixes you will come across on the ward are **mega-**, **milli-**, **micro-** and **nano-**.

Thus in practice, drug strengths and dosages can be expressed in various ways.

- Benzylpenicillin is sometimes expressed in terms of mega units (1 mega unit means 1 million units of activity). Each vial contains benzylpenicillin 600 mg, which equals 1 mega unit.

- Small volumes of liquids are often expressed in millilitres (mL), e.g lactulose, 10 mL to be given three times a day.
- Drug strengths are usually expressed in milligrams (mg), e.g. furosemide (frusemide) 40 mg tablets.
- When the amount of drug in a tablet or other formulation is very small, strengths are expressed as micrograms or even nanograms, e.g. digoxin 125 microgram tablets; alfacalcidol 250 nanogram tablets.

Tip In prescriptions the words 'micrograms' and 'nanograms' should be written in full. However, the abbreviations mcg (for micrograms) and ng (nanograms) are still sometimes used, so care must be taken when reading handwritten abbreviations. Confusion can occur, particularly between mg and ng. The abbreviation μg (for micrograms) should not be used, as it may be confused with mg or ng.

EQUIVALENCES

The SI base units are too large for everyday clinical use, so they are subdivided into multiples of 1000.

EQUIVALENCES OF WEIGHT

1 kilogram (kg) = 1,000 grams (g)
1 gram (g) = 1,000 milligrams (mg)
1 milligram (mg) = 1,000 micrograms (mcg)
1 microgram (mcg) = 1,000 nanograms (ng)

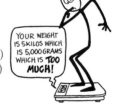

YOUR WEIGHT IS 5 KILOS WHICH IS 5,000 GRAMS WHICH IS **TOO MUCH!**

EQUIVALENCES OF VOLUME

1 litre (L) = 1,000 millilitres (mL)

EQUIVALENCES OF AMOUNT OF SUBSTANCE

1 mole (mol) = 1,000 millimoles (mmol)
1 millimole (mmol) = 1,000 micromoles (mcmol)

Moles and millimoles are the terms used by chemists when measuring quantities of certain substances or chemicals; they are more accurate than using grams. For a fuller explanation, see Chapter 5, 'Moles and millimoles'.

Examples of these equivalences include:

0.5 kg = 500 g
0.25 g = 250 mg
0.2 mg = 200 micrograms
0.5 L = 500 mL
0.25 mol = 250 mmol

1 Kg
1,000g
1,000,000 mg
1,000,000,000 mcg
1,000,000,000,000 ng

1 l
1,000 ml

1 mole
1 mol
1,000 mmol
1,000,000 mcmol

CONVERTING FROM ONE UNIT TO ANOTHER

In drug calculations, it is best to work in whole numbers, e.g. 125 micrograms and not 0.125 mg, as fewer mistakes are then made. Avoid using decimals, as the decimal point can be written in the wrong place during calculations. A decimal point in the wrong place can mean errors of 10-fold or even 100-fold. It is always best to work with the smaller unit, to avoid decimals and decimal points, so you need to be able to convert easily from one unit to another. In general:

- To convert from a **larger** unit to a **smaller** unit, **multiply** by multiples of 1,000.
- To convert from a **smaller** unit to a **larger** unit, **divide** by multiples of 1,000.

For each multiplication or division by 1,000 the decimal point moves three places either to the right or to the left, depending upon whether you are converting from a larger unit to a smaller unit or vice versa (see the worked examples below).

When you have to convert from a very large unit to a much smaller unit (or vice versa), you may find it easier to do the conversion in several steps. For example, to convert 0.005 kg to milligrams, first convert to grams:

0.005 kg = 0.005 × 1,000 = 5 g

Next, convert grams to milligrams:

5 g = 5 × 1,000 = 5,000 mg

Remember
When you do conversions like this, the amount remains the same, only the units change. Obviously, it appears more when expressed as a smaller unit, but the amount remains the same. (200 pence is the same as £2, although it may look more.)

WORKED EXAMPLES

1 Convert 0.5 g to milligrams

You are going from a larger unit to a smaller unit, so you have to multiply by 1,000:

   0.5 g × 1,000 = 500 mg

The decimal point moves three places to the right:

   0 . 5 0 0 = 500

2 Convert 2,000 g to kilograms

You are going from a smaller unit to a larger unit, so you have to divide by 1,000:

   2,000 g = $\frac{2,000}{1,000}$ = 2 kg

The decimal point moves three places to the left:

   2 0 0 0 . = 2

3 Convert 1.45 L to millilitres

You are going from a larger unit to a smaller unit, so you have to multiply by 1,000:

   1.45 L × 1,000 = 1,450 mL

The decimal point moves three places to the right:

   1 . 4 5 0 = 1,450

HOW TO WRITE UNITS

The *British National Formulary* makes the following recommendations:

- The unnecessary use of decimal points should be avoided, e.g. 3 mg, **not** 3.0 mg.
- Quantities of 1 gram or more should be expressed as 1.5 g, etc.
- Quantities less than 1 gram should be written in milligrams, e.g. 500 mg, **not** 0.5 g.

- Quantities less than 1 mg should be written in micrograms, e.g. 100 micrograms, **not** 0.1 mg.
- When decimals are unavoidable, a zero should be written in front of the decimal point where there is no other figure, e.g. 0.5 mL **not** .5 mL.
- However, the use of a decimal point is acceptable in a range, e.g. 0.5–1 g.
- 'Micrograms' and 'nanograms' should **not** be abbreviated. Similarly, 'units' should **not** be abbreviated.
- A capital L is used for litre, to avoid confusion (a small l could be mistaken for a figure 1, especially when typed or printed).
- Cubic centimetre (cm^3) is **not** used in medicine or pharmacy: use millilitre (mL) instead.

The following two case reports illustrate examples where bad writing can lead to problems.

PRESCRIBING MICROGRAMS – ONE RULE FOR ALL?

Case report

On admission to hospital, a patient taking thyroxine replacement therapy presented her general practitioner's referral letter which stated that her maintenance dose was 0.025 mg once daily. The clerking house officer incorrectly converted this dose and prescribed 250 micrograms rather than the 25 micrograms required. A dose was administered before the error was detected by the ward pharmacist the next morning.

Comment

The hospital that submitted this error has a standard that microgram doses are prescribed as such and not as fractions of milligrams. However, no such requirements are laid down in primary care.

In complying with the hospital standard, the house officer made an error in converting the dose from that stated by the GP. Steps are now being taken to promote this standard through the local joint prescribing strategy working party in an effort to educate GPs. Standardization of prescribing practice between primary and secondary care would do much to reduce the potential for medication errors at the interface between the two sectors.

Taken from *Pharmacy in Practice* 1994; 4: 124

This example highlights several errors:

- the wrong units were originally used – milligrams instead of micrograms
- a number containing a decimal point was used
- conversion from one unit to another was incorrectly carried out.

THIS UNIT ABBREVIATION IS DANGEROUS

Case report

Patient received 50 units of insulin instead of the prescribed stat dose of 5 units. A junior doctor requiring a patient to be given a stat dose of 5 units Actrapid insulin wrote the prescription appropriately but chose to incorporate the abbreviation for 'units' that occasionally sees use on written requests for units of blood. Thus the prescription read: 'Actrapid insulin 5 ⊙ stat'.

The administering nurse misread the abbreviation used and interpreted the prescription as 50 units of insulin. This was administered to the patient who of course became profoundly hypoglycaemic and required urgent medical intervention.

Comment

The use of the symbol ⊙ to indicate units of blood is an old fashioned practice which is now in decline. This case serves to illustrate the catastrophic effect that the inappropriate use of this abbreviation can have – it led to misinterpretation by the nursing staff and resulted in harm to the patient. We would strongly recommend that this practice be discouraged and would like to see local prescribing guidelines giving specific mention to the dangers of this practice. The word 'units' should always be written in full, whether ordering drug doses expressed in this quantity or units of blood.

A large question mark must be drawn against the competency of the individual nurse and the checking system that allows such a dose of insulin to be administered.

This case also serves to reiterate the point we have made previously that nurse administration procedures cannot be relied upon to detect significant errors in drug dosing.

Taken from *Pharmacy in Practice* 1995; 5: 131

This example illustrates that abbreviations should not be used. As recommended, the word 'units' should not be abbreviated.

PROBLEMS

Question 1   Convert 0.0125 kilograms to grams.

Question 2   Convert 250 nanograms to micrograms.

Question 3   Convert 3.2 litres to millilitres.

Question 4   Convert 0.0273 moles to millimoles.

Question 5   Convert 3,750 grams to kilograms.

Question 6   Convert 0.05 grams to micrograms.

Question 7   Convert 25,000 milligrams to kilograms.

Question 8   Convert 4.5×10^{-6} grams to nanograms.

Question 9   You have an ampoule of digoxin 0.5 mg in 2 mL. Calculate the volume in micrograms/mL.

Question 10 You have an ampoule of fentanyl 0.05 mg/mL. Calculate the amount (in micrograms/mL) in a 2 mL ampoule.

ANSWERS TO PROBLEMS

Question 1   12.5 grams

Question 2   0.25 micrograms

Question 3   3,200 millilitres

Question 4   27.3 millimoles

Question 5   3.75 kilograms

Question 6   50,000 micrograms

Question 7   0.025 kilograms

Question 8   4,500 nanograms. Note that the 10^{-6} is a power. The -6 indicates that it is a negative power, i.e. the number is divided by 10 six times. In reality, we would move the decimal point six places to the left, i.e. $= 0.0000045$ g

When converting from a larger unit to a smaller unit, you multiply by 1,000. Thus for each conversion, multiply by 1,000, i.e. the decimal point moves three places to the right.

$$0.0000045 \text{ g} = 0.0045 \text{ mg}$$
$$= 4.5 \text{ micrograms}$$
$$= 4,500 \text{ nanograms}$$

Question 9 250 micrograms/mL. To convert milligrams to micrograms you are going from a larger unit to a smaller unit; so you multiply by 1,000:

0.5 mg × 1,000 = 500 micrograms

Thus you have 500 micrograms in 2 mL. Divide by 2 to find out how much is in 1 mL:

$$\frac{500}{2} = 250 \text{ micrograms}$$

Question 10 100 micrograms in a 2 mL ampoule. To convert milligrams to micrograms you are going from a larger unit to a smaller unit; so multiply by 1,000:

0.05 mg × 1,000 = 50 micrograms

Thus you have 50 micrograms in 1 mL, so to find out how much is in a 2 mL ampoule, multiply by 2:

50 micrograms × 2 = 100 micrograms

KEY POINTS

Equivalences of weight
- 1 kilogram (kg) = 1,000 grams (g).
- 1 gram (g) = 1,000 milligrams (mg).
- 1 milligram (mg) = 1,000 micrograms (mcg).
- 1 microgram (mcg) = 1,000 nanograms (ng).

Equivalences of volume
- 1 litre (L) = 1,000 millilitres (mL).

Equivalences of amount of substance
- 1 mole (mol) = 1,000 millimoles (mmol).
- 1 millimole (mmol) = 1,000 micromoles (mcmol).
- Milligrams, micrograms and nanograms should be written in full to avoid confusion.
- Avoid decimals – a decimal point written in the wrong place can mean 10-fold or even 100-fold errors.

Converting units
- It is always best to work with the smaller unit, to avoid the use of decimals.
- When converting, the amount remains the same, only the unit changes.
- Remember to look at the units carefully; converting from one unit to another may involve two steps.
- To convert from a **larger** unit to a **smaller** unit, **multiply** by 1,000.
- To convert from a **smaller** unit to a **larger** unit, **divide** by 1,000.

3 Dosage calculations

OBJECTIVES

At the end of this chapter, you should be familiar with the following:

- Calculating the number of tablets or capsules required
- Calculating dosages based on body weight or surface area
- Calculating divided doses
- Checking your answer – does it seem reasonable?

Dosage calculations are the basic everyday type of calculations you will be doing on the ward. They include calculating number of tablets or capsules required, divided doses, simple drug dosages and dosages based on patient parameters, e.g. weight and body surface area. It is important that you are able to do these calculations confidently, as mistakes may have serious consequences for the patient, resulting in the patient receiving the wrong dose. After completing this chapter, not only should you be able to do the calculations, but also know how to decide whether your answer is reasonable or not.

CALCULATING THE NUMBER OF TABLETS OR CAPSULES REQUIRED

On the drug round, you will usually have available the strength of tablets or capsules for the dose prescribed on a patient's drug chart, e.g. dose prescribed is furosemide (frusemide) 40 mg; tablets available are furosemide (frusemide) 40 mg. However, there may be instances when the strength of the tablets or capsules available does not match the dose prescribed. Therefore you will have to calculate how many tablets or capsules to give the patient.

WORKED EXAMPLE

A patient is prescribed 75 micrograms of levothyroxine (thyroxine) but the strength of the tablets available is 25 micrograms. How many tablets are required?

This is a very simple calculation. The answer involves finding how many 25s are in 75, or in other words 75 divided by 25:

$$= \frac{75}{25} \text{ or } \frac{3}{1} = 3 \text{ tablets}$$

In most cases, it is a simple sum you can do in your head, but even so, it is a drug calculation – so care must always be taken.

A general formula can be derived:

$$\text{number required} = \frac{\text{amount prescribed}}{\text{amount in each tablet or capsule}}$$

WORKED EXAMPLE

A patient is prescribed 2 g of flucloxacillin to be given orally but the drug is only available in 500 mg capsules. How many capsules do you give?

This is slightly more complicated than our earlier example, as the dose prescribed and the medication available are in different units.

Step 1

The first step is to convert everything to the same units. We could either convert the 500 mg into grams, or we could convert the 2 g into milligrams. However, it's preferable to convert the grams to milligrams as this avoids decimal points. Remember it's best not to work with decimal points, as a decimal point in the wrong place can mean a 10-fold or even a 100-fold error.

To convert grams to milligrams, multiply by 1,000:

$$2 \text{ g} = 2 \times 1,000 \text{ mg} = 2,000 \text{ mg}$$

Step 2

The calculation is now similar to our earlier example. The answer involves finding how many 500s are in 2,000 or in other words 2,000 divided by 500:

$$\frac{2,000}{500} \text{ or } \frac{4}{1} = 4 \text{ capsules}$$

Once again, although it is a simple sum you can do in your head, it's still a drug calculation – so care must always be taken.

For dosage calculations involving liquids and injections, see 'Calculating drug dosages' (p. 51).

PROBLEMS

Question 1   500 mg is prescribed, tablets are 250 mg each: how many tablets will you give?

Question 2   1 mg is prescribed, tablets are 500 micrograms: how many tablets will you give?

CALCULATING DRUG DOSAGES BASED ON BODY WEIGHT OR SURFACE AREA

Sometimes the dose required is calculated on the basis of a patient's body weight (mg/kg) or surface area (mg/m^2). This particularly applies to cytotoxics and other drugs that require an accurate individual dose. To find the body surface area for a patient, you will need to know that patient's weight and height. Then the body surface area can be calculated, using a formula or nomogram (see Appendix 3).

WORKED EXAMPLES

Weight

The dose required is 3 mg/kg and the patient weighs 68 kg. This means that for every kilogram (kg) of a patient's weight, you will need 3 mg of drug. In this example, the patient weighs 68 kg, so this patient will need 68 lots of 3 mg of drug, i.e. you simply multiply the dose by the patient's weight.

3 mg/kg = 3 × 68 = 204 mg

Thus the patent will need a total dose of 204 mg.

This can be summarized as:

total dose required = dose/kg × patient's weight

Surface area

The dose required is $500 \ mg/m^2$ and the patient's body surface area equals $1.89 \ m^2$. This means that for every square metre (m^2) of a patient's surface area, you will need 500 mg of drug. The dose is given in mg/m^2, so you just multiply the dose by the patient's surface area (obtained from a formula or nomogram – see Appendix 3):

total dose required = dose/m^2 × body surface area

The patient's body surface area is 1.89 m², so this patient will need 1.89 lots of 500 mg of drug:

500 mg/m² = 500 × 1.89 = 945 mg

Thus the patient will need a total dose of 945 mg.

PROBLEMS

Work out the following dosages:

Question 3   Dose = 1.5 mg/kg, patient's weight = 73 kg

Question 4   Dose = 8 mg/kg, patient's weight = 64.5 kg

Question 5   Dose = 60 mg/kg, patient's weight = 12 kg

Question 6   Dose = 0.4 mL/kg, patient's weight = 62 kg

Question 7   Dose = 50 mg/m², patient's surface area = 1.94 m²

Question 8   Dose = 120 mg/m², patient's surface area = 1.55 m²

Question 9   Dose = 400 micrograms/kg, patient's weight = 54 kg
i)   What is the total dose in micrograms?
ii) What is the total dose in mg?

Question 10 Dose = 5 micrograms/kg/min, patient's weight = 65 kg. What is the dose in micrograms/min? (You will meet this type of calculation with intravenous infusions – see later).

Question 11 Dose = 3 micrograms/kg/min, patient's weight = 85 kg. What is the dose in micrograms/min?

Question 12 Dose = 500 micrograms/kg/min, patient's weight = 78 kg. What is the dose in mg/min?

CALCULATING DIVIDED DOSES

Sometimes the dose of a drug is given as a total daily dose (TDD), which has to be given in divided doses (usually three or four times a day).

It is important that you can tell the difference between the total daily dose (TDD) and individual doses. If not interpreted properly, then the patient is at risk of receiving the TDD as an individual dose, thus receiving three or four times the normal dose (which could have disastrous results).

This can be a problem with paediatric doses, as some of the doses are given in reference books as total daily doses (see Chapter 9, 'Paediatric dosage calculations').

To illustrate this point, consider the following example:

Ibuprofen 1200 mg daily given **three** times a day.

It is **not** 1200 mg to be given three times a day, but 1200 mg in three divided doses, i.e.

$$\frac{1200}{3} = 400 \text{ mg three times a day}$$

The patient is at risk of receiving three times the intended dose. It is therefore very important that doses are read and interpreted properly. Always **read the wording carefully**.

To calculate divided doses, simply divide the total daily dose by the number of required doses. For example,

Cefuroxime IV 2.25 g in divided doses every 8 hours.

8 hourly is equal to 3 doses in 24 hours (6 hourly would be equal to 4 doses). Therefore, in this case, divide the total daily dose by 3. In this case, it would be better to convert 2.25 g to milligrams, as each dose will have to be measured in milligrams:

2.25 g = 2.25 × 1,000 = 2,250 mg

Then divide by 3 to find the amount needed for each dose:

$$\frac{2,250}{3} = 750 \text{ mg}$$

You will need to give cefuroxime IV 750 mg every 8 hours (three times a day).

Sometimes it may be necessary to calculate hourly volumes for infusions. In this case, simply divide the total volume by the number of hours over which the infusion is to be given. For example,

500 mL sodium chloride 0.9% infusion over 8 hours.

To find the hourly volume, divide 500 by 8:

$$\frac{500}{8} = 62.5 \text{ mL}$$

Knowing the hourly volume is very useful in IV calculations. It is used in the formula to calculate infusion drip rates (see Chapter 7, 'Infusion rate calculations').

CALCULATING DRUG DOSAGES

There are several ways of solving this type of calculation. It is best to learn one way and stick to it. The easiest way is by proportion: what you do to one side of an equation, do the same to the other side.

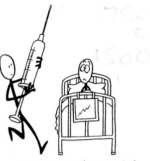

Whatever the type of calculation you are doing, it is always best to make what you've got equal to 1 and then multiply by what you want. This can be called the **one unit** rule. This may sound a bit confusing, but it should appear clearer after working through the worked example.

ARE YOU SURE YOU'VE CALCULATED THE DOSE CORRECTLY ?

Also, when what you've got and what you want are in different units, you need to convert everything to the same units. When converting to the same units, it is best to convert to whole numbers to avoid decimal points as fewer mistakes are then made. If possible, it is a good idea to convert everything to the units of the answer.

WORKED EXAMPLE

You need to prepare an infusion of digoxin containing 0.75 mg. Digoxin comes in 2 mL ampoules of 250 micrograms/mL. What volume (in mL) is needed?

Step 1

The units of what you've got (500 micrograms/2 mL) and what you want (0.75 mg) are different. Converting everything to micrograms will avoid decimal points.

$$0.75 \text{ mg} = 0.75 \times 1{,}000 = 750 \text{ micrograms}$$

Step 2

Calculate how much one unit is of what you have, i.e.

500 micrograms in 2 mL, therefore

$$1 \text{ microgram} = \frac{2}{500} \text{ mL}$$

This is the **one unit** rule.

Step 3

You need to know how much digoxin to draw up for 750 micrograms, therefore multiply the amount from Step 2 by 750:

$$750 \text{ micrograms} = \frac{2}{500} \times 750 = 3 \text{ mL}$$

Answer: You will need to draw up 3 mL of digoxin.

A simple formula can be used to calculate drug dosages:

$$\frac{\text{amount you want}}{\text{amount you've got}} \times \text{volume it's in}$$

Once again, before entering numbers in the formula, you must convert everything to the same units. Thus:

amount you want   = 750 micrograms
amount you've got = 500 micrograms
volume it's in   = 2 mL

Substitute the numbers in the formula:

$$\frac{750}{500} \times 2 = 3 \text{ mL}$$

Answer: You will need to draw up 3 mL of digoxin.

You can apply this method to whatever type of calculation you want (not just micrograms and milligrams).

The following case report illustrates the importance of ensuring that your calculations are right.

A SECOND CHANCE FOR DOCTORS?

Case report

A female baby, born seven weeks prematurely, died at 28 hours old when a junior doctor miscalculated a dose of intravenous morphine resulting in the administration of a 100 times overdose. The doctor is reported to have worked out the dose on a piece of paper and then checked it on a calculator but the decimal point was inserted in the wrong place and 15 instead of 0.15 milligrams was prescribed. The dose was then prepared and handed to the senior registrar who administered it without double checking the calculation and, despite treatment with naloxone, the baby died 55 minutes later.

Comment

At the inquest into this case the coroner recorded an open verdict, believing that the death was caused by the overdose but being unable to state so 'beyond reasonable doubt'. A number of points were also made by the coroner which we feel should be considered in this column. Perhaps the most far reaching of these is the coroner's recommendation to the General Medical Council that they advise all doctors to check the drug doses they prepare with a qualified colleague. The medical profession must surely be the only discipline that does not have a requirement for secondary checking by colleagues and this anomaly must be regarded as a contributory factor to many serious medication errors. As long ago as 1991, in the wake of incidents involving the maladministration of cytotoxic drugs, a recommendation was issued by the Trent region medical officer that, 'in the case of certain drugs it should be a requirement that two qualified doctors check the drug label and dosage before the drug is administered' Whether the GMC acts on this recommendation remains to be seen – there are obviously practical issues around the feasibility of implementing such a proposal.

We believe that hospital pharmacists, through local drug administration policies and teaching of junior doctors and medical students, should actively encourage the development of a culture in which it is accepted practice for junior doctors to obtain a second check of drug dosing. This requirement should apply particularly in critical areas such as chemotherapy, paediatrics and all intravenous therapy. Must this second check be obtained from a qualified doctor? Surely, in the interest of patient safety a second check could be given by a qualified nurse or pharmacist. As multiskilling of healthcare professionals develops there must be scope for legislating the checking of accuracy across the existing professional boundaries. We would welcome colleagues' comments through the letters column of this journal.

The coroner was also extremely critical of the arithmetical capabilities of junior medical staff and advised a review of educational standards. Similar criticism has previously been published in the medical literature[1,2] where, for example, success rates in converting concentrations to drug doses were as low as 16 per cent and numerical skill was notably poorer amongst junior medical staff compared to seniors and anaesthetists. Again, we feel that pharmacists should be much more involved with the training of medical staff in practical areas such as drug dosage calculation, preparation and administration.

Finally, in the aftermath of this incident, it is reported that the strength of morphine ampoules stocked in the special care baby unit has been reduced. We have commented previously on the responsibility we feel that pharmacists have to actively manage the stocks held in clinical areas with regard to the potential risk of overdose or error. This tragic case provides a further illustration of that responsibility.[3,4]

References

1 Baldwin L. Calculating drug doses. *BMJ* 1995; 310: 1154.
2 Rolfe S, Harper NJN. Ability of hospital doctors to calculate drug doses. *BMJ* 1995; 310: 1173–1174.
3 Cousins DH, Upton DR. Medication errors. Error 33. Two deaths resulting from narcotic overdose. *Pharmacy in Practice* 1995; 5: 130,132.
4 Cousins DH, Upton DR. Medication errors. Error 59. Regulate supply to minimize risk. *Pharmacy in Practice* 1996; 6: 254.

Taken from *Pharmacy in Practice* 1997; 7: 368–369

CHECKING YOUR ANSWER – DOES IT SEEM REASONABLE?

When doing this sort of calculation, it is good practice to have a rough idea of the answer first, so you can check your final calculated answer. To illustrate this point, consider the earlier worked example:

> You have digoxin 500 micrograms in 2 mL, and you want digoxin 750 micrograms.

Obviously, the final volume you want will be more than 2 mL, but less than 4 mL, (4 mL = 1,000 micrograms). So the answer will be between 2 and 4 mL. If the answer you get is outside this range, then your answer is wrong and you should re-check your calculations.

As you can see, having a rough idea of the answer before you do your calculation, means that you can decide as to whether the answer you get is reasonable or not.

Sometimes, it may not be possible to guess your answer (as with our worked example). However, it is possible to estimate your answer by rounding up or down numbers enabling easy calculations (see 'Estimation of answers', p. 27).

The following guide may be useful in helping you to decide as to whether your answer is reasonable or not. Any answer outside these ranges probably means that you have calculated the wrong answer.

THE MAXIMUM YOU SHOULD GIVE A PATIENT

- Tablets: not more than 4 for any one dose. (An exception to this is prednisolone. Some doses of prednisolone may mean the patient taking up to ten tablets at any one time. Even with prednisolone, it is important to check the dose and the number of tablets.)

- Liquids: anything from 5 mL to 20 mL for any one dose.
- Injections: anything from 1 mL to 10 mL for any one dose.

 Tip Re-check your answer. If you are in any doubt about any calculation, **stop and get help**.

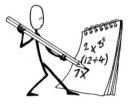

Always write your calculations down on paper

The following two case reports illustrate the importance of checking numbers before administration.

BE ALERT TO HIGH NUMBERS OF DOSE UNITS

An unusual request from a ward led to the discovery of a serious error.

Case report 1

A male patient was prescribed a stat dose of 2 g amiodarone for conversion of atrial fibrillation. Although it is still not known whether this dose was chosen deliberately or prescribed in error, there is evidence to support the use of a 2 g oral regimen.[1,2] What concerned the reporting hospital was that the nurse administered 10 × 200 mg tablets to the patient without any reference or confirmation that this was indeed what was intended. This use of amiodarone is at present outside the product licence and would not have been described in any of the literature available on the ward.

The patient subsequently died but at the time of writing no causal effect from this high dose of amiodarone had been established.

Case report 2

A female patient aged approximately 65 was prescribed 2,500 units of dalteparin sodium subcutaneously once a day under the hospital's post-thoracoscopy DVT prophylaxis protocol. The prescribed dose was misread and two nurses checking each other gave five pre-filled syringes i.e. 25,000 units to the patient in error. So much heparin was required that another patient's supply had to be used as well and the error came to light when the ward made a request to pharmacy for 25,000 unit doses of dalteparin. When the error was discovered the patient's coagulation status was checked immediately and fortunately she came to no harm.

Comment

It seems inconceivable to us that such high numbers of dose units could be administered to patients without the nurses involved at least querying that something might be wrong. The case of five pre-filled syringes being administered at once is probably the most extreme case we have come across of this nature. Both cases were reported by the same hospital, which has raised understandable concerns about the lack of awareness of 'usual' drug doses.

Pharmacists must ensure that local medicines management policies include guidelines that require doses to be confirmed if administration is found to potentially involve more than three or four dose units.

References

1. Blanc J-J, Voinov Q Maarek M. Comparison of oral loading dose of propafenone and amiodarone for converting recent-onset atrial fibrillation. *American Journal of Cardiology* 1999; 84: 1029–1032.

2. Andrivet P et al. A clinical study of amiodarone as a single oral dose in patients with recent-onset atrial tachyarrhythmia. *European Heart Journal* 1994; 15: 1396–1402.

Taken from *Pharmacy in Practice* 2001; 6: 194

PROBLEMS

Question 13 You need to give 1 g of erythromycin orally. You have erythromycin suspension 250 mg in 5 mL. How much of the suspension do you need to give?

Question 14 You need to give a patient 125 micrograms of digoxin orally. You have digoxin elixir 50 micrograms/mL supplied with a dropper pipette. How much do you need to draw up?

Question 15 You need to give a slow IV injection of salbutamol 250 micrograms. Salbutamol injection comes as a 50 micrograms/mL ampoule. What volume (in mL) do you need to draw up?

Question 16 You have pethidine injection 100 mg in 2 mL. The patient is prescribed 75 mg. How much do you draw up?

Question 17 You have to give cefotaxime IV to a baby weighing 5.6 kg at a dose of 100 mg/kg daily in four divided doses. You have 500 mg vials of cefotaxime injection, and each vial has to be reconstituted to 2 mL. How much do you need for each dose?

Question 18 You need to give a dose of trimethoprim suspension to a child weighing 18.45 kg at a dose of 4 mg/kg. You have trimethoprim suspension 50 mg in 5 mL. What dose do you need to give and how much of the suspension do you need?

Question 19 You need to give a very slow IV injection of aminophylline 325 mg using a syringe driver over 30 min. Aminophylline injection comes as 250 mg in 10 mL ampoules. What volume (in mL) do you need to draw up?

Question 20 You need to give aciclovir (acyclovir) as an infusion at a dose of 5 mg/kg every 8 h. The patient weighs 76 kg and aciclovir (acyclovir) is available as 250 mg vials. How many vials do you need for each dose?

Question 21 A 50 kg woman is prescribed aminophylline as an infusion at a dose of 0.5 mg/kg/hour. Aminophylline injection comes as 250 mg in 10 mL ampoules. How much is required if the infusion is to run for 12 hours?

Question 22 You need to prepare an infusion of co-trimoxazole at a dose of 120 mg/kg per day in four divided doses for a patient weighing 68 kg. Co-trimoxazole is available as 5 mL ampoules at a strength of 96 mg/mL
   i) What volume of co-trimoxazole do you need for each dose?
   ii) How many ampoules do you need for each dose?
   iii) How many ampoules do you need for 24 hours?
   iv) Before administration, co-trimoxazole must be diluted further: 1 ampoule diluted to 125 mL. Therefore what volume should each dose be given in?

ANSWERS TO PROBLEMS

Question 1 Two 250 mg tablets.

Question 2 Two 1 microgram tablets.

Question 3 Dose = 1.5 mg/kg, patient's weight = 73 kg. Therefore to calculate the total dose required, multiply:

$$1.5 \times 73 = 109.5$$

Thus you will need 109.5 mg (rounding up = 110 mg).

Question 4 516 mg

Question 5   720 mg

Question 6   24.8 mL (25 mL)

Question 7   97 mg

Question 8   186 mg

Question 9   **i)** 21,600 micrograms;   **ii)** 21.6 mg (22 mg)

Question 10   325 micrograms/min

Question 11   255 micrograms/min

Question 12 $500 \times 78 = 39,000$ micrograms/min

$$\frac{39,000}{1,000} = 39 \text{ mg/min}$$

Question 13   20 mL

Question 14   2.5 mL

Question 15   5 mL

Question 16   1.5 mL

Question 17   Total daily dose = weight $\times$ dose

$$5.6 \times 100 = 560 \text{ mg}$$

This needs to be given in four divided doses, therefore to find out how the amount needed for each dose, divide by 4:

$$\frac{560}{4} = 140 \text{ mg}$$

You have cefotaxime 500 mg in 2 mL:

Thus $1 \text{ mg} = \dfrac{2}{500} \text{ mL}$

Therefore for 140 mg, you will need:

$$\frac{2}{500} \times 140 = 0.56 \text{ mL}$$

Using the formula:

$$\frac{\text{amount you want}}{\text{amount you've got}} \times \text{volume it's in}$$

where in this case:

amount you want = 140 mg
amount you've got = 500 mg
volume it's in   = 2 mL

Substitute the numbers in the formula:

$$\frac{140}{500} \times 2 = 0.56 \text{ mL}$$

Question 18   Total amount required = weight × dose

= 18.45 × 4 = 73.8 mg

Volume required = 7.4 mL

Question 19   13 mL

Question 20   Dose required = 76 × 5 = 380 mg, so you will need two vials of 250 mg

Question 21   Dose required for the patient = 50 × 0.5 = 25 mg/hour. Therefore for 12 h, you will need, 25 × 12 = 300 mg. You have 250 mg in 10 mL:

Therefore 1 mg would equal $\frac{10}{250}$ mL (one unit rule)

Thus, 300 mg = $\frac{10}{250}$ × 300 = 12 mL

Answer: 12 mL

Question 22   **i)** Total daily dose = weight × dose

= 120 × 68 = 8,160 mg

However, it is to be given in four divided doses, so for each dose, you will need:

$\frac{8,160}{4}$ = 2,040 milligrams

You have co-trimoxazole injection containing 96 mg/mL:

Thus 1 mg = $\frac{1}{96}$ mL

Therefore for 2,040 mg you will need:

$\frac{1}{96}$ × 2,040 = 21.25 mL

ii) Each ampoule equals 5 mL. To work out how many ampoules are needed, divide the total volume required by the volume for each ampoule, i.e.

$\frac{21.25}{5}$ = 4. 25

Therefore you will need five ampoules (25 mL) for each dose, drawing up 21.25 mL and discarding the remainder.

iii) Since it is to be given in four divided doses; to calculate how many ampoules are needed for 1 day, multiply the amount for each dose by four, i.e. 5 × 4 = 20 ampoules.

iv) 1 ampoule must be diluted to 125 mL, thus for 4.25 ampoules, you will need:

$$4.25 \times 125 = 531.25 \text{ mL}$$

Therefore give in 1 litre sodium chloride infusion 0.9%.

KEY POINTS

Calculating the number of tablets or capsules required

$$\text{number required} = \frac{\text{amount prescribed}}{\text{amount in each tablet/capsule}}$$

Dosages based on patient parameters

- Weight (dose/kg): dose × body weight (kg).
- Surface area (dose/m²) dose × body surface area (m²).

Calculating doses

$$\frac{\text{amount you want}}{\text{amount you've got}} \times \text{volume it's in}$$

- Take care when reading doses, either prescribed or found in the literature.
- Total daily dose (TDD) is the total dose and needs to be divided by the number of doses per day to give a single dose.
- To be sure that your answer is correct, it is best to calculate from first principles (for example, using the 'one unit rule').
- If using a formula, make sure that the figures are entered correctly.
- Ensure that everything is in the same units.
- Always re-check your answer – if in any doubt, stop and get help.
- Ask yourself: does my answer seem reasonable?

Percent and percentages

4

OBJECTIVES

At the end of this chapter, you should be familiar with the following:

- Percent and percentages
- Converting fractions to percentages and vice versa
- Converting decimals to percentages and vice versa
- Calculations involving percentages
- Drug calculations involving percentages
- How to use the percentage key on your calculator

The percent or percentage is a common way of expressing the amount of something, and is very useful for comparing different quantities.

It is unlikely that you will need to calculate the percentage of something on the ward. It is more likely that you will need to know how much drug is in a solution given as a percentage, e.g. an infusion containing potassium 0.3%.

PERCENT AND PERCENTAGES

As stated before, a convenient way of expressing drug strengths is by using the percent.

We will be dealing with how percentages are used to describe drug strengths or concentrations in the next chapter ('Drug strengths or concentrations').

The aim of this chapter is to explain the concept of percent and how to do simple percentage calculations. It is important to understand percent before moving on to percentage concentrations.

Percent means 'part in a hundred' or a 'proportion of a hundred', and the symbol for percent is %. So 30% means 30 parts in 100.

Percentages are often used to give a quick indication of a specific quantity and are very useful when making comparisons.

If you consider a town where 5,690 people live and the number of people unemployed is 853, it is very difficult to visualize exactly how many or what proportion of people are unemployed.

It is much easier to say that in a town of 5,690 people, 15% of them are unemployed.

If we consider another town of 11,230 people where 2,246 people are unemployed, it is very difficult, at a glance, to see which town has the greater proportion of unemployed.

But when the numbers are given as percentages, it is much easier to compare: the first town has 15% unemployment, whereas the second town has 20%.

Percentages can be very useful, and so is being able to convert to a percentage. It is easier to compare numbers or quantities when they are given as percentages.

CONVERTING FRACTIONS TO PERCENTAGES AND VICE VERSA

To convert a fraction to a percentage, you simply **multiply** by 100, i.e.

$$\frac{2}{5} = \frac{2}{5} \times 100 = 40\%$$

Conversely, to convert a percentage to a fraction, **divide** by 100, i.e.

$$40\% = \frac{40}{100} = \frac{4}{10} = \frac{2}{5}$$

If possible, always reduce the fraction to its lowest terms before making the conversion.

CONVERTING DECIMALS TO PERCENTAGES AND VICE VERSA

To convert a decimal to a percentage, once again you simply **multiply** by 100, i.e.

$$0.4 = 0.4 \times 100 = 40\%$$

Remember, to multiply by 100 you move the decimal point **two places to the right**.

To convert a percentage to a decimal, you **divide** by 100, i.e.

$$\frac{40}{100} = 0.4$$

To divide by 100 you move the decimal point **two places to the left**.

So, to convert fractions and decimals to percentages or vice versa, you simply multiply or divide by 100.

Thus:

$$25\% = \frac{25}{100} = \frac{1}{4} = 0.25 \quad \text{(a quarter)}$$

$$33\% = \frac{33}{100} = \frac{1}{3} = 0.33 \quad \text{(approximately a third)}$$

$$50\% = \frac{50}{100} = \frac{1}{2} = 0.5 \quad \text{(a half)}$$

$$66\% = \frac{66}{100} = \frac{2}{3} = 0.66 \quad \text{(approximately two-thirds)}$$

$$75\% = \frac{75}{100} = \frac{3}{4} = 0.75 \quad \text{(three-quarters)}$$

The next step is to look at how to find the percentage of something. The following worked example should show how this is done.

CALCULATIONS INVOLVING PERCENTAGES

The first type of calculation we are going to look at is how to find the percentage of a given quantity or number.

WORKED EXAMPLE

How much is 28% of 250?

There are several ways of solving this type of calculation.

Method 1

With this method you are working in percentages.

Step 1

When doing percentage calculations, the number or quantity you want to find the percentage of, is always equal to 100%. In this example, 250 is equal to 100% and you want to find out how much is 28%. So,

250 = 100%

(Thus you are converting the number to a percentage).

Step 2

Calculate how much is equal to 1%, i.e. divide by 100 (you are using the one unit rule)

$$1\% = \frac{250}{100}$$

Step 3

Multiply by the percentage required (28%):

$$28\% = \frac{250}{100} \times 28 = 70$$

Answer: 28% of 250 = 70

Method 2

In this method you are working in fractions or decimals and not percentages.

Step 1

To convert the percentage to a fraction or decimal, divide by 100, i.e.

$$\frac{28}{100} \text{ or } 0.28$$

Step 2

Multiply by the original number (250):

$$\frac{28}{100} \times 250 = 70$$

which is the same as:

$$0.28 \times 250 = 70$$

Thus you are finding out how much the fraction or decimal is of the original number.

Answer: 28% of 250 = 70

From both of these methods, a simple formula can be devised:

$$\frac{\text{number}}{100} \times \text{percentage required}$$

In this example:

number = 250
percentage required = 28%

Substitute the numbers in the formula:

$$\frac{250}{100} \times 28 = 70$$

Answer: 28% of 250 = 70

Tip Whatever method you use, you always **divide** by 100.

However, you may want to find out what percentage a number is of another larger number, especially when comparing numbers or quantities. So this is the second type of percentage calculation we are going to look at.

WORKED EXAMPLE

What percentage is 630 of 9,000?

In this case, it is best to work in percentages since it is that you want to find.

Step 1

Once again, the number or quantity you want to find the percentage of is always equal to 100%.

In this example, 9,000 is equal to 100% and you want to find out the percentage of 630. So,

9,000 = 100%

(thus you are converting the number to a percentage).

Step 2

Calculate the percentage for 1 (i.e. divide by 9,000, using the one unit rule)

$$\frac{100\%}{9,000}$$

Step 3

Multiply by the number you wish to find the percentage of, i.e. the smaller number (630).

$$\frac{100}{9,000} \times 630 = 7\%$$

Answer: 630 is 7% of 9,000.

Once again, a simple formula can be devised:

$$\frac{100}{\text{larger number}} \times \text{smaller number} \quad \text{or} \quad \frac{\text{smaller number}}{\text{larger number}} \times 100$$

Tip In this case, **multiply** by 100.

PERCENT AND PERCENTAGES – SUMMARY

- To convert a fraction to a percentage, multiply by 100 (move the decimal point two places to the right).
- To convert a percentage to a fraction, divide by 100 (move the decimal point two places to the left).
- To convert a decimal to a percentage, multiply by 100 (move the decimal point two places to the right).
- To convert a percentage to a decimal, divide by 100 (move the decimal point two places to the left).
- To find the percentage of a number, always divide by 100:

$$\frac{\text{number}}{100} \times \text{percentage required}$$

- To find what percentage one number is of another, always multiply by 100:

$$\frac{100}{\text{larger number}} \times \text{smaller number} \quad \text{or} \quad \frac{\text{smaller number}}{\text{larger number}} \times 100$$

PROBLEMS

Work out the following:

Question 1   30% of 3,090

Question 2   84% of 42,825

Question 3   56.25% of 800

Question 4   60% of 80.6

Question 5   17.5% of 285.76

What percentage are the following?

Question 6   60 of 750

Question 7   53,865 of 64,125

Question 8   29.61 of 47

Question 9   53.69 of 191.75

Question 10 48 of 142

DRUG CALCULATIONS INVOLVING PERCENTAGES

The principles here can easily be applied to drug calculations. As before, it is unlikely that you will need to find the percentage of something, but these calculations are included here to help you gain an understanding of percent and percentages, especially where drugs are concerned. Once again, always convert everything to the same units before solving the calculation.

WORKED EXAMPLE

What volume (in mL) is 60% of 1.25 litres?

Step 1

Convert 1.25 litres into millilitres (mL), since the required answer is in millilitres (mL):

1.25 litres = 1.25 × 1,000 = 1,250 mL

Step 2

As before, the quantity you want to find the percentage of is always equal to 100%, i.e.

1,250 mL = 100%

Thus you are converting the volume to a percentage.

Step 3

Calculate the volume (in mL) that equals 1% by dividing by 100, using the one unit rule

$1\% = \dfrac{1,250}{100}$

Step 4

Multiply by the percentage required (60%)

$60\% = \dfrac{1,250}{100} \times 60 = 750 \text{ mL}$

Answer: 60% of 1.25 litres equals 750 mL

Alternatively, you can use the formula:

$\dfrac{\text{number}}{100} \times \text{percentage required}$

rewriting it as:

$\dfrac{\text{what you've got}}{100} \times \text{percentage required}$

where:

what you've got = 1,250 mL
percentage required = 60%

Substitute the numbers in the formula:

$\dfrac{1,250}{100} \times 60 = 750 \text{ mL}$

Answer: 60% of 1.25 litres is 750 mL

Now consider the following example.

WORKED EXAMPLE

What percentage is 125 mg of 500 mg?

Step 1

In this case, everything is already in the same units milligrams (mg). If you are working in different units, you should convert everything to the same units – usually those of the answer, but always to the units that avoid decimal points.

Step 2

As always, the quantity you want to find the percentage of is equal to 100%, i.e.

500 mg = 100%

Thus you are converting the quantity or amount to a percentage.

Step 3

Calculate the percentage for 1 mg of what you have by dividing by 500, using the one unit rule, i.e.

$$1 \text{ mg} = \frac{100}{500} \%$$

Step 4

However, you want to know the percentage for 125 mg, so multiply by 125, i.e.

$$125 \text{ mg} = \frac{100}{500} \times 125 = 25\%$$

Answer: 125 mg is equal to 25% of 500 mg

Alternatively, you can use the formula:

$$\frac{100}{\text{larger number}} \times \text{smaller number}$$

where:

smaller number = 125 mg
larger number = 500 mg

Substitute the numbers in the formula:

$$\frac{100}{500} \times 125 = 25\%$$

Answer: 125 mg is equal to 25% of 500 mg

DRUG CALCULATIONS INVOLVING PERCENTAGES – SUMMARY

- To find the percentage of something:

$$\frac{\text{what you've got}}{100} \times \text{percentage required}$$

- To find what percentage one quantity is of another:

$$\frac{\text{smaller number}}{\text{larger number}} \times 100 \qquad \frac{100}{\text{large number}} \times \text{small No}$$

PROBLEMS

Work out the following:

Question 11 How much is 15% of 3 litres?

Question 12 How much is 63% of 2.5 litres?

Question 13 How much is 28% of 500 g?

Question 14 How much is 98% of 3 kg?

Question 15 How much is 27.6% of 500 mL?

What percentage are the following:

Question 16 230 mL of 500 mL?

Question 17 48 g of 750 g?

Question 18 320 mg of 800 mg?

Question 19 64.5 g of 250 g?

Question 20 750 mg of 5 g? (beware of units!)

Question 21 64.5 mg of 1 g? (beware of units!)

HOW TO USE THE PERCENTAGE KEY ON YOUR CALCULATOR

Your calculator may have a percentage button [%]. Using this [%] button is a quick way to work out percentages on the calculator. However, it is important that the numbers and the [%] button are pressed in the right sequence; otherwise it is quite easy to get the wrong answer! Let's go back to our original example:

How much is 28% of 250?

You could easily find the answer by the long method, i.e.

$$\frac{250}{100} \times 28$$

Key in the sequence

[2][5][0] [÷] [1][0][0] [×] [2][8] [=]

to give an answer of 70.

When using the [%] button, you need to enter in the following way:

enter	[2][8]	display = 28
enter	[×]	display = 28
enter	[2][5][0]	display = 250
enter	[%]	display = 70 (answer)
enter	[=]	display = 1960

Depending upon what kind of calculator you have, pressing the [=] may give the wrong answer! What happens is that by pressing the [=] button, you are multiplying by the percentage again, i.e. 28 × 28% of 250, giving a nonsensical answer!

Now let's look at our second example:

What percentage is 630 of 9,000?

Once again, you can easily find the answer by:

$$\frac{630}{9,000} \times 100$$

Key in the sequence:

[6][3][0] [÷] [9][0][0][0] [×] [1][0][0] [=]

to give an answer of 7%.

But when using the [%] button, you need to enter in the following way:

enter	[6][3][0]	display = 630
enter	[÷]	display = 630
enter	[9][0][0][0]	display = 9000
enter	[%]	display = 7% (answer)
enter	[=]	display = 1960

Once again, pressing the [=] key may give the wrong answer!

By pressing [=], you are dividing by 9,000 again, i.e.

$$\frac{630}{9,000 \times 9,000} \times 100$$

Thus when using your calculator for a percentage calculation, **do not** press the [=] button.

It's also important to enter the numbers in the right sequence. If you don't, you will again get the wrong answer:

enter [9][0][0][0] display = 9000
enter [÷]   display = 630
enter [6][3][0]   display = 630
enter [%]   display = 1428.5714

What happens if you enter [=]?

enter [=]   display = 2.2675736

To explain this, look at the long method of solving this problem:

9,000 = 100%

Therefore:

$$\frac{1}{9,000} = 100\,\%$$

Thus:

$$630 = \frac{100}{9,000} \times 630\,\% \qquad \text{OR} \qquad \frac{630}{9,000} \times 100\,\%$$

You can see that it is 630 divided by 9,000, and not the other way round.

Therefore it is important to enter the numbers the right way round on your calculator. An easy way to remember is: **enter the smaller number first**.

It is also important to remember to enter or press the [%] button last, otherwise you will get the wrong answer, i.e. in our first example: How much is 28% of 250?

enter [2][8]   display = 28
enter [%]   display = 28
enter [×]   display = 28
enter [2][5][0]   display = 250
enter [=]   display = 7000

You are simply multiplying 28 by 7,000.

In both examples, entering the numbers in the wrong sequence will give the wrong answer. Try experimenting with your own calculator; you will soon see how many different answers you can get!

So, to summarize, if you want to use the [%] button on your calculator, remember the following sequence:

1 Enter the numbers in the right sequence.
   • If you are finding the percentage of something, **multiply** the two numbers, (it doesn't matter in which order you enter the numbers).

- If you are finding the percentage one number is of another, **divide** the **smaller** number (enter first) by the **larger** number (enter second).
- In this case, the sequence of numbers is important.

2 Always enter or press the [%] button **last**.

3 Do **not** enter or press the [=] button.

4 Refer to your calculator manual to see how your own calculator uses the [%] button.

5 Don't forget to clear your calculator (press the [CE] button) when you have finished, otherwise the numbers left in your calculator may be carried over to your next sum.

Although using the [%] button is a quick way of finding percentages, you have to use it properly, so it may be best to ignore it and do the calculations the long way.

> **Tip** Get to know how to use your calculator – read the manual! If you don't know how to use your calculator properly, then there is the potential for errors because you won't know if the answer you've got is correct or not.

ANSWERS TO PROBLEMS

CALCULATIONS INVOLVING PERCENTAGES

Question 1   927

Question 2   35,973

Question 3   450

Question 4   48.36

Question 5   50.008 (50)

Question 6   8%

Question 7   84%

Question 8   63%

Question 9   28%

Question 10 33.8%

DRUG CALCULATIONS INVOLVING PERCENTAGES

Question 11 0.45 litres (450 mL)

Question 12 1.575 litres (1,575 mL)

Question 13 140 g

Question 14 2.94 kg (2,940 g)

Question 15 138 mL

Question 16 46%

Question 17 6.4%

Question 18 40%

Question 19 25.8%

Question 20 15%

Always work in the same units. It is best to work in whole numbers, so in this case it is best to work in milligrams since this is the smaller unit. Convert the larger unit (grams) to the smaller unit (milligrams):

$$5 \times 1,000 = 5,000 \text{ mg}$$
$$5,000 \text{ mg} = 100\%, \quad \text{thus } 1 \text{ mg} = \frac{100}{5,000} \%$$

Therefore:

$$750 \text{ mg} = \frac{100}{5,000} \times 750 = 15\%$$

Answer: 750 mg is 15% of 5 g

You could also use the formula:

$$\frac{100}{\text{larger number}} \times \text{smaller number}$$

where:

smaller number = 750 mg
larger number = 5,000 mg (5 g)

Substitute the numbers in the formula:

$$\frac{100}{5,000} \times 750 = 15\%$$

Answer: 750 mg is 15% of 5 g

Question 21 6.45% (beware of units: convert 1 g to 1,000 mg)

KEY POINTS

Percent

- Percent means 'part of a hundred' or a 'proportion of a hundred'.
- The symbol for percent is %, so (for example) 30% means 30 parts of 100.
- Percent is often used to give a quick indication of a specific quantity and is very useful when making comparisons.

Percentages and fractions

- To convert a **fraction** to a **percentage**, **multiply** by 100.
- To convert a **percentage** to a **fraction**, divide by 100.

Percentages and decimals

- To convert a **decimal** to a **percentage**, **multiply** by 100 (move the decimal point two places to the right).
- To convert a **percentage** to a **decimal**, **divide** by 100 (move the decimal point two places to the left).

Thus:

$$25\% = \frac{25}{100} = \frac{1}{4} = 0.25 \quad \text{(a quarter)}$$

$$33\% = \frac{33}{100} = \frac{1}{3} = 0.33 \quad \text{(approximately a third)}$$

$$50\% = \frac{50}{100} = \frac{1}{2} = 0.5 \quad \text{(a half)}$$

$$66\% = \frac{66}{100} = \frac{2}{3} = 0.66 \quad \text{(approximately two-thirds)}$$

$$75\% = \frac{75}{100} = \frac{3}{4} = 0.75 \quad \text{(three-quarters)}$$

- To find the percentage of a number, always **divide** by 100:

$$\frac{\text{number}}{100} \times \text{percentage required}$$

- To find what percentage one number is of another, always **multiply** by 100:

$$\frac{100}{\text{larger number}} \times \text{smaller number} \quad \text{or} \quad \frac{\text{smaller number}}{\text{larger number}} \times 100$$

Drug calculations involving percentages

- To find the percentage of something:

$$\frac{\text{what you've got}}{100} \times \text{percentage required}$$

- To find what percentage one quantity is of another:

$$\frac{\text{smaller number}}{\text{larger number}} \times 100$$

Moles and millimoles

OBJECTIVES

At the end of this chapter, you should be familiar with the following:

- What moles and millimoles are
- Calculations involving mole and millimoles

Everyday references may be made to moles and millimoles in relation to electrolyte levels, blood glucose, serum creatinine or other test results. These are measurements carried out by chemical pathology and the units used are usually millimoles or micromoles. The unit millimole is also encountered with infusions when electrolytes have been added.

For example:

Mr J. Brown   sodium = 138 mmol/L
An infusion contains 20 mmol potassium chloride

Before you can interpret such results or amounts, you will need to be familiar with this rather confusing unit, the **mole**.

In this chapter we try to explain what moles and millimoles are, and how to do calculations involving millimoles.

WHAT ARE MOLES AND MILLIMOLES?

The concept of moles and millimoles is difficult to understand; you need to be familiar with basic chemistry. It's important to know what they are and how they are derived.

MOLES

Counting atoms

All elements are made up from atoms. Atoms are too small to be counted or weighed individually. The mole is the unit used by chemists to make counting and measuring of atoms a lot easier. So what is a mole? A mole represents a number, just like the word 'dozen' represents the number 12.

A mole is the number of atoms in 12 grams of carbon (^{12}C). This turns out to be a huge number, approximately 6×10^{23}. When this is written out in full, it is equal to:

600,000,000,000,000,000,000,000

a very large number indeed. It is called **Avogadro's number** in honour of the Italian scientist Amedeo Avogadro (1776–1856).

The usual way of counting atoms is by weighing them. Each element has an atomic mass or weight (based on the average mass of an atom of that element). So if you know how much of an element you have (by weighing) and the atomic mass (from tables) you have a way of calculating how many atoms you are working with.

Chemists are not the only the people who 'count by weighing'. Bank clerks use the same idea when they count coins by weighing them. For example, 100 1p coins weigh 356 g; it is quicker to weigh 356 g of 1p coins than to count 100 coins.

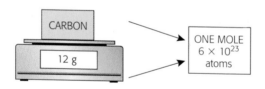

12 g of carbon = 1 mole or 6×10^{23} atoms

1 g of carbon = $\frac{1}{12}$ mole or $\frac{1}{12} \times 6 \times 10^{23}$ atoms

10 g of carbon = $\frac{10}{12}$ mole or $\frac{10}{12} \times 6 \times 10^{23}$ atoms

Since 1 mole is equal to 12 g of carbon, it follows that:

1 mole = the atomic mass in grams

Counting molecules

Now consider a molecule, for example sodium chloride (NaCl). The individual parts of the molecule are called ions. Sodium chloride is made up of two ions: sodium (Na^+) and chloride (Cl^-).

Na Cl = molecule

Na^+ Cl^- = ions

Hence 1 mole of sodium chloride contains (or provides) 1 mole of sodium and 1 mole of chloride.

Table 7 on page 80 shows atomic and molecular masses; from this we can find the relative atomic masses of sodium and chloride:

sodium (Na)   23
chloride (Cl)   35.5

The molecular mass is the sum of the atomic masses, i.e. in this case:

23 + 35.5 = 58.5

So the molecular mass of sodium chloride is 58.5.

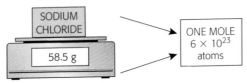

58.5 g of sodium chloride = 1 mole or 6 × 10²³ atoms

1 g of sodium chloride = $\frac{1}{58.5}$ mole or $\frac{1}{58.5}$ × 6 × 10²³ atoms

10 g of sodium chloride = $\frac{10}{58.5}$ mole or $\frac{10}{58.5}$ × 6 × 10²³ atoms

Since 1 mole is equal to 58.5 g of sodium chloride, it follows that:

1 mole = the molecular mass in grams

What about carbon dioxide (CO_2)? Here the individual parts of the molecule are atoms, not ions. The '2' after the 'O' in the chemical formula means two atoms of oxygen, so one molecule of carbon dioxide consists of one carbon atom (C) and two oxygen atoms (O).

CO_2 = C + 2O

Hence 1 mole of carbon dioxide contains 1 mole of carbon atoms and 2 moles of oxygen atoms.

MILLIMOLES

Moles are too big for everyday clinical use, so the unit **millimoles** is used instead.

1 millimole is equal to one-thousandth (i.e. 1/1,000) of a mole.

We know 1 mole is the atomic mass or molecular mass in grams, so it follows that:

1 millimole is the atomic mass or molecular mass in milligrams.

So, in the above explanation, you can substitute millimoles for moles and milligrams for grams.

SUMMARY

- The **mole** is a unit used by chemists to count atoms and molecules.
- A **mole** of any substance is the amount which contains the same number of particles of the substance as there are atoms in 12 g of carbon (C^{12}) — known as **Avogadro's number**.

Amount	1 mole of Carbon chloride	1 mole of Sodium chloride	1 mole of Sodium chloride
	CONTAINS	CONTAINS	CONTAINS
Number	6×10^{23} carbon atoms	6×10^{23} sodium atoms	6×10^{23} sodium chloride molecules
	HAVE MASS	HAVE MASS	HAVE MASS
Mass	12 g of carbon	23 g of sodium	58.5 g of sodium chloride

- For elements or atoms, 1 mole = the atomic mass in grams.
- For molecules, 1 mole = the molecular mass in grams.
- 1 millimole is equal to 1/1,000 of a mole, so 1 millimole is the atomic mass or molecular mass in milligrams.

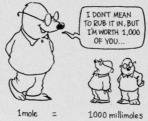

I DON'T MEAN TO RUB IT IN, BUT I'M WORTH 1,000 OF YOU...

1 mole = 1000 millimoles

CALCULATIONS INVOLVING MOLES AND MILLIMOLES

In this chapter we can only provide a quick and simple explanation of moles and millimoles. As we are not chemists and won't be doing calculations involving chemical equations, we are not concerned with detailed explanations. For our purposes:

	sodium chloride 1 mole (58.5 g)	would give	sodium 1 mole (23 g)	+	chloride 1 mole (35.5 g)
or	1 millimole (58.5 mg)		1 millimole (23 mg)		1 millimole (35.5 mg)

The following are examples and problems to see if you can understand the concept of millimoles. It is unlikely that you will encounter calculations such as these on the ward, but it is useful to know how they are done and can be used for reference if necessary.

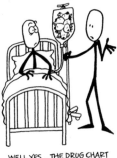

WELL, YES... THE DRUG CHART
DID SAY 100 millimoles / litre BUT
I COULD ONLY SQUEEZE IN 10!

Table 7 Atomic and molecular masses

Atom or molecule	Atomic symbol	Mass
Calcium	Ca	40
Calcium chloride		147
Calcium gluconate		448.5
Carbon	C	12
Chloride	Cl	35.5
Dextrose/glucose		180
Hydrogen	H	1
Magnesium	Mg	24
Magnesium chloride		203
Magnesium sulphate		246.5
Oxygen	O	16
Potassium	K	39
Potassium chloride		74.5
Sodium	Na	23
Sodium bicarbonate		84
Sodium chloride		58.5
Sodium citrate		194
Sodium phosphate		358

The reason why sometimes the molecular mass does not always equal the sum of the atomic masses of the individual atoms is that water forms a part of the molecule. For example, calcium chloride is *not* just $CaCl_2$ but is actually $CaCl_2.2H_2O$.

CONVERSION OF MILLIGRAMS (MG) TO MILLIMOLES (MMOL)

Sometimes it may be necessary to calculate the number of millimoles in an infusion or injection, or to convert mg/litre to mmol/litre.

WORKED EXAMPLE 1

How many millimoles of sodium are there in a 500 mL infusion containing 1.8 mg/mL sodium chloride?

Step 1

We already know that 1 millimole of sodium chloride yields 1 millimole of sodium and 1 millimole of chloride. So it follows that the amount (in milligrams) equal to 1 millimole of sodium chloride will give 1 millimole of sodium.

In this case, we need to calculate the total amount (in milligrams) of sodium chloride and convert this to millimoles to find out the number of millimoles of sodium.

Step 2

Calculate the total amount of sodium chloride.

You have an infusion containing 1.8 mg/mL, so in 500 mL, you have:

$1.8 \times 500 = 900$ mg sodium chloride

Step 3

From the table:

molecular mass of sodium chloride (NaCl) = 58.5

So 1 millimole of sodium chloride (NaCl) weighs 58.5 mg and this amount will give 1 millimole of sodium (Na).

Step 4

Next calculate the number of millimoles in the infusion. First work out the number of millimoles for 1 mg of sodium chloride, then the number for the total amount.

58.5 mg sodium chloride will give 1 millimole of sodium, so 1 mg will give:

$\dfrac{1}{58.5}$ millimoles of sodium

So, 900 mg will give:

$$\frac{1}{58.5} \times 900 = 15.4 \text{ mmol (or 15 mmol approx.)}$$

Answer: There are 15.4 mmol (approximately 15 mmol) of sodium in a 500 mL infusion containing 1.8 mg/mL sodium chloride.

A formula can be used:

$$\frac{\text{total number}}{\text{of millimoles}} = \frac{\text{mg/ml}}{\text{mg of substance containing 1 mmol}} \times \frac{\text{volume}}{\text{(mL)}}$$

where, in this case:

mg/mL =1.8
mg of substance containing 1 mmol = 58.5
volume (mL) = 500

Substituting the numbers in the formula:

$$\frac{1.8}{58.5} \times 500 = 15.38 \text{ mmol (or 15 mmol approx.)}$$

Answer: There are 15.4 mmol (approximately 15 mmol) of sodium in a 500 mL infusion containing 1.8 mg/mL sodium chloride.

If you are given the total amount in mg/litre, the calculations are the same. In this example, the total amount per litre would be 1,800 mg/litre.

WORKED EXAMPLE 2

How many millimoles of sodium are there in a 500 mL infusion containing sodium chloride 1,800 mg/litre?

Step 1

You have 1,800 mg in 1 litre. Therefore for a 500 mL infusion, you will have:

1,800 mg   in   1 litre (1.000 mL)

$$\frac{1,800}{1,000} \quad \text{in} \quad 1 \text{ mL}$$

$$500 \text{ mL} = \frac{1,800}{1,000} \times 500 = 900 \text{ mg}$$

Step 2

1 millimole of sodium chloride yields 1 millimole of sodium and 1 millimole of chloride. So it follows that the amount (in

milligrams) equivalent to 1 millimole of sodium chloride will give 1 millimole of sodium.

In this case, calculate the total amount (in milligrams) of sodium chloride and convert this to millimoles to find out the number of millimoles of sodium.

Step 3

From the tables, we can find that the molecular mass of sodium chloride (NaCl) is 58.5. So 1 millimole of sodium chloride (NaCl) will weigh 58.5 mg and this amount will give 1 millimole of sodium (Na).

Step 4

Next calculate the number of millimoles in the infusion. First work out the number of millimoles for 1 mg of sodium chloride, then the number for the total amount. 58.5 mg sodium chloride will give 1 millimole of sodium, so 1 mg will give:

$\frac{1}{58.5}$ millimoles of sodium

So, 900 mg will give:

$\frac{1}{58.5} \times 900 = 15.4$ mmol (or 15 mmol approx.)

Answer: There are 15.4 mmol (approximately 15 mmol) of sodium in a 500 mL infusion containing 1.8 mg/mL sodium chloride.

The formula we used earlier can be rewritten:

total number of millimoles =

$$\frac{mg/litre}{mg \text{ of substance containing 1 mmol} \times 1,000} \times volume \text{ (ml)}$$

where, in this case:

mg/litre = 1,800
mg of substance containing 1 mmol = 58.5
volume = 500

Multiplying by 1,000 simply converts the mg/litre strength to a mg/mL strength.

Substitute the numbers in the formula:

$\frac{1,800 \times 500}{58.5 \times 1,000} = \frac{90,000}{58,500} = 15.38$ mmol (or 15 mmol approx.)

Answer: There are 15.4 mmol (approximately 15 mmol) of sodium in a 500 mL infusion containing 1.8 mg/mL sodium chloride.

MOLES AND MILLIMOLES 1 – SUMMARY

Conversion of milligrams (mg) to millimoles (mmol)

- To convert mg/mL to millimoles:

  total number of millimoles =

  $$\frac{mg/ml}{mg \text{ of substance containing 1 mmol}} \times volume \text{ (mL)}$$

- To convert mg/litre to millimoles:

  total number of millimoles =

  $$\frac{mg/litre}{mg \text{ of substance containing 1 mmol} \times 1,000} \times volume \text{ (mL)}$$

PROBLEMS

Work out the following:

Question 1 How many millimoles of sodium are there in a 500 mL infusion containing 27 mg/mL sodium chloride?

Question 2 How many millimoles of sodium are there in a 10 mL ampoule containing 200 mg/mL sodium chloride?

Question 3 How many millimoles of sodium, potassium and chloride are there in a 500 mL infusion containing 9 mg/mL sodium chloride and potassium chloride 3 mg/mL?

Question 4 How many millimoles of glucose are there in a litre infusion containing 50 g/litre?

Question 5 How many millimoles of sodium are there in a litre infusion containing sodium bicarbonate 27.4 g/litre?

Question 6 You are asked to draw up 35 mmol of potassium and to add this to a litre infusion. You have an ampoule containing 2 g of potassium in 10 mL. How much do you need to draw up?

Question 7 You are asked to draw up 15 mmol of potassium and to add this to a litre infusion. You have an ampoule containing 1 g of potassium in 5 mL. How much do you need to draw up?

CONVERSION OF PERCENTAGE STRENGTH (% W/V) TO MILLIMOLES (MMOL)

Sometimes it may be necessary to convert percentages to the number of millimoles.

WORKED EXAMPLE 3

How many millimoles of sodium are there in 1 litre of sodium chloride 0.9% infusion?

Step 1

As before, 1 millimole of sodium chloride will give 1 millimole of sodium and 1 millimole of chloride. So, the amount (in milligrams) equivalent to 1 millimole of sodium chloride will give 1 millimole of sodium.

Step 2

To calculate the number of milligrams there are in 1 millimole of sodium chloride, either refer to tables or work from first principles using atomic masses.

From tables:

molecular mass of sodium chloride (NaCl) = 58.5

So 1 millimole of sodium chloride (NaCl) weighs 58.5 mg and this amount will give 1 millimole of sodium (Na).

Step 3

Calculate the total amount of sodium chloride present:

0.9% = 0.9 g in 100 mL
   = 900 mg in 100 mL

Thus for a 1 litre (1,000 mL) infusion, the amount equals:

$\frac{900}{100} \times 1,000 = 9,000$ mg or 9 g

Step 4

In Step 2, we found that 58.5 mg sodium chloride will give 1 millimole of sodium.

So it follows that:

1 mg of sodium chloride will give $\frac{1}{58.5}$ millimoles of sodium.

So 9,000 mg sodium chloride =

$$\frac{1}{58.5} \times 9,000 = 153.8\ (154)\ \text{mmol of sodium}$$

Answer: 1 litre of sodium chloride 0.9% infusion contains 154 mmol of sodium (approx.).

A formula can be devised:

total number of mmol =

$$\frac{\text{percentage strength (\% w/v)}}{\text{mg of substance containing 1 mmol}} \times 10 \times \text{volume (mL)}$$

where in this case:

percentage strength (% w/v) = 0.9
mg of substance containing 1 mmol = 58.5
volume = 1,000

Multiplying by 10 simply converts percentage strength (g/100 mL) to mg/mL, so that everything is in the same units.
Substituting the numbers in the formula:

$$\frac{0.9}{58.5} \times 10 \times 1,000 = 153.8\ (154)\ \text{mmol of sodium}$$

Answer: 1 litre of sodium chloride 0.9% infusion contains 154 mmol of sodium (approx.).

MOLES AND MILLIMOLES 2 – SUMMARY

● To convert of percentage strength (% w/v) to millimoles

total number of mmol =

$$\frac{\text{percentage strength (\% w/v)}}{\text{mg of substance containing 1 mmol}} \times 10 \times \text{volume (mL)}$$

PROBLEMS

Work out the following:

Question 8 How many millimoles of sodium are there in a 1 litre infusion of glucose 4% and sodium chloride 0.18%?

Question 9 How many millimoles of calcium and chloride are there in a 10 mL ampoule of calcium chloride 10%? (calcium chloride = $CaCl_2$)

Question 10 How many millimoles of sodium are there in a 10 mL ampoule of sodium chloride 30%?

Question 11 How many millimoles of calcium are there in a 10 mL ampoule of calcium gluconate 10%?

Question 12 How many millimoles of sodium are there in a 200 mL infusion of sodium bicarbonate 8.4%?

ANSWERS TO PROBLEMS

Question 1 1 millimole of sodium chloride will give 1 millimole of sodium and 1 millimole of chloride. So the amount (in milligrams) for 1 millimole of sodium chloride will give 1 millimole of sodium. From Table 7 on page 80, the molecular mass of sodium chloride = 58.5. So 58.5 mg (1 millimole) of sodium chloride will give 1 millimole of sodium.

Thus:

1 mg of sodium chloride will give $\dfrac{1}{58.5}$ millimoles of sodium

Now work out the total amount of sodium chloride in a 500 mL infusion.

You have 27 mg/mL, so for 500 mL:

$27 \times 500 = 13{,}500$ mg

Next work out the number of millimoles for the infusion:

1 mg will give $\dfrac{1}{58.5}$ millimoles

13,500 mg will give $\dfrac{1}{58.5} \times 13{,}500 = 230.8$ (231) mmol

Answer: There are 231 mmol (approx) of sodium in a 500 mL infusion containing sodium chloride 27 mg/mL.

Using the formula:

total number of millimoles =

$$\frac{\text{mg/mL}}{\text{mg of substance containing 1 mmol}} \times \text{volume (mL)}$$

where, in this case:

mg/mL = 27
mg of substance containing 1 mmol = 58.5
volume = 500

Substitute the numbers in the formula:

$$\frac{27}{58.5} \times 500 = 230.8 \ (231) \ \text{mmol}$$

Answer: There are 231 mmol (approx) of sodium in a 500 mL infusion containing sodium chloride 27 mg/mL.

Question 2   34.2 mmol (34 mmol, approx.) of sodium

Question 3
Sodium	76.9 mmol	(77 mmol, approx.)
Potassium	20.2 mmol	(20 mmol, approx.)
Chloride	97.2 mmol	(97 mmol, approx.)

1 millimole of potassium chloride gives 1 millimole of potassium and 1 millimole of chloride.

1 millimole of sodium chloride gives 1 millimole of sodium and 1 millimole of chloride.

To find the total amount of chloride, add the amount for the sodium and potassium together.

Question 4   277.8 mmol (278 mmol, approx.) of glucose

Question 5   326.2 mmol (326 mmol, approx.) of sodium

Question 6   1 millimole of potassium chloride gives 1 millimole of potassium and 1 millimole of chloride. From Table 7, the molecular mass of potassium chloride is 74.5.

Thus 1 millimole of potassium chloride = 74.5 mg.

Therefore 35 mmol = $74.5 \times 35 = 2{,}607.5$ mg

To work out the volume required:

You have 2 g (2,000 mg) in 10 mL; thus 1 mg = $\frac{10}{2{,}000}$ mL

Therefore for 2,607.5 mg, you will need:

$$\frac{10}{2{,}000} \times 2{,}607.5 = 13.04 \ \text{mL}$$

Answer: You will need to draw up 13 mL.

Using the formula:

total number of millimoles =

$$\frac{\text{mg/mL}}{\text{mg of substance containing 1 mmol}} \times \text{volume (mL)}$$

where, in this case, the unknown is the volume you need to draw up.

So the formula can be rewritten as:

volume (mL) =

$$\frac{\text{mg of substance containing 1 mmol}}{\text{mg/mL}} \times \frac{\text{total number}}{\text{of millimoles}}$$

Where, in this case:

mg of substance containing 1 mmol = 74.5
mg/mL = 200
total number of millimoles = 35

Substitute the numbers in the formula:

$$\frac{74.5}{200} \times 35 = 13.04 \ (13) \text{ mL}$$

Answer: You will need to draw up 13 mL.

Question 7   You will need to draw up 5.6 mL

Question 8   We can ignore the glucose since it contains no sodium; simply consider the infusion as sodium chloride 0.18%.

1 millimole of sodium chloride will give 1 millimole of sodium and 1 millimole of chloride.

So the amount (in milligrams) for 1 millimole of sodium chloride will give 1 millimole of sodium.

From Table 7, the molecular mass of sodium chloride is 58.5.

So 58.5 mg (1 millimole) of sodium chloride will give 1 millimole of sodium.

Now work out the number of millimoles for 1 mg of sodium chloride:

58.5 mg sodium chloride will give 1 millimole of sodium.

1 mg sodium chloride will give $\frac{1}{58.5}$ millimoles of sodium

Next, calculate the total amount of sodium chloride present:

0.18% = 0.18 g or 180 mg per 100 mL

Therefore in 1 litre there are:

180 × 10 = 1,800 mg sodium chloride

Now calculate the number of millimoles for 1,800 mg sodium chloride:

$$1{,}800 \text{ mg} = \frac{1}{58.5} \times 1{,}800 = 30.8 \text{ (31) mmol}$$

Answer: 1 litre of glucose 4% and sodium chloride 0.9% infusion contains 31 mmol of sodium (approx.).

Using the formula:

total number of mmol =

$$\frac{\text{percentage strength (\% w/v)}}{\text{mg of substance containing 1 mmol}} \times 10 \times \text{volume (mL)}$$

where:

percentage strength (% w/v) = 0.18
mg of substance containing 1 mmol = 58.5
volume = 1,000

Substituting the numbers in the formula:

$$\frac{0.18}{58.5} \times 10 \times 1{,}000 = 30.8 \text{ (31) mmol of sodium}$$

Answer: 1 litre of glucose 4% and sodium chloride 0.9% infusion contains 31 mmol of sodium (approx.).

Question 9 In this case 1 millimole of calcium chloride will give 1 millimole of calcium and **2 millimoles** of chloride. So the amount (in milligrams) equivalent to 1 millimole of calcium chloride will give 1 millimole of calcium and 2 millimoles of chloride.

From Table 7, the molecular mass of calcium chloride is 147. So 147 mg (1 millimole) of calcium chloride will give 1 millimole of calcium and 2 millimoles of chloride.

Now calculate how much calcium chloride there is in a 10 mL ampoule containing calcium chloride 10%:

10% = 10 g in 100 mL, therefore in 10 mL:
1 g or 1,000 mg calcium

Calcium:

1 millimole of calcium is equivalent to 147 mg of calcium chloride. Therefore 1 mg calcium chloride is equal to:

$$\frac{1}{147} \text{ mmol of calcium}$$

However, you have 1,000 mg of calcium chloride, so:

$$1,000 \text{ mg} = \frac{1}{147} \times 1,000 = 6.8 \text{ mmol (7 mmol, approx.)}$$

Chloride:

2 millimoles of chloride is equal to 147 mg of calcium chloride, so 1 mg calcium chloride is equivalent to:

$\frac{2}{147}$ mmol of chloride.

However, you have 1,000 mg of calcium chloride, so:

$$1,000 \text{ mg} = \frac{2}{147} \times 1,000 = 13.6 \text{ mmol (14 mmol, approx.)}$$

Answer: There are 7 millimoles of calcium and 14 millimoles of chloride in a 10 mL ampoule of calcium chloride 10% (approx.).

Using the formula:

total number of mmol =

$$\frac{\text{percentage strength (\% w/v)}}{\text{mg of substance containing 1 mmol}} \times 10 \times \text{volume (mL)}$$

Calcium:

percentage strength (% w/v) = 10
mg of substance containing 1 mmol = 147
volume = 10

Substituting the numbers in the formula:

$$\frac{10}{147} \times 10 \times 10 = 6.8 \text{ mmol (7 mmol, approx.)}$$

Chloride:

percentage strength (% w/v) = 10
mg of substance containing 1 mmol = 73.5
volume = 10

NB: mg of substance containing 1 mmol = 73.5. This is because 2 mmol of chloride = 147 mg, thus:

1 mmol chloride $= \frac{147}{2} = 73.5$ mg

Substituting the numbers in the formula:

$$\frac{10}{73.5} \times 10 \times 10 = 13.6 \text{ mmol (14 mmol, approx.)}$$

Answer: There are 7 millimoles of calcium and 14 millimoles of chloride in a 10 mL ampoule of calcium chloride 10% (approx.).

Question 10 51.28 mmol (51 mmol, approx.)

Question 11 2.23 mmol (2 mmol, approx.)

Question 12 200 mmol

KEY POINTS

Moles

- The mole is a unit used by chemists to count atoms and molecules.
- A mole of any substance is the amount which contains the same number of particles of the substance as there are atoms in 12 g of carbon (C^{12}) – known as Avogadro's number.
- For elements or atoms, 1 mole = the atomic mass in grams.
- For molecules, 1 mole = the molecular mass in grams.

Millimoles

- Moles are too big for everyday use, so we use millimoles.
- 1 millimole is equal to one-thousandth (1/1,000) of a mole.
- If 1 mole is the atomic mass or molecular mass in grams, then 1 millimole is the atomic mass or molecular mass in milligrams.

Conversion of milligrams (mg) to millimoles (mmol)

- To convert mg/mL to millimoles:

    total number of millimoles =

    $$\frac{mg/mL}{mg \text{ of substance containing 1 mmol}} \times \text{volume (in mL)}$$

- To convert mg/litre to millimoles:

    total number of millimoles =

    $$\frac{mg/litre}{mg \text{ of substance containing 1 mmol} \times 1,000} \times \text{volume (in mL)}$$

Conversion of percentage strength (% w/v) to millimoles

total number of mmol =

$$\frac{\text{percentage strength (\% w/v)}}{mg \text{ of substance containing 1 mmol}} \times \text{volume (in mL)}$$

Drug strengths or concentrations

OBJECTIVES

At the end of this chapter, you should be familiar with the following:

- Percentage concentration
- Concentrations in mg/mL
- '1 in ...' concentrations or ratio strengths
- Drugs measured in units: heparin and insulin
- Molarity and molar solutions

There are various ways of expressing how much actual drug is present in a medicine. These medicines are usually liquids for oral or parenteral administration, but also include preparations for topical use.

This aim of this chapter is to explain the various ways in which drug strengths can be stated.

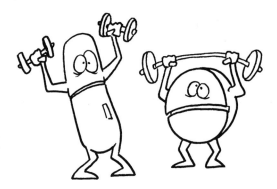

PERCENTAGE CONCENTRATION

One method of describing concentration is to use the percentage as a unit (see Chapter 4). The most common one you will come across is the **percentage concentration, w/v** (weight in volume). This is used when a solid is dissolved in a liquid and means the number of grams dissolved in 100 mL.

% w/v = number of grams in 100 mL

For example, 5% w/v means 5 g in 100 mL).

Another type of concentration you might come across is the **percentage concentration, w/w** (weight in weight). This is used when a solid is mixed with another solid, e.g. creams and ointments, and means the number of grams in 100 g.

% w/w = number of grams in 100 g

For example, 5% w/w means 5 g in 100 g.

Another concentration is the **percentage concentration, v/v** (volume in volume). This is used when a liquid is mixed or diluted with another liquid, and means the number of millilitres (mL) in 100 mL.

% v/v = number of mL in 100 mL

For example, 5% v/v means 5 mL in 100 mL.

The most common percentage concentration you will encounter is the percentage w/v, so that's the one considered here.

The percentage concentration has nothing to do with the size of the container. For example, glucose 5% infusion means that there are 5 g of glucose dissolved in each 100 mL of fluid and this will remain the same if it is a 500 mL bag or a 1 litre bag.

To find the total amount of drug present in a bottle or infusion bag, you must take into account the size or volume of the bottle or infusion bag.

WORKED EXAMPLE 1: TO CALCULATE THE TOTAL AMOUNT OF DRUG IN A SOLUTION

How much sodium bicarbonate is there in a 200 mL infusion sodium bicarbonate 8.4% w/v?

The calculations used with percentage concentrations are similar to those seen earlier (Chapter 4).

Step 1

Convert the percentage to the number of grams in 100 mL, i.e.

8.4% w/v = 8.4 g in 100 mL

(You are converting the percentage to a specific quantity.)

Step 2

Calculate how many grams there are in 1 mL, i.e. divide by 100 (using the one unit rule, see p. 51).

$\frac{8.4}{100}$ g in 1 mL

Step 3

However, you have a 200 mL infusion. So to find out the total amount present, multiply how much is in 1 mL by the volume you've got (200 mL).

$\frac{8.4}{100} \times 200 = 16.8$ g in 200 mL

Answer: There are 16.8 g of sodium bicarbonate in 200 mL of sodium bicarbonate 8.4% w/v infusion.

A simple formula can be devised, based on one used in an earlier chapter:

$\frac{\text{number}}{100} \times$ percentage required

This can be rearranged to give:

$\frac{\text{percentage}}{100} \times$ number

where:

percentage is the percentage of what you've got
number is the total volume you've got

Therefore the formula can be rewritten as:

total amount (g) $= \frac{\text{percentage}}{100} \times$ total volume (mL)

In the present example:

percentage = 8.4
total volume (mL) = 200

Substituting the numbers in the formula:

total amount (g) $= \frac{8.4}{100} \times 200 = 16.8$ g

Answer: There are 16.8 g of sodium bicarbonate in 200 mL of sodium bicarbonate 8.4% w/v infusion.

WORKED EXAMPLE 2: TO CALCULATE DOSAGES FROM PERCENTAGE CONCENTRATIONS

You have salbutamol nebulizer solution 0.5%. What volume is required for a 2.5 mg dose?

Step 1

Write down what 0.5% exactly represents. It means 0.5 g in 100 mL.

Step 2

Convert 0.5 g to mg by multiplying by 1,000 (the dose required is in mg):

$0.5 \text{ g} = 0.5 \times 1{,}000 = 500 \text{ mg}$

Step 3

Of what you've got, work out the volume for 1 mg, thus:

500 mg in 100 mL

$1 \text{ mg} = \dfrac{100}{500} \text{ mL (one unit rule)}$

Step 4

Now work out the volume required for the dose needed, i.e.

$2.5 \text{ mg} = \dfrac{100}{500} \times 2.5 = 0.5 \text{ mL}$

Answer: The volume required is 0.5 mL.

Alternatively, you can use a formula you encountered earlier when calculating drug dosages (p. 52).

$$\dfrac{\text{amount you want}}{\text{amount you've got}} \times \text{volume it's in}$$

Once again, before substituting numbers in the formula, convert everything to the same units:

0.5% = 0.5 g in 100 mL OR 500 mg in 100 mL

In this situation, the 'volume it's in' is therefore 100 mL. There is no need to worry about the volume of the bottle, ampoule or whatever; always convert the percentage to an amount in 100 mL. Therefore the formula can be rewritten as:

$$\dfrac{\text{amount you want}}{\text{amount you've got}} \times 100$$

Here:

amount you want = 2.5 mg
amount you've got = 500 mg

Substituting the numbers in the formula:

$$\frac{2.5}{500} \times 100 = 0.5 \text{ mL}$$

Answer: The volume required is 0.5 mL.

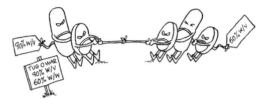

PERCENTAGE CONCENTRATIONS – SUMMARY

- Percentage 'weight in volume' (% w/v) = number of grams per 100 g.
- Percentage 'weight in weight' (% w/w) = number of mL per 100 mL.
- Percentage 'volume in volume' (% v/v) = number of grams per 100 mL.

PROBLEMS

Calculate the following:

Question 1   How many grams of sodium chloride are there in a litre infusion of sodium chloride 0.9%?

Question 2   How many grams of potassium, sodium and glucose are there in a litre infusion of potassium 0.3%, sodium chloride 0.18% and glucose 4%?

Question 3   How many grams of sodium chloride are there in a 500 mL infusion of sodium chloride 0.45%?

Question 4   You need to give a continuous infusion containing calcium gluconate 4 g. You have 10 mL ampoules of calcium gluconate 10%. How much do you need to draw up?

CONCENTRATIONS IN MG/ML

Another way of expressing the amount or concentration of drug in a solution, usually for oral or parenteral administration, is mg/mL, i.e. number of milligrams of drug per mL of liquid. This is the most common way of expressing the amount of drug in a solution.

- For oral liquids, it is usually expressed as the number of milligrams in a standard 5 mL spoonful, e.g. erythromycin 250 mg in 5 mL.
- For injections, it is usually expressed as the number of milligrams per 1 mL or the number of milligrams per volume of the ampoule, (1 mL, 2 mL, 5 mL, 10 mL and 20 mL), e.g. furosemide (frusemide) 10 mg/mL and gentamicin 80 mg in 2 mL.

NB: Strengths can also be expressed in micrograms/mL, e.g. hyoscine injection 600 micrograms/mL.

Only mg/mL will be considered here, but the principles learnt here can be applied to other concentrations or strengths, e.g. micrograms/mL.

Sometimes it may be useful to convert percentage concentrations to mg/mL concentrations.

Some examples:

lidocaine (lignocaine) 0.2%	= 0.2 g per 100 mL
	= 200 mg per 100 mL
	= 2 mg per mL (2 mg/mL)
sodium chloride 0.9%	= 0.9 g per 100 mL
	= 900 mg per 100 mL
	= 9 mg per mL (9 mg/mL)
glucose 5%	= 5 g per 100 mL
	= 5,000 mg per 100 mL
	= 50 mg per mL (50 mg/mL)

This will give the strength of the solution irrespective of the size of the bottle, infusion bag, etc.

An easy way of finding the strength in mg/mL is by simply multiplying the percentage by 10. This can be explained using lidocaine (lignocaine) 0.2% as an example:

You have lidocaine (lignocaine) 0.2%. This is equivalent to 0.2 g in 100 mL. Divide by 100 to find out how much is in 1 mL:

$$\frac{0.2}{100} \text{ g/mL}$$

Multiply by 1,000 to convert grams to milligrams:

$$\frac{0.2}{100} \times 1,000 \text{ mg/mL}$$

Simplify to give:

$$0.2 \times 10 = 2 \text{ mg/mL}$$

Therefore you simply multiply the percentage by 10.

With our earlier examples:

lidocaine (lignocaine) 0.2% = 0.2 × 10 = 2 mg/mL
sodium chloride 0.9% = 0.9 × 10 = 9 mg/mL
glucose 5% = 5 × 10 = 50 mg/mL

Consequently, to convert a mg/mL concentration to a percentage, you simply divide by 10.

Once again, using lidocaine (lignocaine) as an example:

You have lidocaine (lignocaine) 2 mg/mL. Percentage means 'per 100 mL', so multiply by 100, i.e.

2 mg/mL × 100 = 200 mg/100 mL (2 × 100)

Percentage (w/v) means 'the number of grams per 100 mL', so you will have to convert milligrams to grams by dividing by 1,000, i.e.

$$\frac{2 \times 100}{1,000} = \frac{2}{10} = 0.2\%$$

Therefore you simply divide the mg/mL concentration by 10.
With our earlier examples,

lidocaine (lignocaine) 2 mg/mL = 2 ÷ 10 = 0.2%
sodium chloride 9 mg/mL = 9 ÷ 10 = 0.9%
glucose 50 mg/mL = 50 ÷ 10 = 5%

Once again, calculations with mg/mL concentrations are the same as seen earlier with dosage calculations.

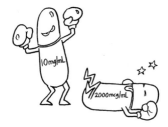

CONCENTRATIONS IN MG/ML – SUMMARY

- mg/mL = number of mg per 1 mL.
- To convert a percentage to a mg/mL concentration – multiply by 10.
- To convert a mg/mL concentration to a percentage – divide by 10.

PROBLEMS

Calculate the strengths (mg/mL) for the following:

Question 5 Sodium chloride infusion 0.45%

Question 6 Metronidazole infusion 0.5%

Question 7 Potassium chloride 0.2%, sodium chloride 0.18% and glucose 4%

'1 IN . . . ' CONCENTRATIONS OR RATIO STRENGTHS

This final type of concentration is only used occasionally, and is written as '1 in . . .', e.g. 1 in 10,000, and is sometimes known as a **ratio strength**. It means 1 gram in however many mL.

For example:

1 in 1,000 means 1 g in 1,000 mL
1 in 10,000 means 1 g in 10,000 mL

Therefore it can be seen that 1 in 10,000 is weaker than 1 in 1,000. So, higher the number, the weaker the solution.

TUBERCULIN STRENGTHS

Tuberculin is an exception to this. Strengths are sometimes written in a '1 in . . .' notation.
For example:

1 in 10,000   (10 units/mL)
1 in 1,000   (100 units/mL)
1 in 100   (1,000 units/mL)

It is **not** 1 g in 10,000 mL, etc., but simply a dilution: 1 mL diluted 10,000 times, so it is important that you don't get confused between the two notations.
Undiluted tuberculin contains 100,000 units per mL.
A 1 in 10,000 dilution is therefore equal to:

$$\frac{100,000}{10,000} \text{ units/mL} = 10 \text{ units/mL}$$
(1 mL diluted 10,000 times)

A 1 in 1,000 dilution is therefore equal to:

$$\frac{100,000}{1,000} \text{ units/mL} = 100 \text{ units/mL}$$
(1 mL diluted 1,000 times).

A 1 in 100 dilution is therefore equal to:

$$\frac{100,000}{100} \text{ units/mL} = 1,000 \text{ units/mL}$$

(1 mL diluted 100 times).

It is better to write the concentration as 10 units/mL instead of 1 in 10,000 to avoid confusion; but the old notation is still used.

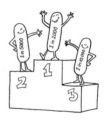

'1 IN ...' CONCENTRATIONS OR RATIO STRENGTHS – SUMMARY

- '1 in ...' concentration:

    '1 in ...' = 1 g in however many mL

PROBLEMS

Question 8 Adrenaline (epinephrine) is sometimes combined with lidocaine (lignocaine) when used as a local anaesthetic, usually as a 1 in 200,000 strength. How much adrenaline (epinephrine) is there in a 20 mL vial?

Question 9 Sometimes adrenaline (epinephrine) eye drops may be written as 'adrenaline (epinephrine) 1 in 100'. What percentage strength is this?

DRUGS MEASURED IN UNITS: HEPARIN AND INSULIN

Some drugs, such as insulin and heparin, are made from animal or biosynthetic sources. The purity of drugs like these can vary, so standard measurements for these drugs are expressed in terms of **units** rather than weight.

HEPARIN

The strengths available are:

1,000 units/mL	1 mL, 5 mL, 10 mL ampoules
5,000 units/mL	1 mL, 5 mL ampoules
10,000 units/mL	1 mL ampoules
25,000 units/mL	1 mL ampoules

A strength of 25,000 units/mL is also available for subcutaneous use as 0.2 mL ampoules containing 5,000 units.

Heparin is given subcutaneously, two or three times a day, or by continuous intravenous infusion. Infusions are usually given over 24 hours and the dose is adjusted according to laboratory results. Doses can vary, so it is important to know how to calculate how much heparin is needed.

Whatever the dose prescribed, you would choose the most appropriate ampoule(s) for that dose depending upon which strengths of heparin are available.

For example, for a dose of 28,000 units you would choose:

1 × 25,000 units/mL ampoule

and

3 × 1,000 units/mL ampoule OR 1 × 5,000 units/mL – using part of the ampoule

As you can see, there are still some calculations involved with heparin dosages.

Calculations involving units are exactly the same as those seen earlier (see 'Calculating drug dosages', page 51), except that you are working in units instead of milligrams and micrograms.

WORKED EXAMPLE

You need to give heparin as a continuous infusion, 28,000 units in 48 mL normal saline over 24 hours. Assuming that the only strengths of heparin available are 25,000 units/mL and 5,000 units/mL, how much do you need to draw up for the dose prescribed?

Step 1

In this case the dose is 28,000 units.

Therefore you would use:

1 × 25,000 units/mL, 1 mL ampoule

and

1 × 5,000 units/mL, 1 mL ampoule

If ampoules of 1,000 units/mL were available, then you would use 3 × 1,000 units/mL instead.

Step 2

Calculate how much of the 5,000 units/mL ampoule you need:

28,000 units − 25,000 units = 3,000 units

Therefore you need to draw up 3,000 units from the 5,000 units/mL ampoule.

Step 3

Write down what you have, i.e.

5,000 units in 1 mL

Step 4

Work out the volume for 1 unit:

5,000 units in 1 mL

$$1 \text{ unit} = \frac{1}{5,000} \text{ mL (using the one unit rule)}$$

Step 5

Now multiply by the dose required (3,000 units):

$$3,000 \text{ units} = \frac{1}{5,000} \times 3,000 = 0.6 \text{ mL}$$

Answer: You would add 1 × 25,000 units/mL ampoule and 0.6 mL of 1 × 5,000 units/mL to the infusion.

Alternatively, you could use the formula seen earlier in 'Calculating drug dosages':

$$\frac{\text{amount you want}}{\text{amount you've got}} \times \text{volume it's in}$$

Once again, before substituting numbers in the formula, decide as to which ampoule(s) of heparin would be the most appropriate; then, if necessary, calculate how much to draw up.

Thus:

amount you want = 3,000 units
amount you've got = 5,000 units
volume it's in = 1 mL

Substitute the numbers in the formula:

$$\frac{3,000}{5,000} \times 1 = 0.6 \text{ mL}$$

Answer: You would add 1 × 25,000 units/mL ampoule and 0.6 mL of 1 × 5,000 units/mL to the infusion.

Low molecular weight heparins (LMWHs)

Low molecular weight heparins (LMWHs) differ from unfractionated heparin (UFH) in molecular size and weight, method of preparation, and anticoagulant properties. LMWHs have a number of advantages over UFH:

- they have greater bioavailability when given by subcutaneous injection
- they have a longer duration of action, allowing once or twice daily administration
- the anticoagulant response to LMWH is highly correlated with bodyweight, allowing administration of a fixed dose
- laboratory monitoring is not necessary.

Some LMWHs are used in the treatment of deep vein thrombosis (DVT), pulmonary embolism (PE) and unstable coronary artery disease (UCAD). At the time of writing these include dalteparin, enoxaparin and tinzaparin.

Table 8 LMWH

LMWH	Dose for DVT/PE	Dose for UCAD
Dalteparin	200 units/kg, once daily*	120 units/kg, twice daily
Enoxaparin	1 mg/kg, once daily	1.5 mg/kg, twice daily
Tinzaparin	175 units/kg, once daily	Not licensed for this indication

*Maximum of 18,000 units as a single dose, higher doses give twice daily.

Table 9 LMWH 2

LMWH	Strength	Preparations available
Dalteparin (Fragmin)	2,500 units/mL	4 mL amp (10,000 units)
	10,000 units/mL	1 mL amp (10,000 units)
		1 mL syringe (10,000 units)
	12,500 units/mL	0.2 mL syringe (2,500 units)
	25,000 units/mL	0.2 mL syringe (5,000 units)
		0.3 mL syringe (7,500 units)
		0.4 mL syringe (10,000 units)
		0.5 mL syringe (12,500 units)
		0.6 mL syringe (15,000 units)
		0.72 mL syringe (18,000 units)
		4 mL amp (100,000 units)

Table 9 *continued*

LMWH	Strength	Preparations available
Enoxaparin (Clexane)	100 mg/mL (10,000 units/mL)	0.2 mL syringe (2,000 units, 20 mg) 0.4 mL syringe (4,000 units, 40 mg) 0.6 mL syringe (6,000 units, 60 mg) 0.8 mL syringe (8,000 units, 80 mg) 1 mL syringe (10,000 units, 100 mg)
	150 mg/mL (15,000 units/mL)	0.8 mL syringe (12,000 units, 120 mg) 1 mL syringe (15,000 units, 150 mg)
Tinzaparin (Innohep)	10,000 units/mL	0.25 mL syringe (2,500 units) 0.35 mL syringe (2,500 units) 0.45 mL syringe (4,500 units)
	20,000 units/mL	0.5 mL syringe (10,000 units) 0.7 mL syringe (14,000 units) 0.9 mL syringe (18,000 units) 2 mL vial (40,000 units)

WORKED EXAMPLE

A patient weighing 96 kg has been diagnosed with a DVT. A LMWH is indicated to treat the patient. What dose is required?

Dalteparin

Dose = 200 units/kg
Weight = 96 kg
Dose required = 200 × 96 = 19,200 units

This is greater than 18,000 units, therefore give as 9,600 units twice daily – use a 0.4 mL syringe (10,000 units).

Enoxaparin

Dose = 1 mg/kg
Weight = 96 kg
Dose required = 1 × 96 = 96 mg – use a 1 mL syringe (10,000 units, 100 mg)

Tinzaparin

Dose = 175 units/kg
Weight = 96 kg
Dose required = 175 × 96 = 16,800 units – use a 0.9 mL syringe (18,000 units)

The following case report illustrates the point that care must be taken when prescribing and administering LMWHs. Confusion can occur between units and volumes.

BEWARE DOSING ERRORS WITH LOW MOLECULAR WEIGHT HEPARIN

Case report

A retired teacher was admitted to hospital with acute shortage of breath and was diagnosed as having a pulmonary embolus. She was prescribed subcutaneous tinzaparin, in a dose of 0.45 mL from a 20,000 unit per ml prefilled 0.5 ml syringe. Because of confusion over the intended dose, two 0.5 ml prefilled syringes or 20,000 units of tinzaparin were administered in error by the ward nursing staff on four consecutive days. As a result of this cumulative administration error the patient died from a brain haemorrhage which, in the opinion of the pathologist, was due to the overdose of tinzaparin.

It was the prescriber's intention that the patient should receive 9,000 units of tinzaparin each day, but this information was not written on the prescription. The ward sister told a coroner's court hearing that the prescription was ambiguous. The dose was written as 0.45 mL and then 20,000 units, with the rest illegible. Because of this confusion the patient received an overdose and died.

Comment

There is little evidence that low molecular weight heparin products are more effective than unfractionated heparin provided that the unfractionated product is monitored carefully and the dosage adjusted according to laboratory results. However, there are organizational and practical difficulties in administering continuous infusions of unfractionated heparin, requiring daily monitoring and dose adjustment. Unfractionated products have largely been replaced in the majority of UK hospitals by low molecular weight heparin products (certoparin, dalteparin, enoxaparin and tinzaparin). There is an assumption that, by changing to low molecular weight products, all the practical and risk issues associated with the use of the unfractionated heparin products will be eliminated. We have received a number of reports suggesting that the introduction of low molecular weight heparin products have introduced new risk factors that need to be addressed.

These are:

The requirement to know the patient's weight, prior to treatment. Low molecular weight heparin products are dosed on body weight and there are dangers associated with using estimates of body weight or treating all patients with a dose for a 70 kg patient regardless of their actual weight.

It is important that the dose of low molecular weight heparin, in both units and mL, is included on the prescription. This prevents confusion and enables a cross check to be made between units and volume prescribed.

As no laboratory testing is performed to monitor the anticoagulant effect, it is important that the dosing information is confirmed by the pharmacist before syringes of low molecular weight heparin are supplied. Supplying these products as ward stock – avoiding the requirement for a pharmacist to check the dose before treatment is commenced – adds an additional element of risk.

Taken from *Pharmacy in Practice* 2000; 10: 260

INSULIN

Injection devices ('pens'), which hold insulin in a cartridge and deliver the required dose, are convenient to use. The conventional syringe and needle is still the preferred method of insulin administration for many people, and is also required for insulins not available in cartridge form.

There no calculations are involved in the administration of insulin. Insulin comes in 3 mL cartridges or 10 mL vials containing 100 units/mL, and the doses prescribed are written in units/mL. All you have to do is to dial or draw up the required dose using a pen device or an insulin syringe.

Insulin syringes are calibrated as 100 units in 1 mL and are available as 1 mL and 0.5 mL syringes. So if the dose is 30 units, you simply draw up to the 30 unit mark on the syringe.

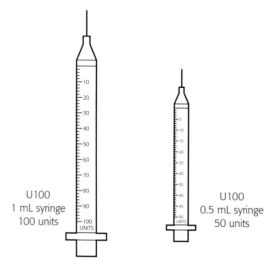

Fig 6.1 Actual size insulin U100 syringes

PROBLEMS

Question 10 You need to give an infusion of heparin containing 27,000 units over 24 hours. Assuming that the only strengths available are 25,000 units/mL and 5,000 units/mL, how much do you need to draw up for the dose prescribed?

Question 11 You need to give an infusion of heparin containing 29,000 units over 24 hours. Assuming that the only strengths available are 25,000 units/mL and 5,000 units/mL. How much do you need to draw up for the dose prescribed?

Question 12 A patient has a DVT and needs be given tinzaparin at a dose of 175 units/kg. The patient weighs 68 kg. What dose do they need, which syringe do you use and what volume do you give?

Question 13 A patient has a DVT and needs be given enoxaparin at a dose of 1.5 mg/kg. The patient weighs 59 kg. What dose do they need, which syringe do you use and what volume do you give?

MOLAR SOLUTIONS AND MOLARITY

Molarity is a term used in chemistry to describe concentrations. (If necessary, refer to Chapter 5, 'Moles and millimoles', to refresh your memory of this concept.) When moles of substances are dissolved in water to make solutions the unit of concentration is molarity, and the solutions are known as molar solutions.

When **1 mole** of a substance is dissolved in **1 litre** of solution, it is known as a 1 molar (1 M) solution. For example, when 1 mole (58.5 g) of sodium chloride (NaCl) is dissolved in 1 litre of water, concentration of the resulting solution is 1 molar (1 M).

- A 1 M solution has 1 mole of the substance dissolved in each litre of solution (equivalent to 1 mmol/mL).
- If 2 moles of a substance are made up to 1 litre (or 1 mole to 500 mL), the solution is said to be a 2 M solution.

WORKED EXAMPLES

If 18 g of sodium citrate (molecular weight = 294) is made up to 200 mL of solution, what is the molarity of the solution?

Step 1

Write down the weight of one mole:

1 mole of sodium citrate = 294 g

Step 2

Calculate the number of moles for 1 g (using the one unit rule):

$\frac{1}{294}$ mole

Step 3

Calculate the number of moles for 18 g:

$\frac{1}{294} \times 18 = \frac{18}{294} = 0.06$ moles

You therefore have 0.06 moles in 200 mL

Step 4

Convert to a molar concentration. To do this, you need to calculate the equivalent number of moles per litre (1,000 mL). You have 0.06 moles in 200 mL, which is equal to:

1 mL $= \frac{0.06}{200}$ moles

Therefore for 1,000 mL:

$\frac{0.06}{200} \times 1,000 = 0.06 \times 5 = 0.3$ moles

Answer: If 18 g of sodium citrate is made up to 200 mL, the resulting solution would have a concentration of 0.3M

Alternatively, a formula can be devised:

concentration (mol/L or m) $= \frac{\text{number of moles}}{\text{volume (L)}}$

The number of moles is calculated from the weight (in g) and the molecular weight, i.e.

$\frac{\text{weight (g)}}{\text{molecular weight}}$

The volume (L) is calculated by dividing the volume (in mL) by 1,000, i.e.

$\frac{\text{volume (mL)}}{1,000}$

Putting this together gives the following formula:

$$\text{concentration (mol/L or m)} = \frac{\text{number of moles}}{\text{volume (L)}} = \frac{\dfrac{\text{weight (g)}}{\text{molecular weight}}}{\dfrac{\text{volume (mL)}}{1,000}}$$

Rewriting this gives:

$$\text{concentration (mol/L or m)} = \frac{\text{weight (g)} \times 1,000}{\text{molecular weight} \times \text{final volume (mL)}}$$

Where, in this case:

weight (g)   = 18
molecular weight   = 294
final volume (mL) = 200

Substitute the figures in the formula:

$$\frac{18 \times 1,000}{294 \times 200} = 0.3 \text{ M}$$

Answer: If 18 g of sodium citrate is made up to 200 mL, the resulting solution would have a concentration of 0.3 M.

The calculation can be done in reverse: how many grams of sodium citrate are needed to make 100 mL of a 0.5 M solution?

Step 1

Write down the final concentration needed and what is signifies:

0.5 M = 0.5 moles in 1,000 mL

Step 2

Work out the number of moles needed for the volume required. You have 0.5 moles in 1,000 mL, so:

$$1 \text{ mL} = \frac{0.5}{1,000} \text{ moles}$$

For 100 mL, you will need:

$$100 \text{ mL} = \frac{0.5}{1,000} \times 100 = \frac{0.5}{10} = 0.05 \text{ moles}$$

Step 3

Convert moles to grams. You know that 1 mole of sodium citrate is equivalent to 294 g:

1 mole = 294 g

Therefore:

0.05 moles = 294 × 0.05 = 14.7 g

Answer: If 14.7 g of sodium citrate is made up to 100 mL, the resulting solution would have a concentration of 0.5 M.

Alternatively, a formula can be devised.

If:

$$\text{concentration (mol/L or m)} = \frac{\text{number of moles}}{\text{volume (L)}}$$

then:

number of moles = concentration (mol/L or m) × volume (L)

We want to go a step further and calculate a weight (in g) instead of number of moles. The number of moles is calculated from the weight (in g) and the molecular weight, i.e.

$$\frac{\text{weight (g)}}{\text{molecular weight}}$$

The volume (L) is calculated by dividing the volume (in mL) by 1,000, i.e.

$$\frac{\text{volume (mL)}}{1,000}$$

Putting this together gives the following formula:

$$\text{number of moles} = \frac{\text{weight (g)}}{\text{molecular weight}}$$

$$= \text{concentration (mol/L or m)} \times \frac{\text{volume (mL)}}{1,000}$$

Re-writing this, gives:

weight (g) =

$$\frac{\text{concentration (mol/L or m)} \times \text{molecular weight} \times \text{final volume (mL)}}{1,000}$$

Where, in this case:

concentration (mol/L or m) = 0.5
molecular weight   = 294
final volume (mL)   = 100

Substitute the figures in the formula:

$$\frac{0.5 \times 294 \times 100}{1,000} = 14.7 \text{ g}$$

Answer: If 14.7 g of sodium citrate is made up to 100 mL, the resulting solution would have a concentration of 0.5 M.

PROBLEMS

Question 14 If 8.4 g of sodium bicarbonate (molecular weight 84) is made up to 50 mL of solution, what is the molarity of the solution?

Question 15 How many grams of sodium citrate (molecular weight 294) are needed to make 250 mL of a 0.1 M solution?

ANSWERS TO PROBLEMS

Question 1 0.9 g in 100 mL; 9 g in 1,000 mL

Question 2 Potassium 0.3 g in 100 mL; 3 g in 1,000 mL. Sodium 0.18 g in 100 mL; 1.8 g in 1,000 mL. Glucose 4 g in 100 mL; 10 g in 1,000 mL

Question 3 0.45 g in 100 mL; 2.25 g in 500 mL

Question 4 Calcium gluconate 10% is equivalent to 10 g in 100 mL. Therefore a 10 mL ampoule contains 1 g calcium gluconate. But you need 4 g, i.e. 4 ampoules = 4 g or 40 mL calcium gluconate 10%.

Using the formula:

$$\frac{\text{amount you want}}{\text{amount you've got}} \times 100$$

where in this case:

amount you want = 4 g
amount you've got = 10 g (10% = 10 g in 100 mL)

Everything is in the same units, so there is no need to change units.

Substitute the numbers in the formula:

$$\frac{4}{10} \times 100 = 40 \text{ mL}$$

Answer: You need to draw up 40 mL, which is equivalent to 4 ampoules.

Question 5 4.5 mg/mL

Question 6 5 mg/mL

Question 7 Potassium 2 mg/mL; sodium chloride 1.8 mg/mL; glucose 40 mg/mL

Question 8 1 in 200,000 means there is 1 g in 200,000 mL. However, you have a 20 mL vial.

First convert 1 g to milligrams:

1,000 mg in 200,000 mL

Next work out how many mg in 1 mL:

$$1 \text{ mL} = \frac{1,000}{200,000} \text{ mg (using the one unit rule)}$$

Now work out how much is in the 20 mL vial:

$$20 \text{ mL} = \frac{1,000}{200,000} \times 20 = 0.1 \text{ mg}$$

Answer: There are 0.1 mg or 100 micrograms of adrenaline (epinephrine) in a 20 mL vial containing 1 in 200,000.

Question 9 1 in 100 means 1 g in 100 mL,

1 g in 100 mL is equal to 1%

Question 10 In this case the dose is 27,000 units. Therefore you would use:

1 × 25,000 units/mL, 1 mL ampoule **and**
1 × 5,000 units/mL, 1 mL ampoule

Calculate how much of the 5,000 units/mL ampoule you need:

27,000 units − 25,000 units = 2,000 units

Therefore you need to draw up 2,000 units from the 5,000 units/mL ampoule.

Write down what you have, i.e. 5,000 units in 1 mL.

Work out the volume for 1 unit (using the one unit rule):

5,000 units in 1 mL

$$1 \text{ unit} = \frac{1}{5,000} \text{ mL}$$

Now multiply by the dose required (2,000 units):

$$2,000 \text{ units} = \frac{1}{5,000} \times 2,000 = 0.4 \text{ mL}$$

Answer: You would add 1 × 25,000 units/mL ampoule and 0.4 mL of 1 × 5,000 units/mL to the infusion.

Using the formula:

$$\frac{\text{amount you want}}{\text{amount you've got}} \times \text{volume it's in}$$

Once again, before substituting numbers in the formula, decide as to which ampoule(s) of heparin would be the most appropriate; then, if necessary, calculate how much to draw up. Thus:

amount you want = 2,000 units
amount you've got = 5,000 units
volume it's in = 1 mL

Substitute the numbers in the formula:

$$\frac{2,000}{5,000} \times 1 = 0.4 \text{ mL}$$

Answer: You would add 1 × 25,000 units/mL ampoule and 0.4 mL of 1 × 5,000 units/mL to the infusion.

Question 11 You would add 1 × 25,000 units/mL ampoule and 0.2 mL of 1 × 5,000 units/mL to the infusion.

Question 12 Dose = 175 units/kg, patient weight = 68 kg, therefore dose required = 175 × 68 = 11,900 units. For a dose of 11,900 units you will need a 0.7 mL (14,000 units) pre-filled syringe.

Volume to be given:

You have 14,000 units in 0.7 mL which is equivalent to:

$$1 \text{ unit in } \frac{0.7}{14,000} \text{ mL}$$

Therefore for 11,900 units, you will need:

$$\frac{0.7}{14,000} \times 11,900 = 0.595 \text{ mL or } 0.6 \text{ mL (rounding up)}$$

In reality, you would round up the dose to 12,000 units and give 0.6 mL as calibrated on the syringe.

Question 13 Dose = 15 mg/kg, patient weight = 59 kg, therefore dose required = 1.5 × 59 = 88.5 mg. For a dose of 88.5 mg you will need a 1 mL syringe (10,000 units, 100 mg)

Volume to be given:

You have 100 mg in 1 mL, which is equivalent to:

$$1 \text{ mg in } \frac{1}{100} \text{ mL}$$

Therefore for 88.5 mg, you will need:

$$\frac{1}{100} \times 88.5 = 0.885 \text{ mL or } 0.9 \text{ mL (rounding up)}$$

In reality, you would round up the dose to 90 mg and give 0.9 mL as calibrated on the syringe.

Question 14 First, write down the weight of 1 mole of sodium bicarbonate: 84 g. Next, calculate the number of moles for 1 g, using the one unit rule:

$$1\text{g would equal } \frac{1}{84} \text{ mole}$$

Then calculate the number of moles for 8.4 g:

$$8.4 \text{ g} = \frac{1}{84} \times 8.4 = \frac{8.4}{84} = 0.1 \text{ moles}$$

You therefore have 0.1 moles in 50 mL.

To convert this to a molar concentration, you need to calculate the equivalent number of moles per litre (1,000 mL). You have 0.1 moles in 50 mL, which is equal to:

$$1 \text{ mL} = \frac{0.1}{50} \text{ moles}$$

Therefore for 1,000 mL:

$$\frac{0.1}{50} \times 1,000 = \frac{100}{50} = 2 \text{ moles}$$

Answer: If 8.4 g of sodium bicarbonate is made up to 50 mL, the resulting solution would have a concentration of 2 M.

Using the formula:

$$\text{concentration (mol/L or m)} = \frac{\text{weight (g)} \times 100}{\text{molecular weight} \times \text{final volume (mL)}}$$

where, in this case:

weight (g) $= 8.4$
molecular weight $= 84$
final volume (mL) $= 50$

Substitute the figures in the formula:

$$\frac{8.4 \times 1,000}{84 \times 50} = 2 \text{ M}$$

Answer: If 8.4 g of sodium bicarbonate is made up to 50 mL, the resulting solution would have a concentration of 2 M.

Question 15 First, write down the final concentration needed and what it signifies:

0.1 M = 0.1 moles in 1,000 mL

Next, work out the number of moles needed for the volume required:

You have: 0.1 moles in 1,000 mL

Therefore in: $1 \text{ mL} = \dfrac{0.1}{1,000}$ moles

For 250 mL, you will need:

$250 \text{ mL} = \dfrac{0.1 \times 250}{1,000} = \dfrac{0.1}{4} = 0.025$ moles

Now convert moles to grams. You know that 1 mole sodium citrate is equivalent to 294 g.

1 mole = 294 g

Therefore:

0.025 moles = 294 3 0.025 = 7.35 g

Answer: If 7.35 g of sodium citrate is made up to 250 mL, the resulting solution would have a concentration of 0.1 M.

Using the formula:

weight (g) =

$$\dfrac{\text{concentration (mol/L or m)} \times \text{molecular weight} \times \text{ final volume (m}}{1,000}$$

where, in this case:

concentration (mol/L or m) = 0.1

molecular weight = 294

final volume (mL) = 250

Substitute the figures in the formula:

$$\dfrac{0.1 \times 294 \times 250}{1,000} = 7.35 \text{ g}$$

Answer: If 7.35 g of sodium citrate is made up to 250 mL, the resulting solution would have a concentration of 0.1 M.

KEY POINTS

Percentage concentration

- % w/v = number of grams in 100 mL. A solid is dissolved in a liquid, thus 5% w/v means 5 g in 100 mL.
- % w/w = number of grams in 100 g. A solid is mixed with another solid, thus 5% w/w means 5 g in 100 g.
- % v/v = number of mL in 100 mL. A liquid is mixed or diluted with another liquid, thus 5% v/v means 5 mL in 100 mL.
- The most common percentage strength encountered is % w/v.
- There is always the same amount of drug present in 100 mL, irrespective of the total volume. Thus in a 5% w/v solution, there is 5 g dissolved in each 100 mL of fluid and this will remain the same if it is a 500 mL bag or a 1 litre bag.
- To find the total amount of drug present, the total volume must be taken into account – there is a total of 25 g present in 500 mL of a 5% w/v solution.

Concentrations in mg/mL

- Defined as the number of mg of drug per mL of liquid.
- Oral liquids are usually expressed as the number of mg in a standard 5 mL spoonful, e.g. erythromycin 250 mg in 5 mL.
- Injections are usually expressed as the number of mg per 1 mL or the number of mg per volume of the ampoule (1 mL, 2 mL, 5 mL, 10 mL or 20 mL), e.g. furosemide (frusemide) 10 mg/mL.
- N.B. Strengths can also be expressed in micrograms/mL:
- To convert percentage concentrations to mg/mL concentrations, multiply the percentage by 10: e.g. lidocaine (lignocaine) 0.2% = 2 mg/mL.
- To convert mg/mL concentrations to percentage concentrations, divide the mg/mL strength by 10: e.g. lidocaine (lignocaine) 2 mg/mL = 0.2%.

'1 in ...' concentrations or ratio strengths

- Defined as: ONE gram in however many mL, for example:
    1 in 1,000 means 1 g in 1,000 mL
    1 in 10,000 means 1 g in 10,000 mL.
- Tuberculin strengths are different – see text.

Heparin and insulin

- The purity of drugs such as insulin and heparin, from animal or biosynthetic sources, varies.
- These drugs are expressed in terms of **units** as a standard measurement, rather than weight.

Molarity and molar solutions

- Molarity is a term used in chemistry to describe concentrations.
- When **1 mole** of a substance is dissolved in **1 litre** of solution, it is known as a **1 molar** (1 M) solution.
- A 1 M solution has 1 mole of the substance dissolved in each litre of solution (equivalent to 1 mmol/mL).
- If 2 moles of a substance are made up to 1 litre (or 1 mole to 500 mL), the solution is said to be a 2 M solution.

Infusion rate calculations

OBJECTIVES

At the end of this chapter you should be familiar with the following:

- Calculating drip rates in drops/min
- Converting dosages to mL/hour
- Converting mL/hour to dosages
- Calculating the length of time for IV infusions

There are two types of infusion rate calculations to be considered:

- drops per minute (drops/min): mainly encountered when infusions are given under gravity, as with fluid replacement
- millilitres per hour (mL/hour): encountered when infusions have to be given accurately or in small volumes using infusion or syringe pumps – particularly if drugs have to be given as infusions.

CALCULATING DRIP RATES IN DROPS/MIN

To set up a manually controlled infusion accurately by eye, you need to be able to count the number of drops per minute. To do this, you have to work out the volume to be infused in terms of drops. This in turn depends upon the giving or administration set being used.

GIVING SETS

There are two types of giving sets:

- The **standard giving set** (SGS) has a drip rate of 20 drops/mL for clear fluids (e.g. sodium chloride or glucose) and 15 drops/mL for blood.
- The **micro-drop giving set** or burette has a drip rate of 60 drops/mL.

The drip rate of the giving set is always written on the wrapper if you are not sure.

In all drip rate calculations, you have to remember that you are simply converting a volume to drops (or vice versa) and hours to minutes.

WORKED EXAMPLE

1 litre of sodium chloride 0.9% ('normal saline') is to be given over 8 hours. What drip rate is required using a standard giving set (SGS) at 20 drops/mL?

Step 1

First convert the volume to a number of drops. To do this, multiply the volume of the infusion by the number of 'drops/mL' for the giving set, i.e.

$1,000 \times 20 = 20,000$ drops

This is the number of drops to be infused, for the giving set being used.

Step 2

Next convert hours to minutes by multiplying the number of hours the infusion is to be given by 60 (60 minutes = 1 hour):

8 hours = $8 \times 60 = 480$ minutes

If the infusion is being given over a period of minutes, then obviously there is no need to convert from hours to minutes.

Now everything has been converted to drops and minutes, i.e. in terms of what you want for your final answer.

Step 3

Write down what you have just calculated, i.e. the total number of drops to be given over how many minutes.

20,000 drops to be given over 480 minutes
(20,000 drops = 480 mins)

Step 4

Calculate the number of drops per minute by dividing the number of drops by the number of minutes, i.e.

20,000 drops over 480 minutes

$\dfrac{20,000}{480} = 41.67$ drops/min

It's impossible to have part of a drop, so round up or down to the nearest whole number:

41.67 = 42 drops/min

Answer: To give a litre (1,000 mL) of sodium chloride 0.9% ('normal saline') over 8 hours, the rate will have to be 42 drops/min using a standard giving set (20 drops/mL).

A formula can be used:

$$\text{drops/min} = \frac{\text{drops/mL of the giving set} \times \text{volume of the infusion (mL)}}{\text{number of hours the infusion is to run} \times 60}$$

where in this case:

drops/mL of the giving set = 20 drops/mL (SGS)
volume of the infusion (in mL) = 1,000 mL
number of hours the infusion is to run = 8 hours
60 = number of minutes in an hour (converts hours to minutes)

Substitute the numbers in the formula:

$$\frac{20 \times 1,000}{8 \times 60} = 41.67 \text{ drops/min (42 drops/min, approx.)}$$

Answer: To give a litre (1,000 mL) of sodium chloride 0.9% ('normal saline') over 8 hours, the rate will have to be 42 drops/min using a standard giving set (20 drops/mL).

CALCULATING INFUSION DRIP RATES (DROPS/MIN) – SUMMARY

$$\text{drops/min} = \frac{\text{drops/mL of the giving set} \times \text{volume of the infusion (mL)}}{\text{number of hours the infusion is to run} \times 60}$$

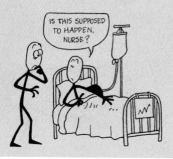

PROBLEMS

Work out the drip rates for the following:

Question 1   500 mL of sodium chloride 0.9% over 6 hours.

Question 2   500 mL of glucose 5% over 8 hours.

Question 3   100 mL of sodium chloride 0.9% over 1 hour.

Question 4   1 litre of glucose 4% and sodium chloride 0.18% over 12 hours.

Question 5   1 unit of blood (500 mL) over 4 hours.

Question 6   1 unit of blood (500 mL) over 6 hours.

Question 7   You are asked to give 3 litres of sodium chloride 0.9% over 24 hours. You only have 1-litre bags of sodium chloride 0.9%. At what rate should each bag run?

CONVERTING DOSAGES TO ML/HOUR

Dosages can be expressed in various ways: mg/min or micrograms/min and mg/kg/minute or micrograms/kg/min. When using infusion pumps, it may be necessary to convert to mL/hour.

The following example show the various steps in this type of calculation, and this can be adapted to any dosage to infusion rate calculation.

WORKED EXAMPLE

You have an infusion of dopamine 800 mg in 500 mL. The dose required is 2 micrograms/kg/min for a patient weighing 68 kg. What is the rate in mL/hour?

Step 1

When answering this type of calculation, it is best to convert the dose required to a volume in mL.

Step 2

First calculate the volume for 1 microgram of drug. It is best to work in micrograms since the dose is in micrograms/kg. If the dose is in milligrams, then calculate the concentration of drug in mg/mL.

800 mg in 500 mL is equal to:

800 mg × 1,000 = 800,000 micrograms in 500 mL

Thus the volume for 1 microgram is:

$$1 \text{ microgram} = \frac{500}{800,000} \text{ mL}$$

Step 3

Now calculate the dose required:

Dose required = Patient's weight × dose prescribed
= 28 × 2 = 136 micrograms/min

If the dose is given as a total dose and not on a weight basis, then miss out this step.

Step 4

The next step is to calculate the volume for the dose required. You have already worked out that 1 microgram of drug equals:

$$1 \text{ microgram} = \frac{500}{800,000} \text{ mL}$$

Thus for the dose of 136 micrograms, the volume is equal to:

$$136 \text{ micrograms} = \frac{500}{800,000} \times 136 \text{ mL} = 0.085 \text{ mL}$$

You can therefore rewrite the dose of 136 micrograms/min as:

0.085 mL/min

You have now converted the dose (136 micrograms) to a volume (0.085 mL).

Step 5

You have just calculated that the rate to be given is:

0.085 mL/min

To calculate the rate in mL/hour, simply multiply by 60 to convert minutes to hours:

0.085 mL/min = 0.085 × 60 = 5.1 mL/hour (5 mL/hour, approx.)

Answer: The rate required is 5 mL/hour.

Using the formula:

$$mL/hour = \frac{\text{total volume to be infused}}{\text{total amount of drug}} \times \text{dose} \times \text{weight} \times 60$$

Tip	• If the dose is in milligrams, then the total amount of drug must be in milligrams.
	• If the dose is in micrograms, then the total amount of drug must be in micrograms.

In this case:

> total volume to be infused = 500 mL
> total amount of drug (micrograms) = 800,000 micrograms
> dose = 2 micrograms/kg/minute
> patient's weight = 68 kg
> 60 minutes = 1 hour

Substitute the numbers in the formula:

$$\frac{500 \times 2 \times 68 \times 60}{800,000} = 5.1 \text{ mL/hour (5 mL/hour, approx.)}$$

Answer: The rate required is 5 mL/hour.

If the dose is given as a total dose and not on a weight basis, then the patient's weight is not needed.

$$\text{mL/hour} = \frac{\text{total volume to be infused}}{\text{total amount of drug}} \times \text{dose} \times 60$$

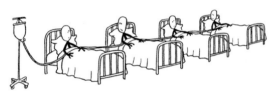

I KNOW THEY'RE SUPPOSED TO CUT COSTS,
BUT THIS IS RIDICULOUS!

CONVERTING DOSAGES TO INFUSION RATES – SUMMARY

● To convert dose/kg/minute to mL/hour:

$$\text{mL/hour} = \frac{\text{total volume to be infused}}{\text{total amount of drug}} \times \text{dose} \times \text{weight} \times 60$$

● To convert dose to mL/hour:

$$\text{mL/hour} = \frac{\text{total volume to be infused}}{\text{total amount of drug}} \times \text{dose} \times 60$$

● If the dose is in milligrams, then the total amount of drug must be in milligrams.
● If the dose is in micrograms, then the total amount of drug must be in micrograms.

Table 10 Infusion rates (ml/hour)

Time Vol	Minutes 10	15	20	30	40	Hours 1	2	3	4	6	8	10	12	16	18	24
10 mL	60	40	30	20												
20 mL	120	80	60	40												
30 mL				60												
40 mL				80	60	40										
50 mL				100	75	50										
60 mL				120	90	60										
80 mL				160	120	80										
100 mL				200	150	100	50	33	25	17						
125 mL				250	188	125	63	42	31	21						
150 mL				300	225	150	75	50	38	25						
200 mL				400	300	200	100	67	50	33	25	20	17	13	11	8
250 mL							125	83	63	42	31	25	21	16	14	10
500 mL									125	83	63	50	42	31	28	21
1000 mL										250	167	125	100	83	63	56	42

NOTE Rates given in the table have been rounded up or down to give whole numbers.

HOW TO USE THIS TABLE

If you need to give a 250 mL infusion over 8 hours, then to find the infusion rate (mL/hour) go down the left-hand (**Volume**) column until you reach 250 mL; then go along the top (**Time**) line until you reach 8 (for 8 hours). Then read off the corresponding infusion rate (mL/hour). In this case it equals 31 mL/hour.

PROBLEMS

Question 8 You have a 500 mL infusion containing 50 mg nitroglycerin. A dose of 10 micrograms/min is required. What is the rate in mL/hour? (Beware of units!)

Question 9 You are asked to give 500 mL of lidocaine (lignocaine) 0.2% in glucose at a rate of 2 mg/min. What is the rate in mL/hour?

Question 10 You have an infusion of dopamine 800 mg in 500 mL. The dose required is 3 micrograms/kg/min for a patient weighing 80 kg. What is the rate in mL/hour? (Beware of units!)

Question 11 A 63 kg patient is prescribed aminophylline as an infusion at a dose of 0.5 mg/kg per hour over 12 hours. Aminophylline injection comes as 250 mg in 10 mL ampoules and should be given in a 500 mL infusion bag.
i) What dose and volume of aminophylline is required?
ii) What is the rate in mL/hour?

Question 12 You need to give aciclovir (acyclovir) as an infusion at a dose of 5 mg/kg every 8 hours. The patient weighs 86 kg and aciclovir (acyclovir) is available as 500 mg vials. Each vial needs to be reconstituted with 20 mL water for injection and diluted further to 100 mL. The infusion should be given over 60 minutes.
i) What dose and volume of aciclovir (acyclovir) is required?
ii) What is the rate in mL/hour for each dose?

Question 13 Glyceryl trinitrate is to be given at a starting rate of 150 micrograms/min. You have an infusion of 50 mg in 50 mL glucose 5%. What is the rate in mL/hour? (Beware of units!)

Question 14 You have an infusion of furosemide (frusemide) 250 mg in 250 mL sodium chloride 0.9%. The patient is to receive a dose of 1.5 mg/min. What is the rate in mL/hour?

Question 15 You are asked to give an infusion of salbutamol. You have an ampoule containing salbutamol 5 mg in 5 mL, which has to be added to a 500 mL infusion of sodium chloride 0.9%. The rate at which it has to be given is 5 micrograms/min.
i) What is the concentration (micrograms/mL) of salbutamol?
ii) What is the rate in mL/hour?

Question 16 You are asked to give an infusion of dobutamine to a patient weighing 73 kg at a dose of 5 micrograms/kg/min. You have an infusion of 500 mL sodium chloride 0.9% containing 250 mg of dobutamine.
i) What is the dose required (micrograms/min)?
ii) What is the concentration (micrograms/mL) of dobutamine?
iii) What is the rate in mL/hour?

Question 17 You are asked to give an infusion of isosorbide dinitrate 50 mg in 500 mL of glucose 5% at a rate of 2 mg/hour.
i) What is the rate in mL/hour?
ii) The rate is then changed to 5 mg/hour. What is the new rate in mL/hour?

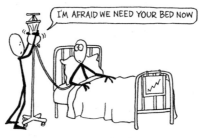

INCREASING THE INFUSION RATE

CONVERTING ML/HOUR TO DOSAGES

Sometimes it may be necessary to convert mL/hour back to the dose: mg/min or micrograms/min and mg/kg/min or micrograms/kg /min: for example, when checking that an infusion pump is giving the correct dose. Nurses changing shifts, especially on critical care wards, check that the pumps are set correctly at the beginning of each shift.

WORKED EXAMPLE

An infusion pump containing 250 mg dobutamine in 50 mL is running at a rate of 3.5 mL/hour. You want to convert to micrograms/kg/min to check that the pump is set correctly. The patient's weight is 70 kg.

Step 1

In this type of calculation, convert the volume being given to the amount of drug, and then work out the amount of drug being given per minute, or per kilogram of the patient's weight.

Step 2

Convert the amount of drug (dobutamine) from milligrams to micrograms. The final answer wanted is in micrograms (micrograms/kg/min), so convert everything to micrograms.

250 mg = 250 × 1,000 = 250,000 micrograms

Obviously, if the dose is already in milligrams, you can miss out this step.

Step 3

You have just worked out that you have 250,000 micrograms of dobutamine in 50 mL. Now you have to work out the amount in 1 mL:

250,000 micrograms in 50 mL

$\dfrac{250,000}{50}$ micrograms in 1 mL

Step 4

The rate at which the pump is running is 3.5 mL/hour. You have just worked out the amount in 1 mL (Step 2), so for 3.5 mL:

$$3.5 \text{ mL/hour} = \dfrac{250,000}{50} \times 3.5 \text{ micrograms/hour}$$

So the rate (mL/hour) has been converted to the amount of drug being given over an hour.

Step 5

In Step 4, it was calculated that the rate was:

$$\dfrac{250,000}{50} \times 3.5 \text{ micrograms/hour}$$

Now calculate the rate per minute by dividing by 60 (to convert hours to minutes):

$$\dfrac{250,000 \times 3.5}{50 \times 60} \text{ micrograms/min}$$

Step 6

The final step in the calculation is to work out the rate according to the patient's weight (70 kg). If the dose is not given in terms of the patient's weight, then miss out this final step.

$$\dfrac{250,000 \times 3.5}{50 \times 60 \times 70} = 4.11 \text{ microgram/kg/min}$$

This can be rounded down to 4 micrograms/kg/min.

Now check your answer against the dose written on the drug chart to see if the pump is delivering the correct dose. If your answer does not match the dose written on the drug chart, then re-check your calculation. If the answer is still the same, then inform the doctor and, if necessary, calculate the correct rate.

Using the formula:

mg or micrograms/kg/min =

$$\dfrac{\text{rate (mL/hour)} \times \text{amount of drug (mg or micrograms)}}{60 \times \text{weight (kg)} \times \text{volume (mL)}}$$

where in this case:

> rate = 3.5 mL/hour
> amount of drug (micrograms) = 250,000 micrograms
> weight (kg) = 70 kg
> volume (mL) = 50 mL
> 60 converts hours to minutes

Substitute the numbers in the formula:

$$\frac{3.5 \times 250,000}{60 \times 70 \times 50} = 4.11 \text{ microgram/kg/min}$$

This can be rounded down to 4 micrograms/kg/min.

If the dose is either micrograms/min or mg/min, then the formula is now rewritten as:

mg or micrograms/min =

$$\frac{\text{rate (mL/hour)} \times \text{amount of drug (mg or micrograms)}}{60 \times \text{volume (mL)}}$$

Tip If the dose is in milligrams, then the total amount of drug must be in milligrams.

If the dose is in micrograms, then the total amount of drug must be in micrograms.

CONVERTING ML/HOUR TO DOSAGES – SUMMARY

- To convert mL/hour to mg or micrograms/kg/min:

  mg or micrograms/kg/min =

  $$\frac{\text{rate (mL/hour)} \times \text{amount of drug (mg or micrograms)}}{60 \times \text{weight (kg)} \times \text{volume (mL)}}$$

- To convert mL/hour to mg or micrograms/min:

  mg or micrograms/min =

  $$\frac{\text{rate (mL/hour)} \times \text{amount of drug (mg or micrograms)}}{60 \times \text{volume (mL)}}$$

- If the dose is in milligrams, then the amount of drug must be in milligrams.
- If the dose is in micrograms, then the amount of drug must be in micrograms.

PROBLEMS

Convert the following infusion pump rates to a dose in micrograms/kg/min:

Question 18 You have dopamine 200 mg in 50 mL and the pump is running at 4 mL/hour. The prescribed dose is 3 micrograms/kg/min. The patient's weight is 89 kg.
  i) What dose is the pump delivering?
  ii) If the dose is wrong, at what rate should the pump be set?

Question 19 You have dobutamine 250 mg in 50 mL and the pump is running at 5.6 mL/hour. The prescribed dose is 6 micrograms/kg/min. The patient's weight is 64 kg.
  i) What dose is the pump delivering?
  ii) If the dose is wrong, at what rate should the pump be set?

Question 20 You have dopexamine 50 mg in 50 mL and the pump is running at 2.3 mL/hour. The prescribed dose is 6 micrograms/kg/min. The patient's weight is 78 kg.
  i) What dose is the pump delivering?
  ii) If the dose is wrong, at what rate should the pump be set?

Convert the following infusion pump rates to a dose in mg/min:

Question 21 You have a 100 mL infusion containing 250 mg of furosemide (frusemide) being given by an infusion pump at a rate of 50 mL/hour. The maximum rate at which furosemide (frusemide) can be given is 4 mg/min. At what rate is the pump delivering (mg/min)?

Question 22 You have a 500 mL infusion of lidocaine (lignocaine) 0.2% being given by an infusion pump at a rate of 90 mL/hour. The prescribed dose is 3 mg/min. What dose is the pump delivering (mg/min)?

Question 23 You have a 500 mL infusion containing 2 mg of isoprenaline being given by an infusion pump at a rate of 45 mL/hour. The prescribed dose is 3 micrograms/min. At what rate is the pump delivering (micrograms/min)?

CALCULATING THE LENGTH OF TIME FOR INTRAVENOUS (IV) INFUSIONS

MANUALLY CONTROLLED INFUSIONS

Sometimes it may be necessary to calculate the number of hours an infusion should run at a specified rate. Also, it is a good way of checking your calculated drip rate for an infusion.

For example:

> You are asked to give a litre of 5% glucose over 8 hours. You have calculated that the drip rate should be 42 drops/min (using a standard giving set, 20 drops/mL).

To check your answer, you can calculate how long the infusion should take at the calculated drip rate of 42 drops/min. The answer should be 8 hours. If your answer does not correspond to this figure, you have made an error and should re-check your calculation.

Alternatively, you can use this type of calculation to check the drip rate of an infusion already running.

For example:

> If an infusion is supposed to run over 6 hours, and the infusion is nearly finished after 4 hours, you can check the drip rate by calculating how long the infusion should take using that drip rate If the calculated answer is less than 6 hours, then the original drip rate was wrong and the doctor should be informed, if necessary.

WORKED EXAMPLE

The doctor prescribes 1 litre of 5% glucose to be given over 8 hours. The drip rate for the infusion is calculated to be 42 drops/min. You wish to check the drip rate, how many hours is the infusion going to run? (Remember there are 20 drops/mL with a standard giving set).

Step 1

In this calculation, you first convert the volume being infused to drops; then calculate how long it will take at the specified rate.

Step 2

First, convert the volume to drops by multiplying the volume of the infusion by the number of drops/mL for the giving set.

$1,000 \times 20 = 20,000$ drops

Step 3

From the rate, calculate how many minutes it will take for 1 drop, i.e.

42 drops per minute

1 drop = $\frac{1}{42}$ min

Step 4

Calculate how many minutes it will take to infuse the total number of drops:

1 drop = $\frac{1}{42}$ min

20,000 drops = $\frac{1}{42} \times 20,000 = 476$ min

Step 5

Convert minutes to hours by dividing by 60:

476 min = $\frac{476}{60} = 7.94$ hour

How much is 0.94 of an hour? Multiply by 60 to convert part of an hour back to minutes:

0.94 × 60 = 56.4 min = 56 min (approx.)

Answer: 1 litre of glucose 5% at a rate of 42 drops/min will take approximately 8 hours to run (7 hours and 56 minutes).

A formula can be used:

$$\text{number of hours the infusion is to run} = \frac{\text{volume of the infusion}}{\text{rate (drops/min)} \times 60} \times \text{drip rate of giving set}$$

where in this case:

volume of the infusion = 1,000 mL
rate (drops/min) = 42 drops/min
drip rate of giving set = 20 drops/mL
60 converts minutes to hours

Substitute the numbers in the formula:

$\frac{1,000}{42 \times 60} \times 20 = 7.94$ hours

0.94 hours = 56 minutes (approx.)

Answer: 1 litre of glucose 5% at a rate of 42 drops/min will take approximately 8 hours to run (7 hours 56 minutes).

INFUSION OR SYRINGE PUMPS

The same method can be applied to infusion or syringe pumps. If we use our original example:

You are asked to give a litre of 5% glucose over 8 hours. You have calculated that the infusion rate should be 125 mL/hour.

To check your answer, you can calculate how long the infusion should take at the calculated infusion rate of 125 mL/hour. The answer should be 8 hours. If your answer does not correspond to this figure, you have made an error and should re-check your calculation.

Once again, you can use this type of calculation to check the rate of an infusion already running. As before, if an infusion is supposed to run over 6 hours and is nearly finished after 4 hours, calculating how long the infusion should take using the rate set on the pump can check that rate was originally correct.

WORKED EXAMPLE

The doctor prescribes 1 litre of 5% glucose to be given over 8 hours. The rate for the infusion is calculated to be 125 mL/hour. You wish to check the calculated rate. How many hours is the infusion going to run?

This is a simple calculation. You divide the total volume by the rate to give you the time over which the infusion is to run.

calculated rate = 125 mL/hour   volume = 1,000 mL

$$\frac{1,000}{125} = 8 \text{ hours}$$

Answer: 1 litre of glucose 5% at a rate of 125 mL/hour will take 8 hours to run.

A simple formula can be used:

$$\text{number of hours the infusion is to run} = \frac{\text{volume of the infusion}}{\text{rate (mL/hour)}}$$

where in this case:

volume of the infusion = 1,000 mL
rate (mL/hour) = 125 mL/hour

Substitute the numbers in the formula:

$$\frac{1,000}{125} = 8 \text{ hours}$$

Answer: 1 litre of glucose 5% at a rate of 125 mL/hour will take 8 hours to run.

ADDING A DRUG TO THE INFUSION

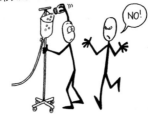

CALCULATING THE TIME AN INFUSION IS GOING TO RUN – SUMMARY

Manually controlled infusions

$$\text{number of hours the infusion is to run} = \frac{\text{volume of the infusion}}{\text{rate (drops/min)} \times 60} \times \text{drip rate of giving set}$$

Infusion or syringe pumps

$$\text{number of hours the infusion is to run} = \frac{\text{volume of the infusion}}{\text{rate (mL/hour)}}$$

PROBLEMS

Question 24 A 1 litre infusion of sodium chloride 0.9% is being given over 12 hours, with a standard giving set. The rate at which the infusion is being run is 28 drops/min. How long will the infusion run at the specified rate?

Question 25 A 500 mL infusion of sodium chloride 0.9% is being given over 4 hours with a standard giving set. The rate at which the infusion is being run is 42 drops/min. How long will the infusion run at the specified rate?

Question 26 A unit of blood (500 mL) is being given over 6 hours with a standard giving set. The rate at which the infusion is being run is 21 drops/min. How long will the infusion run at the specified rate?

Question 27 A patient is currently on a heparin infusion. At 3 pm you hear the pump start bleeping, indicating a blockage, and press the 'stop' button. The SHO walks on to the ward and asks you how much heparin the patient has had so far today. The rate set on the pump was 2 mL/hour and has not altered since it was set up at 8 am. The patient was prescribed 25,000 units in 50 mL sodium chloride 0.9%.

ANSWERS TO PROBLEMS

CALCULATING IV INFUSION RATES (DROPS/MIN)

Question 1 First convert the volume to a number of drops. To do this, multiply the volume of the infusion by the number of drops per mL for the giving set, i.e.

$$500 \times 20 = 10{,}000 \text{ drops}$$

Next convert hours to minutes by multiplying the number of hours the infusion is to be given by 60 (60 minutes = 1 hour).

$$6 \text{ hours} = 6 \times 60 = 360 \text{ minutes}$$

Write down what you have just calculated, i.e. the total number of drops to be given over how many minutes:

$$10{,}000 \text{ drops} = 360 \text{ minutes}$$

Calculate the number of drops per minute by dividing the number of drops by the number of minutes, i.e. divide 10,000 by 360. You have 10,000 drops over 360 minutes. Thus:

$$\text{drops/min} = \frac{10{,}000}{360} = 27.78 \text{ drops/min}$$
$$(28 \text{ drops/min, approx.})$$

Answer: To give 500 mL of sodium chloride 0.9% over 6 hours, the rate will have to be 28 drops/min using a standard giving set (20 drops/mL).

Using the formula:

$$\text{drops/min} = \frac{\text{drops/mL of the giving set} \times \text{volume of the infusion}}{\text{number of hours the infusion is to run} \times 60}$$

where in this case:

drops/mL of the giving set = 20 drops/mL (SGS)
volume of the infusion (in mL) = 500 mL
number of hours the infusion is to run = 6 hours

Substitute the numbers in the formula:

$$\frac{20 \times 500}{6 \times 60} = 27.78 \text{ drops/min (28 drops/min, approx.)}$$

Answer: To give 500 mL of sodium chloride 0.9% over 6 hours, the rate will have to be 28 drops/min using a standard giving set (20 drops/mL).

Question 2 20.8 drops/min (21 drops/min) using a standard giving set (20 drops/mL).

Question 3 33.3 drops/min (33 drops/min) using a standard giving set (20 drops/mL).

Question 4 27.7 drops/min (28 drops/min) using a standard giving set (20 drops/mL).

Question 5 31.25 drops/min (31 drops/min) using a standard giving set (15 drops/mL).

Question 6 20.8 drops/min (21 drops/min) using a standard giving set (20 drops/mL).

Question 7 3 litres over 24 hours, thus:

$$1 \text{ litre over } \frac{24}{3} = 8 \text{ hours}$$

Answer: 41.67 drops/min (42 drops/min) using a standard giving set (20 drops/mL).

CONVERTING DOSAGES TO ML/HOUR

Question 8 First convert the amount of drug from milligrams to micrograms, (the dose is in micrograms; so it is best to work in micrograms).

nitroglycerin 50 mg = 50 × 1,000 = 50,000 micrograms

Next, calculate the volume for 1 microgram of nitroglycerin:

$$50,000 \text{ micrograms in 500 mL; } 1 \text{ microgram} = \frac{500}{50,000} \text{ mL}$$

Thus for the dose of 10 micrograms/min, the rate is equal to:

$$10 \text{ micrograms/min} = \frac{500}{50,000} \times 10 = 0.1 \text{ mL/min}$$

You have just calculated that the rate to be given = 0.1 mL/min. To calculate the rate in mL/hour, simply multiply by 60 to convert minutes to hours:

0.1 mL/min = 0.1 × 60 = 6 mL/hour

Answer: The rate required is 6 mL/hour.

Using the formula:

$$\text{mL/hour} = \frac{\text{total volume to be infused}}{\text{total amount of drug}} \times \text{dose} \times 60$$

where:

    total volume to be infused = 500 mL
    total amount of drug (micrograms) = 50,000 micrograms
    dose = 10 micrograms/min

Substitute the numbers in the formula:

$$\frac{500 \times 10 \times 60}{50,000} = 6 \text{ mL/hour}$$

Answer: The required rate is 6 mL/hour.

Question 9 60 mL/hour

Question 10 9 mL/hour

Question 11 **i)** The dose required for the patient is:

    $63 \times 0.5 = 31.5$ mg/hour

Therefore for 12 hours, you will need:

    $31.5 \times 12 = 378$ mg

You have 250 mg in 10 mL Therefore(using the one unit rule) 1 mg is equivalent to:

$$\frac{10}{250} \text{ mL}$$

Thus:

$$378 \text{ mg} = \frac{10}{250} \times 378 = 15.12 \text{ mL}$$
$$= 15 \text{ mL (rounded down)}$$

Answer: Add 15 mL (378 mg) to a 500 mL infusion bag.

ii) As the infusion is to run over 12 hours, calculate the hourly rate:

    500 mL to be given over 12 hours

Therefore the hourly rate is:

$$\frac{500}{12} \text{ mL} = 41.67 \text{ mL/hour} = 42 \text{ mL/hour (rounded up)}$$

Answer: 42 mL/hour.

Question 12   **i)** First calculate the dose required:

$$5 \times 86 = 430 \text{ mg}$$

Next, calculate the volume of the reconstituted vial required:

$$500 \text{ mg} = 20 \text{ mL}$$
$$1 \text{ mg} = \frac{20}{500} \text{ mL}$$

Therefore for 430 mg:

$$430 \text{ mg} = \frac{20}{500} \times 430 = \frac{430}{25} = 17.2 \text{ mL}$$
$$= 17.2 \text{ mL or } 17 \text{ mL (rounded down)}$$

Answer: Add 17 mL (430 mg) to a 100 mL infusion bag

ii) As the infusion is to run over 60 minutes (= 1 hour), no further calculation is needed.

Answer: 100 mL/hour

Question 13   Beware of units – convert 50 mg to micrograms (= 50,000 micrograms).

Answer: 9 mL/hour

Question 14   90 mL/hour

Question 15   **i)** You have 5 mg in 500 mL. Calculate the number of milligrams in 1 mL by dividing by 500:

$$\frac{5}{500} = \frac{1}{100} \text{ mg in 1 mL}$$

Convert milligrams to micrograms by multiplying by 1,000:

$$\frac{1}{100} \times 1,000 = 10 \text{ micrograms/mL}$$

Answer: 10 micrograms/mL

ii) 30 mL/hour

Question 16   **i)** The dose required is:

dose (5 micrograms/kg/min) × patient's weight (73 kg)
$$= 5 \times 73 = 365 \text{ micrograms/min}$$

ii) Convert 250 mg to micrograms (multiply by 1,000). You have 250,000 micrograms in 500 mL. To find the concentration (micrograms/mL), divide by 500:

$$\frac{250,000}{500} = 500$$

Answer: 500 micrograms/mL

iii) 43.8 mL/hour (44 mL/hour)

Question 17 **i)** The rate is 2 mg/hour. Converting mg to mL, you have 50 mg in 500 mL. Therefore:

$$1 \text{ mg} = \frac{500}{50} = 10 \text{ mL}$$

Thus:

$$2 \text{ mg/hour} = 10 \times 2 = 20 \text{ mL/hour}$$

Answer: The rate is 20 mL/hour

ii) 50 mL/hour

CONVERTING ML/HOUR TO DOSAGES

Question 18 **i)** Convert the amount of drug to micrograms (same units):

$$200 \text{ mg} = 200 \times 1,000 = 200,000 \text{ micrograms}$$

You have 200,000 micrograms in 50 mL, so you have:

$$\frac{200,000}{50} \text{ micrograms in 1 mL}$$

The rate at which the pump is running is 4 mL/hour.

ii) You have just worked out the amount of dopamine in 1 mL, therefore in 4 mL:

$$\frac{200,000}{50} \times 4 \text{ micrograms/hour}$$

To convert the rate to micrograms/min, divide by 60:

$$\frac{200,000 \times 4}{50 \times 60} \text{ micrograms/min}$$

To find out the rate in terms of the patient's weight, divide by the weight (89 kg):

$$\frac{200,000 \times 4}{50 \times 60 \times 89} = 2.99 \text{ micrograms/kg/min}$$
$$(3 \text{ micrograms/kg/min})$$

Answer: The dose is correct (3 micrograms/kg/min) and no adjustment is necessary.

Using the formula:

$$\frac{\text{micrograms/}}{\text{kg/min}} = \frac{\text{rate (mL/hour)} \times \text{amount of drug (micrograms)}}{60 \times \text{weight (kg)} \times \text{volume (mL)}}$$

where:

rate = 4 mL/hour
amount of drug (micrograms) = 200,000 micrograms
weight (kg) = 89 kg
volume (mL) = 50 mL

Substitute the numbers in the formula:

$$\frac{4 \times 200,000}{60 \times 89 \times 50} = 2.99 \text{ micrograms/kg/min}$$
$$(3 \text{ micrograms/kg/min})$$

Answer: The dose is correct (3 micrograms/kg/min) and no adjustment is necessary.

Question 19 **i)** Convert the amount of drug to micrograms (same units):

250 mg = 250 × 1,000 = 250,000 micrograms

You have 250,000 micrograms in 50 mL, so you have:

$$\frac{250,000}{50} \text{ micrograms in 1 mL}$$

ii) The rate at which the pump is running is 5.6 mL/hour. You have just worked out the amount in 1 mL. So in 5.6 mL:

$$\frac{250,000}{50} \times 5.6 \text{ micrograms/hour}$$

To convert the rate to micrograms/min, divide by 60:

$$\frac{250,000}{50 \times 60} \times 5.6 \text{ micrograms/min}$$

To find out the rate in terms of the patient's weight, divide by the weight (64 kg):

$$\frac{250,000 \times 5.6}{50 \times 60 \times 64} = 7.29 \text{ micrograms/kg/min}$$
$$(7 \text{ micrograms/kg/min})$$

Answer: 7.29 micrograms/kg/min
(7 micrograms/kg/min, rounded down).
The dose being delivered by the pump
set at a rate of 5.6 mL/hour is too high.
Inform the doctor and adjust the rate of
the pump.

Using the formula:

$$\frac{\text{micrograms/}}{\text{kg/min}} = \frac{\text{rate (mL/hour)} \times \text{amount of drug (micrograms)}}{60 \times \text{weight (kg)} \times \text{volume (mL)}}$$

where:

> rate = 5.6 mL/hour
> amount of drug (micrograms) = 250,000 micrograms
> weight (kg) = 64 kg
> volume (mL) = 50 mL

Substitute the numbers in the formula:

$$\frac{5.6 \times 250,000}{60 \times 64 \times 50} = 7.29 \text{ micrograms/kg/min}$$
$$(7 \text{ micrograms/kg/min})$$

Answer: 7.29 micrograms/kg/min
(7 micrograms/kg/min, rounded down). The dose being delivered by the pump set at a rate of 5.6 mL/hour is too high. Inform the doctor and adjust the rate of the pump.

Changing the rate of the pump

In this case, the calculation is done the other way round, starting with the dose. The dose required is 6 micrograms/kg/min. The patient's weight is 64 kg, so the dose for the patient is:

> 6 × 64 = 384 micrograms/min

To find the dose per hour, multiply by 60:

> 384 × 60 = 23,040 micrograms/hour

You have 50/250,000 micrograms/mL of dobutamine (worked out previously). Therefore to find the volume for the dose, multiply by 23,040:

$$\frac{50 \times 23,040}{250,000} = 4.608 \text{ mL/hour}$$

Answer: The rate at which the pump should have been set is 4.6 mL/hour and not 5.6 mL/hour.

Using the formula:

$$\frac{\text{micrograms/}}{\text{kg/min}} = \frac{\text{rate (mL/hour)} \times \text{amount of drug (micrograms)}}{60 \times \text{weight (kg)} \times \text{volume (mL)}}$$

In this case, the unknown is the rate (mL/hour). So the formula needs to be rewritten:

rate (mL/hour) =

$$\frac{\text{dose (micrograms/kg/min)} \times \text{weight (kg)} \times \text{volume (mL)} \times 60}{\text{amount of drug (micrograms)}}$$

where:

dose (micrograms/kg/min) = 6 micrograms/kg/min
weight (kg) = 64 kg
volume (mL) = 50 mL
amount of drug (micrograms) = 250,000 micrograms

Substitute the numbers in the formula:

$$\frac{6 \times 64 \times 50 \times 60}{250,000} = 4.6 \text{ mL/hour}$$

Answer: The rate at which the pump should have been set is 4.6 mL/hour and not 5.6 mL/hour.

Question 20 **i)** The dose on the prescription chart is 6 micrograms/kg/min.
ii) The dose is correct: no adjustment is necessary.

Question 21 You have 250 mg furosemide (frusemide) in 100 mL. First, work out the amount of furosemide (frusemide) in 1 mL:

250 mg in 100 mL

$$\frac{1}{100} \text{ mL} = 250 \text{ mg}$$

The pump is delivering at a rate of 50 mL/hour, so work out the amount of furosemide (frusemide) the pump is delivering per hour:

$$50 \text{ mL} = \frac{250 \times 50}{100} = 125 \text{ mg/hour}$$

Next, divide by 60 to find the amount per minute:

$$\frac{125}{60} = 2.08 \text{ mg/min (2 mg/min)}$$

Answer: The pump is delivering furosemide (frusemide) at a rate of 2 mg/min, which is within the recommended rate of 4 mg/min.

Using the formula:

$$\text{mg/min} = \frac{\text{rate (mL/hour)}}{60 \times \text{volume (mL)}} \times \text{amount of drug (mg)}$$

where:

rate = 50 mL/hour
amount of drug (milligrams) = 250 mg
volume (mL) = 100 mL

Substitute the numbers in the formula:

$$\frac{50 \times 250}{60 \times 100} = 2.08 \text{ mg/min (2 mg/min)}$$

Answer: The pump is delivering furosemide (frusemide) at a rate of 2 mg/min, which is within the recommended rate of 4 mg/min.

Question 22 The pump is delivering at a rate of 3 mg/min, which is the same as the prescribed dose.

Question 23 Convert the amount of isoprenaline to micrograms, as the dose is in micrograms:

isoprenaline 2 mg = 2 × 1,000 = 2,000 micrograms

Now calculate the rate as before.

Answer: The pump is delivering at a rate of 3 micrograms/min, which is the same as the prescribed dose.

CALCULATING THE LENGTH OF TIME FOR IV INFUSIONS

Question 24 First, convert the volume to drops by multiplying the volume of the infusion by the number of drops/mL for the giving set:

1,000 × 20 = 20,000 drops

Next, calculate how many minutes it will take for 1 drop, i.e.

28 drops per minute

$$\frac{1}{28} \text{ drop} = 1 \text{ min}$$

Calculate how many minutes it will take to infuse the total number of drops:

$$20,000 \text{ drops} = \frac{1 \times 20,000}{28} = 714 \text{ min}$$

Convert minutes to hours by dividing by 60:

$$714 \text{ min} = \frac{714}{60} = 11.9 \text{ hours}$$

11.9 hours = 11 hours 54 min (approximately 12 hours)

Answer: 1 litre of sodium chloride at a rate of 28 drops/min will take approximately 12 hours to run.

Using the formula:

$$\text{number of hours the infusion is to run} = \frac{\text{volume of the infusion}}{\text{rate (drops/min)} \times 60} \times \text{drip rate of giving set}$$

where:

volume of the infusion = 1,000 mL
rate (drops/min) = 28 drops/min
drip rate of giving set = 20 drops/mL

Substitute the numbers in the formula:

$$\frac{1,000 \times 20}{28 \times 60} = 11.9 \text{ hours}$$

11.9 hours = 11 hours 54 min (approximately 12 hours)

Answer: 1 litre of sodium chloride at a rate of 28 drops/min will take approximately 12 hours to run.

Question 25 238 minutes (3 hours, 58 minutes), approximately 4 hours.

Question 26 357 minutes (5 hours, 57 minutes), approximately 6 hours.

Question 27 You know the infusion has been running from 8 am until 3 pm, i.e. for 7 hours. Next, calculate the volume given by multiplying the rate by the time over which the infusion has been running:

rate = 2 mL/hour, therefore volume given = 2 × 7 = 14 mL

Next, calculate the dose given for the volume given. You have 25,000 units in 50 mL. Therefore (using the one unit rule):

$$\frac{1}{50} \text{ mL} = 25,000$$

Thus:

$$14 \text{ mL} = \frac{25,000 \times 14}{50} = 7,000 \text{ units}$$

Answer: The patient has received 7,000 units of heparin.

KEY POINTS

Giving sets

- The standard giving set (SGS) has a drip rate of 20 drops/mL for clear fluids (e.g. sodium chloride or glucose) and 15 drops/mL for blood.
- The micro-drop giving set or burette has a drip rate of 60 drops/mL.

Drip rate calculations (drops/min)

- In all drip rate calculations, you have to remember that you are simply converting a volume to drops (or vice versa) and hours to minutes.

$$\text{drops/min} = \frac{\text{drops/mL of the giving set} \times \text{volume of the infusion (mL)}}{\text{number of hours the infusion is to run} \times 60}$$

Converting dosages to mL/hour

- If the dose is in milligrams, then the total amount of drug must be in milligrams.
- If the dose is in micrograms, then the total amount of drug must be in micrograms.
- In this type of calculation, it is best to convert the dose required to a volume in millilitres.
- Doses expressed on a weight basis, i.e. dose/weight per minute:

$$\text{mL/hour} = \frac{\text{total volume to be infused}}{\text{total amount of drug}} \times \text{dose} \times \text{weight} \times 60$$

- Doses expressed as a total dose, i.e. dose/min:

$$\text{mL/hour} = \frac{\text{total volume to be infused}}{\text{total amount of drug}} \times \text{dose} \times 60$$

Converting mL/hour to dosages

- Sometimes it may be necessary to convert mL/hour back to the dose: mg/min or micrograms/min and mg/kg/min or micrograms/kg/min.
- If the dose is in milligrams, then the total amount of drug must be in milligrams.
- If the dose is in micrograms, then the total amount of drug must be in micrograms.
- Doses expressed on a weight basis, i.e. dose/weight per minute:

mg or micrograms/kg/min =

$$\frac{\text{rate (mL/hour)} \times \text{amount of drug (mg or micrograms)}}{60 \times \text{weight (kg)} \times \text{volume (mL)}}$$

- Doses expressed as a total dose, i.e. dose/min

  mg or micrograms/min =

  $$\frac{\text{rate (mL/hour)} \times \text{amount of drug (mg or micrograms)}}{60 \times \text{volume (mL)}}$$

Calculating the length of time for iv infusions

- Sometimes it may be necessary to calculate the number of hours an infusion should run at a specified rate. Also, it is a good way of checking your calculated drip rate for an infusion.

Manually controlled infusions

$$\text{number of hours the infusion is to run} = \frac{\text{volume of the infusion}}{\text{rate (drops/min)} \times 60} \times \text{drip rate of giving set}$$

Infusion or syringe pumps

$$\text{number of hours the infusion is to run} = \frac{\text{volume of the infusion}}{\text{rate (mL/hour)}}$$

Infusion devices   8

OBJECTIVES

At the end of this chapter you should be familiar with the following:
- Infusion pumps
- Classification of infusion devices
- Syringe drivers

INFUSION PUMPS

In general, infusion pumps are capable of accurate delivery of solution over a wide range of volumes and flow rates, and may be designed for specialist application, e.g. for neonatal use.

Two main types of infusion pumps are available: gravity controllers, including drip-rate and volumetric controllers; and pumped systems, which include drip-rate pumps, volumetric pumps, syringe pumps and pumps for ambulatory use.

GRAVITY CONTROLLERS

There are two types: drip-rate and volumetric controllers. Both types of device rely on gravity to provide flow, and both detect and count the drops falling through a drop chamber. They have limited accuracy and use, and are only really suitable for low-risk infusions.

PUMPED SYSTEMS

Syringe pumps

These are low volume, high accuracy devices designed to infuse at low flow rates and are typically calibrated for delivery in millilitres per hour, typically 0.1 to 99 ml/hour. Many pumps will accept different sizes and different brands of syringe, but the pumps must be set up for the particular type and size of syringe. Care must be taken when setting up to ensure that the pump operates safely.

Volumetric pumps

These are the preferred pumps for medium and large flow rate and large volume infusions; although some are designed specially to operate at low flow rates for neonatal use. All are mains/battery powered, with rate being selected in millilitres per hour (mL/hour).

Volumetric pumps usually incorporate a wide range of features, required for neonatal and high-risk infusions, including an air-in-line detector and comprehensive alarm systems.

Typically, most volumetric pumps will perform satisfactorily at rates down to 5 mL/hour. If you wish to infuse at lower rates, you should check the suitability of the pump with manufacturer's literature.

All volumetric pumps are designed to use a specific giving set. Using any set other than the correct one will result in reduced accuracy and poor alarm responses.

Drip-rate pumps

The flow rate is selected in drops per minute. A drop sensor attached to the drip chamber counts drops, and the pump then infuses the set drip rate into the patient.

Controls are few and simple, with only rudimentary alarms to warn of any deviation from the set rate. Air-in-line detection and occlusion response is poor, with high pressures being reached. These pressures are so high that in practice the alarm would probably never activate during an infusion, or during extravasation.

As a result, the UK Department of Health Medicines Device Agency (MDA) **does not recommend** this type of pump. No manufacturer currently offers them for sale in the UK, but they are still in use in hospitals.

Patient-controlled analgesia (PCA)

Most of the pumps used for PCA are designed specifically for this application and are mains/battery operated. They are typically syringe pumps, as the total volume of drug to be infused can usually be conveniently contained in a single-use syringe. Some PCA pumps are based on volumetric designs. The difference between a PCA pump and a normal syringe pump is the provision of a facility to enable patients to deliver a bolus dose themselves. Clinical staff may programme a PCA pump to deliver a pre-set bolus on demand, with a pre-set lockout time between boluses. In addition to the bolus delivered on patient demand, PCA pumps may also be programmed to deliver a basal rate (continuous low rate) infusion.

Once it is programmed, access to control of the pump is usually only permitted by a key or software code, but in some cases limited patient access is allowed in order to change some parameters.

A feature of most PCA pumps is a memory log, which can be either accessed through the display, or downloaded via a printer or computer. This enables the clinician to determine when, and how often, the patient has made a demand and what total volume of drug has been infused over a given time.

Anaesthesia pumps

These are syringe pumps designed for use in anaesthesia or sedation and must be used only for this purpose. They should be clearly labelled ' For anaesthesia only' and should be restricted to operating and high-dependency areas.

These specialized pumps are designed to have features that allow greater ease in changing rates and doses during an infusion. They usually allow high rates in order to deliver large bolus doses (as for induction). Other sophistications may be built in, such as automatic dose and time-profiling linked to particular drugs.

Pumps for ambulatory use

These are designed as small (pocket or pouch sized) battery-powered devices, which are intended to be worn by the user. Because of the size of the devices, the available battery capacity is low and continuous pumping is not feasible. Most ambulatory pumps, therefore, give an output in the form of a small bolus delivered every few minutes. Two types are available:

- Syringe drivers (see later).
- Miniature volumetric pumps. These use removable reservoirs that contain the solution within the pump. Some may offer a large variety of programming options. Those pumps having bolus on demand, as well as basal rate, are also suitable for PCA applications.

CLASSIFICATION OF INFUSION DEVICES

All pumps are now classified according to their performance. Pumps may be labelled as:

Suitable only for low risk infusions
Suitable only for high risk and low risk infusions
Suitable only for neonatal, high risk and low risk infusions
PCA infusion device
For anaesthesia only

- Administration is considered safe provided a high-risk drug is administered using a high-performance pump.

- An infusion is potentially unsafe when a high-risk drug is administered with a lower performance pump.
- All infusions to neonates require a neonatal pump.

Most modern pumps are now programmable: you must ensure that the pump is configured or programmed properly before use.

The following case report illustrates that care must be taken when setting up infusion pumps.

DRUG ADMINISTRATION RATE ERRORS: INCORRECT HEPARIN INFUSION RATE

Case report

A patient was prescribed 25,000 units of intravenous (IV) heparin over 12 hours. The dose was administered over 2 hours instead of 12 hours. (There appeared to have been a fault setting the correct rate of administration.) The patient's heparin therapy was discontinued until his KCCT results returned to the accepted levels.

Comment

Errors involving the incorrect setting of IV pumps are among the most common errors reported. These errors involve volumetric infusion pumps as well as syringe driver and patient controlled analgesic pumps. Due to the wide variety of uses for these devices, errors in setting the correct drug administration rates may involve narcotic analgesics, insulin, heparin, cardiovascular drugs and cancer chemotherapy agents. Although a fault with the equipment is frequently cited, testing the pumps after an error has occurred rarely shows that they are in fact faulty. In the vast majority of cases the fault is due to operator error.

There are many manufacturers of IV infusion pumps and there is a wide variety of models available. It is essential that a regular programme of in-service training sessions are conducted for all staff (including medical staff) using this type of equipment. These sessions should be run by hospital staff: it is inappropriate that infusion pump manufacturers provide the only form of in-service education on their equipment (usually when new equipment is purchased).

In-service training sessions should review all the various types of pumps in the hospital, their indication for use and operation, as well as common problems encountered. Staff should be updated every three years on topics relating to IV infusion pumps. Pharmacists (particularly those working in aseptic dispensing units) should have a thorough knowledge of the types and operation of IV pumps available in their hospital. They should be able to advise and help ward staff use this type of equipment.

A planned preventative maintenance policy on all IV pumps should also be operated in all hospitals to ensure that the small percentage of errors attributed to equipment failure is reduced.

As a multidisciplinary committee the Drugs & Therapeutics Committee should take responsibility for drug administration equipment as well as drug selection. Written policies should be available to guide practitioners as to which drugs require an infusion pump of a particular type. Particular attention should be given to the use of the appropriate IV administration set for the individual drug and IV pump.

Taken from *Pharmacy in Practice* 1993; 3: 467

SYRINGE DRIVERS

These pumps are designed to deliver drugs accurately over a certain period of time (usually 24 hours). They have the advantage of being small and compact, so they can easily be carried by the patient, and avoid the need for numerous injections throughout the day. These pumps are useful for potent drugs or small doses of drugs that have to be administered accurately, such as opiates, insulin, chemotherapy, hormones and anti-emetics.

They can typically accept syringes between 2 and 10 mL and are able to achieve very low rates of delivery. Rate is set in terms of millimetres per hour or millimetres per day, that is, linear travel of syringe plunger against time. Calculations that depend on the syringe used may be required to convert from flow rate to linear travel per unit time.

Various devices suitable for continuous subcutaneous infusion are available. It is not possible to give details of them all here. Most are battery operated but they may differ in their method of operation, particularly for setting the delivery rate.

The Graseby syringe drivers type MS16A (blue panel) and type MS26 (green panel), are described here because they are widely used. This does not imply that these two models are any better than the others. It should be noted that syringe drivers are undergoing continual development and improvement.

There are two types of Graseby syringe drivers:

- MS16A (blue panel): designed to deliver drugs at an hourly rate.
- MS26 (green panel): designed to deliver drugs at a daily rate (i.e. over 24 hours).

To avoid confusion between the two pumps, the MS16A is clearly marked with '1HR' (highlighted in pink) in the bottom right-hand corner; the MS26 has '24HR' (highlighted in orange/brown) instead.

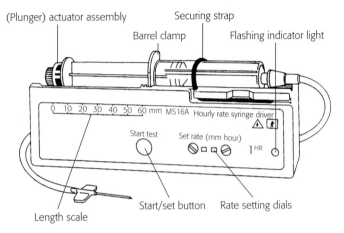

Fig. 8.1 Graseby Medical MS16A hourly rate syringe driver. From: *The Royal Marsden Hospital Manual of Clinical Nursing Procedures*, 5th edition, 2000, Oxford, Blackwell Science.

CALCULATING THE DOSE

The amount required is the total dose to be given over 24 hours.

- If the dose is prescribed in mg/hour, then you have to calculate the total amount for 24 hours by multiplying by 24. For example, if the dose is 3 mg/hour, then:

  total amount required for 24 hours = 3 × 24 = 72 mg

- If the dose is prescribed every 4 hours (or whatever), multiply the dose by the number of times the dose is given in 24 hours. For example, if the dose is 20 mg every 4 hours the dose is being given 6 times in 24 hours (divide 24 by the dosing frequency, i.e. 24 divided by 4 = 6). So:

  total amount required for 24 hours = 20 × 6 = 120 mg

- If the dose is prescribed as mg/day (24 hours), then no calculation is necessary, i.e. if the dose is 60 mg/day (24 hours), then:

  total amount required for 24 hours = 60 mg

SETTING THE RATE

The syringe fluid length (L) is defined as the length from the bottom of the plunger to the end of the syringe. Always set up a syringe driver to make L about 50 mm with diluent before priming the infusion set. Priming will take about 2 mm of this total, leaving 48 mm of fluid to be transfused over 24 hours. This makes the arithmetic of setting easier. When infusions do not require a priming volume, L should be set at 48 mm. The volume varies from one brand of syringe to another, but the dose and the distance L are the important factors, not the volume.

MAKE SURE THAT THE INFUSION DEVICE IS SET UP PROPERLY.

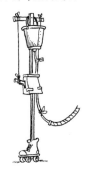

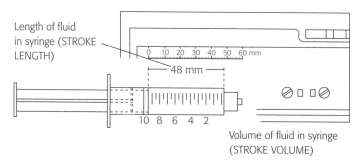

Length of fluid in syringe (STROKE LENGTH)

48 mm

Volume of fluid in syringe (STROKE VOLUME)

Fig. 8.2 Measurement of fluid length in syringe against millimetre scale on the syringe driver

- Graseby MS16A (blue panel): mm/hour

$$\text{rate} = \frac{\text{distance } L \text{ in mm (48)}}{\text{infusion time in hours}} = 2 \text{ mm/hour}$$

So the dial should read:

02 mm/hour

- Graseby MS26 (green panel): mm/24 hours

$$\text{rate} = \frac{\text{distance } L \text{ in mm (48)}}{\text{infusion time in days (1)}} = 48 \text{ mm/24 hours}$$

So the dial should read:

48 mm/24 hours

The following case report illustrates that care must be taken when setting up syringe drivers.

ANOTHER FATAL ERROR WITH A SYRINGE DRIVER

Case report

An 84-year-old man died after receiving his 24-hour dose of diamorphine in 3 hours after two experienced nurses incorrectly set the administration rate on a Graseby infusion pump.

The error involved a brand new Graseby MS16A pump and occurred in June 1995 well after the publication of Hazard Warnings from the Department of Health and new pump labels had been issued by Graseby Medical in August 1994. The prescription required the pump to be set to give 15 mg of diamorphine over 24 hours via the subcutaneous route. With a standard 10 ml syringe filled to 8 ml this represented 48 mm in 24 hours or 2 mm per hour. The pump was subsequently set up at 20 mm per hour (both nurses assumed that a setting of 20 on the pump represented 2 mm). As a result of this error the total dose was administered in 2.4 hours instead of 24 hours. The syringe was started at 3 pm and the error was found at 6 pm. The ward staff administered three bolus doses of naloxone, but the patient only made a partial recovery and died some time later in his sleep.

The coroner's verdict was that the patient died from natural causes since his primary diagnosis was cancer of the liver and pancreas with widespread metastases and this lead to an obstruction of the pulmonary artery. Both nurses were suspended but later reinstated and reprimanded. They were subsequently retrained and a new procedure for syringe drivers was implemented in the hospital. The wards are now required to keep a record of all syringe drivers in use and the setting up of all syringe drivers is checked and signed by trained ward staff.

Comment

We regret to have to report yet another incident with a Graseby syringe driver. We refer readers to the requirement from the Department of Health for hospitals to introduce new policies and procedures to control the use of infusion devices. One of the requirements is for hospital managers to ensure that an effective training and assessment programme for users of infusion equipment is in place. However, we also recommended the withdrawal from sale and use of MS16A pumps. We are firmly of the opinion that mm per hour is a very confusing concept for many general ward staff and this unit of measurement should be replaced by ml per hour. We hope that this further report will make Graseby Medical review their marketing strategy of these pumps.

Taken from *Pharmacy in Practice* 1996; 6: 21

KEY POINTS

Using infusion devices

- Use the most appropriate device for the job required.
- Ensure that you know how to use the device – refer to the manual if necessary.
- Most modern pumps are now programmable, so you must ensure that the pump is configured or programmed properly before using it.

Classification of infusion devices

All pumps are now classified according to their performance. Pumps may be labelled as:

- Suitable only for low-risk infusions.
- Suitable only for high-risk and low-risk infusions.
- Suitable only for neonatal, high-risk and low-risk infusions.
- PCA infusion device.
- For anaesthesia only.

Administration is considered safe provided a high-risk drug is administered using a high-performance pump; an infusion is potentially unsafe when a high-risk drug is administered with a lower performance pump. All infusions to neonates require a neonatal pump.

Graseby syringe drivers

There are two types of Graseby syringe drivers:

- MS16A (blue panel): designed to deliver drugs at an hourly rate.
- MS26 (green panel): designed to deliver drugs at a daily rate (i.e. over 24 hours).

To avoid confusion between the two pumps, the MS16A is clearly marked with '1HR' (highlighted in pink) in the bottom right-hand corner; the MS26 has '24HR' (highlighted in orange/brown) instead.

Setting the rate

- Graseby MS16A (blue panel) – mm/hour:

$$\text{set rate} = \frac{\text{distance } L \text{ in mm (48)}}{\text{infusion time in hours}} = 2 \text{ mm/hour}$$

So the dial should read:

02 mm/hour

- Graseby MS26 (green panel) – mm/24 hours:

$$\text{set rate} = \frac{\text{distance } L \text{ in mm (48)}}{\text{infusion time in days (1)}} = 48 \text{ mm/24 hours}$$

So the dial should read:

48 mm/24 hours

Calculation of dose

The amount required is the total dose to be given over 24 hours.

- If the dose is prescribed as mg/hour, multiply by 24 to calculate the total amount for 24 hours. For example, if the dose is 3 mg/hour, then:

total amount required for 24 hours = $3 \times 24 = 72$ mg

- If the dose is prescribed every 4 hours (or whatever), multiply the dose by the number of times the dose is given in 24 hours. For example, if the dose is 20 mg every 4 hours, divide 24 by the dosing frequency, i.e. $\frac{24}{4} = 6$, so:

total amount required for 24 hours = $20 \times 6 = 120$ mg

- If the dose is prescribed as mg/day (24 hours), then no calculation is necessary.

Paediatric dosage calculations

9

OBJECTIVES

At the end of this chapter, you should be familiar with the following:

- Drug use in paediatrics
- Dosing in paediatrics
- Calculating dosages
- Useful approximate values
- Displacement values or volumes
- Administration routes for drugs
- Useful reference books

Children, and particularly neonates, differ in their response to drugs, i.e. absorption, distribution, metabolism of a drug, and its effects and duration of action. When it comes to prescribing and administering medicines, children shouldn't be considered as small adults and care must be taken in calculating doses.

DRUG USE IN PAEDIATRICS

Many drugs used in paediatric practice have not been studied adequately or at all in children, so prescribing for children may not always be easy.

Children should not be considered as scaled-down adults as the difference in dose is not purely dependent upon body mass. Age-related differences in drug handling (pharmacokinetics) and drug sensitivity (pharmacodynamics) occur throughout childhood and account for many of the differences between drug doses at various stages of childhood.

ABSORPTION OF DRUGS

The absorption of drugs in the early days after birth differs to that found later in the neonatal period. This is because factors that affect absorption – stomach acid, bile from the liver and pancreatic enzymes

– are all significantly reduced, but increase during the neonatal period. This can affect how drugs are absorbed – some will have increased absorption and some reduced, depending upon the nature of the drug.

DISTRIBUTION OF DRUGS

During infancy, the percentage of body weight that is water is significantly higher than in older children or adults. As a result, water-soluble drugs are diluted to a greater extent in neonates and larger doses may be required to produce the required plasma concentration.

METABOLISM OF DRUGS

Drugs are usually metabolized or chemically changed by the liver: this is known as **hepatic clearance**. There is a great degree of inter-individual variation in both adults and children.

The rate of hepatic clearance depends on a combination of the maturity of the hepatic enzyme systems and the size of the liver relative to body weight. Generally, as a result of metabolic immaturity, hepatically cleared drugs will be cleared more slowly in neonates and therapy needs to be closely monitored.

In children, the liver is up to 50% greater as a percentage of total body weight than in adults. Once the hepatic pathways are mature, an increased metabolic rate may be seen and higher doses required.

EXCRETION OF DRUGS

The kidneys are relatively immature at birth. Neonates and infants therefore have a reduced ability to eliminate drugs renally and need dose reductions.

DOSING IN PAEDIATRICS

Children's doses have been calculated from adult doses and formulas have been devised (e.g. Clark's rule and Young's rule), but are not accurate for all children as they assume that the child is a miniature adult. As mentioned earlier, many factors affect the way in which drugs act in children, so doses based on adult doses may not be accurate.

So doses related to age are not ideal; doses calculated on a weight or surface area basis are more accurate, as they allow for greater individualization.

However, as clinical knowledge and experience has increased, specialist paediatric books have become available that give accurate doses on a 'dose per weight' basis (e.g. mg/kg) and these sources should be consulted first (a list appears at the end of this chapter).

PROBLEMS ASSOCIATED WITH PAEDIATRIC DOSING

As well as changes in how the body handles drugs, doses may have to be adjusted for the following: fever, oedema, dehydration and gastrointestinal disease. In these cases, the doctor should decide whether a dose needs to be adjusted.

Sometimes it will be difficult to give the dose required because there is no appropriate formulation: for example, giving 33 mg when only a 100 mg tablet is available. In these instances, the pharmacy department should be contacted to see if a liquid preparation is available or can be prepared. If not, the doctor should be informed so that the dose can be modified, or another drug can be prescribed, or another route can be used.

CALCULATING DOSAGES

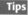 • When doing any calculation, you must make sure that the decimal point is in the right place. A change to the left or right could mean a 10-fold change in the dose, which could be fatal in some cases.
• It is best to work in the smaller units, i.e. 100 micrograms as opposed to 0.1 milligrams. But even so, care must be taken with the number of zeros; a wrong dose can be fatal.
• When calculating any dose, always get your answer checked.

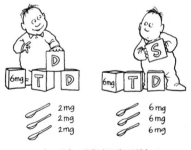

6mg T.D.D. = TOTAL DAILY DOSE OF 6mg
6mg T.D.S. = 6mg 'TER DIE SUMENDUS'
= 6mg THREE TIMES A DAY.

USING BODY WEIGHT

This is the most common method for calculating paediatric dosages.

If you look up doses in paediatric books, it is important to read them correctly. They can either be written as:

- A single dose – to be given as many times as specified.
- Total daily dose (TDD) – to be divided by the number of times the drug is to be given.

For example, ibuprofen can be written as:

5 mg/kg, 3–4 times a day

or as:

20 mg/kg daily (20 mg/kg TDD).

Care must be taken when reading doses.

> **Tip** It's important not to mistake the TDD for a single dose.

WORKED EXAMPLE

A 3-year-old child weighing 13.5 kg has been prescribed ibuprofen at a dose of 5 mg/kg three times a day. Ibuprofen is available as a suspension, 100 mg in 5 mL. How much do you give?

Step 1

To find the dose required, you simply multiply the dose by the weight:

$5 \times 13.5 = 67.5$ mg

Step 2

Next, you now need to calculate how much of the suspension you need for your dose of 67.5 mg.

You have:

100 mg in 5 mL

Therefore (using the one unit rule) :

1 mg in $\dfrac{5}{100}$ mL

But you need 67.5 mg, so:

67.5 mg $= \dfrac{5}{100} \times 67.5 = 3.375$ mL

Therefore you need to give 3.4 mL of the ibuprofen suspension (100 mg in 5 mL) three times a day.

For a more detailed explanation of this method of calculation, see Chapter 3, 'Dosage calculations'.

Obese children

The actual body weight is used in this method of calculation. However, in the case of obese children, the child may receive an artificially high dose because fat tissue plays virtually no part in metabolism. The dose must be estimated on lean or ideal body weight. So, as a rule of thumb, the dose should be reduced by approximately 25% for obese children.

USING BODY SURFACE AREA ESTIMATES

It is more accurate to use body surface area estimates than body weight, since many physical phenomena are more closely related to body surface area.

The dose required is calculated in the same way, but substituting surface area for weight. In this case, the surface area needs to be worked out by use of a formula or a nomogram (see Appendix 3).

The following case reports illustrate that care must be taken with paediatric dosing calculations.

STOP PAEDIATRIC DOSING ERRORS

Case report 1

A 6-week-old baby boy was admitted to hospital for a hernia repair. In the recovery room, a nurse misread a prescription and this resulted in the baby having 4 mg of morphine administered instead of 0.4 mg.

The patient's mother noticed him going blue after his return to the ward. The baby went on to have fits and stopped breathing. He was successfully resuscitated and transferred to the intensive care unit. He was kept in the intensive care unit overnight before going home a few days later.

Case report 2

A 5-year-old boy being treated for lymphoblastic leukaemia was given 4.8 mL of asparaginase instead of the prescribed 0.48 mL by a senior nurse.

A day after the treatment was administered, the patient's father was telephoned by hospital medical staff who told him that his son must be taken immediately from his school to the hospital isolation ward for tests. The boy was tested and monitored for several days and did not exhibit any symptoms as a result of the overdose.

Case report 3

A 4-month-old boy was given morphine overdoses on three separate occasions.

The baby boy had been treated in a hospital special care unit since being born 3 months premature weighing 1 lb 6 oz (624 g). The baby had been receiving regular intravenous doses of morphine, as his mother was a registered heroin addict when she gave birth. The baby was given 10 times the correct dose of morphine on three separate occasions as the nurse administering the injection had misread the decimal point on the prescription. The boy subsequently died. At the inquest the pathologist said that the three morphine overdoses had played no part in the baby's death; the death was attributed to complications arising from the premature birth.

Comments

The cases are concerned with morphine, calculations or decimal points. Intravenous morphine is increasingly used in paediatrics and neonatology as we recognize that babies and children, like adults, feel pain although they may express it in different ways. They deserve similar, powerful and effective medication. Unfortunately, the number of well publicized errors seems also to be increasing.

Morphine may be given by intravenous bolus injection although continuous infusion or PCA is preferred. Calculating the dose to prescribe may prove difficult since doses in microgram/kg will vary with the child's age, must be multiplied by body weight, probably be converted to milligrams and possibly to a concentration to provide a suitably small infusion rate from a syringe pump. We soon see why prescribers can miscalculate – pharmacists do not find it easy!

The nurse, too, may have problems interpreting prescriptions for decimal fractions without a leading zero (for example, .1 rather than 0.1) or when a trailing zero is placed after a whole number (for example, 1.0 rather than 1). Misinterpretation of either may lead to a 10 times overdose. The message is simple (and printed on the back cover of most US paediatric formularies) – always use a leading zero, never use a trailing zero! But we teach that decimal fractions should not be used in prescribing to avoid any confusion with the decimal point – use smaller units instead (for example, 500 micrograms and not 0.5 mg). This, though, may also be a source of error if the prescriber is using one set of units but the medicine is labelled in another. The nurse forced to convert from microgram to milligram may make a 10 fold (or greater) error. And what about using calculators? All too often the answer is a factor of 10 out because the wrong number of zeros had been keyed in and the answer not inspected to check that it is 'in the right ball park'. Simple arithmetic you may say – we all teach our children the pitfalls with calculators, but in hospitals it happens every day.

Now, having made a 10-fold error, are the same mechanisms in place in paediatrics and neonatology to reduce the consequences of the error? Of course not. Children are too frequently therapeutic orphans using unlicensed or off-label medicines formulated for adults. Thus, if only 10 mg ampoules of morphine are stocked on the neonatal unit a 100-fold intravenous bolus overdose can be given to a 2 kg neonate from just one ampoule. Such an error is less likely to happen in adult practice because the large number of ampoules required to give the overdose provides a warning that something is wrong. Smaller 'special' ampoules of morphine are available for neonatal and paediatric use but larger ampoules will be more convenient when preparing 24 hour infusions, even for children – a dilemma.

Some units have prepared detailed weight/ dosage /volume charts to reduce the need for calculation or have provided step-by-step worksheets to help with arithmetic.

Having neonatal or paediatric size preparations is important for drugs like morphine, digoxin, aminophylline and aminoglycosides. Programmable syringe infusion pumps may allow the drug concentration, dose and weight to be keyed in and will then function as a calculator and set infusion rate. Limits can be set to reduce the risk of error and the central intravenous additive service may be able to provide infusions of standard concentration. These sophisticated syringe pumps should be programmed by the pharmacist and carefully checked!

Our medicines protocols may also require attention. Is there always a second, thorough check before administration and is it part of the nurse's responsibility to be aware of safe paediatric doses? Are doctors submitting to the same checking procedures as nurses? If not, they should be. None of us is infallible, especially when tired and stressed.

Neonatology, paediatric intensive care and paediatric oncology are high risk areas for medication error as is the child in a ward with staff not used to dealing with children. Pharmacy resources should be directed at them and, whenever possible, the complexity should be removed from the ward to the pharmacy. For most of us resources do not permit this 'counsel of excellence' but we can be proactive in assessing medicines for their potential to be involved in errors and examine the special processes of prescribing, dispensing and drug administration in paediatrics with a view to reducing their potential for error.

Taken from *Pharmacy in Practice* 1997; 7: 220–221

USEFUL APPROXIMATE VALUES

Table 11 gives average values for various parameters. This method of calculating doses should only be used if a specific dose cannot be found, since it assumes the child is 'average'.

Table 11 Approximate values

Age	Weight kg	Weight lb	Height cm	Height inch	Surface area m²	% of adult dose
Newborn	3.4	7.5	50	20	0.23	12.5
1 month	4.2	9	55	22	0.26	14.5
2 months	4.4	10	51	21	0.28	15
3 months	5.6	12	59	23	0.32	18
4 months	6.5	14	62	24	0.36	20
6 months	7.7	17	67	26	0.4	22
8 months	8.5	19	72	28	0.44	25
1 year	10	22	76	30	0.47	28
18 months	11	24	90	35	0.53	30
3 years	14	31	94	37	0.62	33
5 years	18	40	108	42	0.73	40
7 years	23	51	120	47	0.88	50
10 years	30	66	142	56	1.09	60
12 years	37	81	145	58	1.25	75
14 years	45	110	150	59	1.38	80
16 years	58	128	168	67	1.65	90
Adult						
Male	68	150	173	68	1.8	
Female	56	123	163	64	1.6	

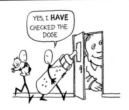

DISPLACEMENT VALUES OR VOLUMES

WHAT IS DISPLACEMENT?

If you take ordinary salt and dissolve it in some water, the resultant solution will have a greater volume than before. The salt appears to 'displace' some water, increasing the volume. This phenomenon is called displacement.

Antibiotic suspensions are good examples to illustrate displacement. For example, to make up 100 mL of amoxicillin suspension, only 68 mL of water needs to be added. The amoxicillin powder must therefore displace 32 mL of water, i.e. $100 - 68 = 32$ mL.

THE IMPORTANCE OF DISPLACEMENT

This phenomenon of displacement can be important in medicine and displacement values or volumes are usually given to freeze-dried injections, particularly antibiotics, which need to be reconstituted before administration.

Displacement volumes vary from drug to drug and may be so small that the increased volume is not considered in calculating doses. However, the total volume may be increased significantly and if this is not taken into account, significant errors in dosage may occur, especially when small doses are involved as with neonates.

For example, suppose cefotaxime is required at a dose of 50 mg/kg, 12 hourly for a baby weighing 3.6 kg. The dose required is $50 \times 3.6 = 180$ mg. The displacement volume for cefotaxime is 0.2 mL for a 500 mg vial, so you need to add 1.8 mL water for injection to give 500 mg in 2 mL. Thus:

$$180 \text{ mg} = \frac{2}{500} \times 180 = 0.72 \text{ mL}$$

If the displacement volume is not taken into account, then you will have:

500 mg in 2.2 mL (2 mL + 0.2 mL displacement volume)

You worked out earlier that that the dose required is 180 mg and this is equivalent to 0.72 mL (assuming you have 500 mg in 2 mL). But actually 0.72 mL equals:

$$\frac{500}{2.2} \times 0.72 = 164 \text{ mg}$$

because the actual volume you have is 2.2 mL, not 2 mL. Thus if the displacement volume is not taken into account, the amount of cefotaxime drawn up is 164 mg and not 180 mg as expected.

Displacement volumes are usually stated in the relevant drug information sheets, or in paediatric dosage books. Tables 12a and b list displacement volumes for some commonly used drugs.

Table 12a Displacement volumes: antibiotics

Drug brand manufacturer	Vial size	Displacement volume†	Diluent volume†	Final volume	Concentration (mg/mL)
Aciclovir					
Zovirax®	250 mg	Negligible	10 mL	10 mL*	25 mg/mL
Glaxo Wellcome	500 mg		20 mL	20 mL*	25 mg/mL
Amoxicillin	250 mg	0.2 mL	4.8 mL	5 mL	50 mg/mL
Amoxil®	500 mg	0.4 mL	9.6 mL	10 mL	50 mg/mL
SKB	1 g	0.8 mL	19.2 mL	20 mL	50 mg/mL
Amphotericin					
Fungizone®	50 mg	Negligible	10 mL	10 mL*	5 mg/mL
Squibb					
Ampicillin					
Penbritin®	500 mg	0.4 mL	9.6 mL	10 mL	50 mg/mL
SKB					
Aztreonam	500 mg	0.3 mL	3.7 mL	5 mL	100 mg/mL
Azactam®	1 g	0.7 mL	9.3 mL	10 mL	100 mg.mL
Squibb	2 g	1.3 mL	8.7 mL	10 mL	200 mg/mL
Benzylpenicillin					
Crystapen®	600 mg	0.4 mL	4.6 mL	5 mL	120 mg/mL
Britannia	1.2 g	0.8 mL	9.2 mL	10 mL	120 mg/mL
Cefamandole					
Kefadol®	1 g	0.7 mL	9.3 mL	10 mL	100 mg/mL
Dista					
Cefazolin					
Kefzol®	500 mg	0.2 mL	1.8 mL	2 mL	250 mg/mL
Lilly	1 g	0.5 mL	2 mL	2.5 mL	400 mg/mL
Cefitoxin					
Mefoxin®	1 g	0.5 mL	9.5 mL	10 mL	100 mg/mL
MSD	2 g	1 mL	19 mL	20 mL	50 mg/mL
Cefotaxime	500 mg	0.2 mL	1.8 mL	2 mL	250 mg/mL
Claforan®	1 g	0.5 mL	3.5 mL	4 mL	250 mg/mL
HMR	2 g	1 mL	9 mL	10 mL	200 mg/mL
Cefradine					
Velosef®	500 mg	0.4 mL	4.6 mL	5 mL	100 mg/mL
Squibb	1 g	0.8 mL	9.2 mL	10 mL	100 mg/mL
Ceftazadime	250 mg	0.2 mL	2.3 mL	2.5 mL	100 mg/mL
Fortum®	500 mg	0.5 mL	4.5 mL	5 mL	100 mg/mL
Glaxo Wellcome	1 g	0.9 mL	9.1 mL	10 mL	100 mg/mL
	2 g	1.8 mL	8.2 mL	10 mL	200 mg/mL
Ceftazadime	500 g	0.4 mL	4.6 mL	5 mL	100 mg/mL
Kefadim®	1 g	0.8 mL	9.2 mL	10 mL	100 mg/mL
Lilly	2 g	1.7 mL	8.3 mL	10 mL	200 mg/mL
Ceftriaxone	250 mg	0.2 mL	4.8 mL	5 mL	50 mg/mL
Rochephin®	1 g	0.8 mL	9.2 mL	10 mL	100 mg/mL
Roche	2 g	1.6 mL	38.4 mL	40 mL	50 mg/mL
Cefuroxime	250 mg	0.2 mL	1.8 mL	2 mL	125 mg/mL
Zinacef®	750 mg	0.5 mL	5.5 mL	6 mL	125 mg/mL
Glaxo Wellcome	1.5 g	1 mL	14 mL	15 mL	100 mg/mL

Table 12a continued

Drug brand manufacturer	Vial size	Displacement volume†	Diluent volume†	Final volume	Concentration (mg/mL)
Chloramphenicol Kemicetine® Pharmacia	1 g	0.8 mL	9.2 mL	10 mL	100 mg/mL
Clarithromycin Klaricid® Abbott	500 mg	Allowed for	10 mL	10 mL*	50 mg/mL
Co-amoxiclav Augmentin® SKB	600 mg 1.2 g	0.5 mL 0.9 mL	9.5 mL 19.1 mL	10 mL 20 mL*	60 mg/mL 60 mg/mL
Co-fluampicil Magnapen® CP Pharmaceuticals	500 mg	0.4 mL	9.6 mL	10 mL	50 mg/mL
Erythromycin Erythrocin® Abbott	1 g	Allowed for	20 mL	20 mL*	50 mg/mL
Flucloxacillin Floxapen® SKB	250 mg 500 mg 1 g	0.2 mL 0.4 mL 0.7 mL	4.8 mL 9.6 mL 19.3 mL	5 mL 10 mL 20 mL	50 mg/mL 50 mg/mL 50 mg/mL
Imipenem Primaxin® MSD	500 mg	Negligible	100 mL	100 mL	5 mg.mL
Meropenem Meropen® AstraZeneca	500 mg 1 g	0.5 mL 0.9 mL	9.5 mL 19.1 mL	10 mL 20 mL	50 mg/mL 50 mg/mL
Piperacillin** Pipril® Lederle	1 g 2 g	0.7 mL 1.5 mL	4.3 mL 8.5 mL	5 mL 10 mL	200 mg/mL 200 mg/mL
Piperacillin + Tazo-bactam Tazocin® Lederle	2.25 g 4.5 g	1.6 mL 3.2 mL	8.4 mL 16.8 mL	10 mL 20 mL	225 mg/mL 225 mg/mL
Sodium fusidate Fucidin® Leo	500 mg	Negligible	10 mL	10 mL*	50 mg/mL
Teicoplanin Targocid® Aventis Pharma	200 mg 400 mg	Allowed for	3 mL 3 mL	Not known	67 mg/mL 133 mg/mL
Ticarcillin Timentin® SKB	1.6 g 3.2 g	1.1 mL 2.2 mL	3.9 mL 7.8 mL	5 mL* 10 mL*	320 mg/mL 320 mg/mL
Vancomycin Vancocin® Lilly	500 mg 1 g	0.4 mL 0.7 mL	9.6 mL 19.3 mL	10 mL 20 mL	50 mg/mL 50 mg/mL

† = Displacement and diluent volumes have been rounded up or down to one decimal place.
* = Further dilution needed.
** = Has now been discontinued.

Table 12b Displacement volumes: other drugs

Drug brand manufacturer	Vial size	Displacement volume†	Diluent volume†	Final volume	Concentration (mg/mL)
Hydrocortisone Solu-Cortef® Pharmacia	100 mg	Negligible	2 mL	2 mL	50 mg/mL
Sodium valproate Epilim® Sanofi-Synthelabo	400 mg	Not given	4 mL	4 mL	95 mg/mL

† = Displacement and diluent volumes have been rounded up or down to one decimal place.

- To calculate doses using displacement volumes:

  volume to be added = diluent volume − displacement volume

  For example, for benzylpenicillin:

  dose required = 450 mg
  displacement volume = 0.4 mL per 600 mg vial
  diluent added = 5 mL
  volume to be added = 5 − 0.4 = 4.6 mL
  final concentration = 120 mg/mL
  volume required = 3.75 mL

MAKE SURE THAT PAEDIATRIC
DOSES ARE CHECKED CAREFULLY

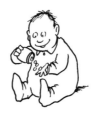

ADMINISTRATION ROUTES FOR DRUGS

Administration routes are largely determined mainly by the age and how ill the child is. In sick premature newborn babies, almost all drugs are given IV, since gastrointestinal function and therefore drug absorption are impaired (IM is not suitable as there is very poor muscle mass).

In older pre-term newborns, full-term newborns and older children, the oral route is suitable. However, for acutely ill children and for children with vomiting, diarrhoea or impaired gastrointestinal function, the parenteral route is recommended.

ORAL ADMINISTRATION

It is not always possible to give tablets or capsules: either the dose required does not exist, or the child cannot swallow tablets or capsules. An oral liquid preparation is therefore necessary, either a ready-made preparation, or one made especially by the pharmacy.

Not all the doses are convenient multiples of 5 mL; in these cases an oral syringe is used.

Many oral syringes are available, usually in the volumes shown in the table. You should choose the oral syringe most appropriate to the dose you are measuring.

Table 13 Oral syringe volumes

Volume (mL)	Graduations (mL)
0.5	0.01
1	0.01 OR 0.1
2.5	0.25
5	0.5
10	0.5
20	1

As with syringes for parenteral use, there is a residual volume of liquid left in the nozzle of the syringe, known as 'dead space' or 'dead volume'. This small volume (0.03 mL) is already taken into account by the manufacturer when calibrating the syringe, so you shouldn't try to administer it.

A part of their design is that it should not be possible to attach a needle to the nozzle of the oral syringe. This prevents the accidental intravenous administration of an oral preparation.

INTRAVENOUS ADMINISTRATION

Giving drugs intravenously is the most common parenteral route. It is now commonplace to use an infusion pump when giving infusions, as opposed to using a paediatric or micro-drop giving set on its own, as pumps are considered to be more accurate and safer.

USEFUL REFERENCE BOOKS

Medicines for Children. Royal College of Paediatrics and Child Health (RCPCH), London, 1999. ISBN 1 900954 38 9

Paediatric Formulary, 5th Edition. Guy's, St Thomas' and Lewisham Hospitals, London, 1999. ISBN 0 95348120 1

Alder Hey Book of Children's Doses ABCD, 6th edition. Alder Hey Children's Hospital, Liverpool, 1994 (with amendments 1996)

Neonatal Formulary 3: The Northern Neonatal Pharmacopoeia, 11th edition. Newcastle Royal Victoria Infirmary, Newcastle upon Tyne. ISBN 0 7279 1547 9

Neonatal Formulary, 7th edition, Hammersmith Hospital NHS Trust, London, August 1999.

Pediatric Injectable Drugs, 6th edition, American Society of Health System Pharmacists, 2002. ISBN 1 58528 012

British National Formulary, Number 45, March 2003, British Medical Association and Royal Pharmaceutical Society of Great Britain, London, 2003. ISBN 0 727 917 722

This list is not exhaustive, and there is probably a local in-house reference produced by your hospital. Check your hospital pharmacy department for details. The latest, most up to date, editions should be consulted.

PROBLEMS

Work out the following dosages, not forgetting to take into account displacement values if necessary.

Question 1 Benzylpenicillin at a dose of 25 mg/kg four times a day to a 9-month-old baby weighing 10 kg. How much do you need to draw up for each dose, assuming that each 600 mg vial is to be reconstituted to 2 mL?

Question 2 Trimethoprim at a dose of 4 mg/kg twice a day to a 9-year-old child weighing 31.7 kg. Trimethoprim suspension comes as a 50 mg in 5 mL suspension. How much do you need to give for each dose?

Question 3 You have to give a dose of ibuprofen to a 5-year-old child weighing 19.8 kg. The dose on the drug chart is 400 mg, four times a day. However, you think that the dose is rather high and you want to check it. A paediatric reference book gives a dose of 20 mg/kg daily in 3–4 divided doses or 5 mg/kg per dose. What do you think the dose for this child should be?

Question 4 You need to give a 4-month-old child 350 mg ceftriaxone IV daily. Ceftriaxone is available as a 1 g vial.
    i) Taking into account displacement volumes, what volume should you add to the vial?
    ii) How much do you need to give for each dose?

Question 5 You need to give cefotaxime IV to a 5-year-old child weighing 18 kg at a dose of 150 mg/kg daily in four divided doses. You have a 1 g cefotaxime vial. How much do you need to draw up for each dose?

Question 6 You need to give ranitidine liquid at a dose of 2 mg/kg to a 9-year-old child weighing 23 kg. You have a 150 mg in 10 mL liquid. How much do you need to give for each dose?

Question 7 Using the appropriate body surface area formula in Appendix 3, and checking with the nomogram, find out the body surface area for a child weighing 18 kg with a height of 108 cm.

Question 8 Using the appropriate body surface area formula in Appendix 3, and checking with the nomogram, find out the body surface area for a child weighing 37 kg with a height of 148 cm.

Question 9 You need to give flucloxacillin IV to a 8-year-old child weighing 19.6 kg. The dose is 12.5 mg/kg four times a day. You have a 500 mg vial that needs to be reconstituted to 10 mL with water for injection. How much do you need to draw up?

Question 10 You need to give aciclovir (acyclovir) to a 12-year-old child with a body surface area of 1.25 m^2 at a dose of 250 mg/m^2 every 8 hours. Aciclovir (acyclovir) comes as a 250 mg vial and should be given as an infusion over 1 hour at a concentration not more than 5 mg/mL. Initially you need to reconstitute each vial with 10 mL water for injection. How much do you need to draw up for each dose, and in what volume would you give the infusion?

ANSWERS TO PROBLEMS

Question 1 First work out the total dose required. The dose is 25 mg/kg and the child's weight is 10 kg, so the total dose is $25 \times 10 = 250$ mg.

Next, look up the displacement value for benzylpenicillin. From Table 12a, the displacement volume is 0.4 mL per 600 mg vial.

Work out how much water for injection you need to add to make a final volume of 2 mL, i.e.

2 mL − 0.4 mL = 1.6 mL

Therefore you need to add 1.6 mL water for injection to each vial to give a final concentration of 300 mg/mL.

The next step is to calculate the volume for 250 mg. There are 300 mg in 1 mL, so:

$$250 \text{ mg} = \frac{1}{300} \times 250 = 0.83 \text{ mL}$$

Answer: You need to draw up a dose of 250 mg (0.83 mL).

Question 2 The dose required is $31.7 \times 4 = 127$ mg. You have 50 mg in 5 mL, so:

$$127 \text{ mg} = \frac{5}{50} \times 127 = 12.7 \text{ mL} = 13 \text{ mL (rounded up)}$$

Answer: You need to give 13 mL of trimethoprim 50 mg in 5 mL.

Question 3 The total daily dose is 20 mg/kg or 5 mg/kg per dose, and the child's weight is 19.8 kg. So:

total daily dose = $20 \times 19.8 = 396$ mg
= 400 mg (rounded up)

If ibuprofen is to be given four times a day (as on the drug chart), then the amount for each dose equals:

$$\frac{400}{4} = 100 \text{ mg}$$

amount per dose = $5 \times 19.8 = 99$ mg
= 100 mg (rounded up)

Therefore the dose should be 100 mg four times a day and not 400 mg as on the drug chart. The total daily dose has been misread as a single dose, and consequently the patient will receive too much drug. This is a common error made by doctors when calculating doses.

Question 4   From the table, the displacement volume for ceftriaxone is 0.8 mL per 1 g vial. Work out how much water for injection you need to add to make a final volume of 10 mL, i.e.

10 mL − 0.8 mL = 9.2 mL

   i) Answer: You need to add 9.2 mL water for injection to each vial to give a final concentration of 100 mg/mL.

   The next step is to calculate the volume for 350 mg. You have 100 mg in 1 mL, so:

$$350 \text{ mg} = \frac{1}{100} \times 350 = 3.5 \text{ mL}$$

   ii) Answer: You need to draw up a dose of 350 mg (3.5 mL).

Question 5   The total daily dose is $18 \times 150 = 2{,}700$ mg, so each dose is:

$$\frac{2{,}700}{4} = 675 \text{ mg}$$

The displacement volume is 0.2 mL for 500 mg, therefore 0.4 mL for 1 g. So add 3.6 mL to a 1 g vial to give 1 g in 4 mL. Thus:

$$675 \text{ mg} = \frac{4}{1{,}000} \times 675 = 2.7 \text{ mL}$$

Answer: You need to draw up 2.7 mL (675 mg).

Question 6   The dose is 2 mg/kg and the child's weight is 23 kg. So the dose required is:

dose × weight = 2 × 23 = 46 mg

You have ranitidine liquid 150 mg in 10 mL, so for 46 mg you will need:

$$\frac{10}{150} \times 46 = 3.06 \text{ mL} = 3 \text{ mL (rounded down)}$$

Answer: You need to give 3 mL of ranitidine liquid 150 mg in 10 mL.

Question 7   Using the formula:

$$m^2 = \sqrt{\frac{\text{height (cm)} \times \text{weight (kg)}}{3600}}$$

The patient's height is 108 cm and the weight is 18 kg, so, substituting these figures in the formula:

$$m^2 = \sqrt{\frac{108 \times 18}{3600}} = \sqrt{\frac{1944}{3600}} = \sqrt{0.54} = 0.735$$

Answer: 0.735 m².

Question 8 Using the formula:

$$m^2 = \sqrt{\frac{height\ (cm) \times weight\ (kg)}{3600}}$$

The patient's height is 148 cm and the weight is 37 kg, so, substituting these figures in the formula:

$$m^2 = \sqrt{\frac{148 \times 37}{3600}} = \sqrt{\frac{5476}{3600}} = \sqrt{1.521} = 1.233$$

Answer: 1.233 m².

Question 9 The dose is:

$$12.5 \times 19.6 = 245\ mg$$

The displacement value is 0.2 mL for 250 mg, thus 0.4 mL for 500 mg. So you need to add 9.6 mL to each vial to give 500 mg in 10 mL. Thus:

$$245\ mg = \frac{10 \times 245}{500} = 4.9\ mL = 5\ mL\ (rounded\ up)$$

Answer: You need to draw up 5 mL.

Question 10 The dose is $250 \times 1.25 = 312.5$ mg, so you need to use 2 vials. The displacement value for aciclovir (acyclovir) is negligible, so add 10 mL water for injection to each vial to give 250 mg in 10 mL. The volume required for each dose is:

$$\frac{10 \times 312.5}{250} = 12.5\ mL$$

so you need to draw up 12.5 mL. The concentration should not be more than 5 mg/mL, and the dose you want is 312.5 mg. To find the volume required, divide the dose by the concentration, i.e.

$$minimum\ volume = \frac{312.5}{5} = 62.5\ mL$$

so you need to use a 100 mL infusion bag.

KEY POINTS

Prescribing in paediatrics

- When it comes to prescribing and administering medicines to children, they shouldn't be considered as small adults and care should be taken in calculating doses.
- Doses related to age are not ideal; doses calculated on a weight or surface area basis are more accurate, as they allow for greater individualization.
- Specialist paediatric books are now available that give accurate doses on a 'dose per weight' basis (e.g. mg/kg).

Displacement values or volumes

- Displacement values or volumes are usually given to freeze-dried injections, particularly antibiotics that need to be reconstituted before administration.
- To calculate doses using displacement volumes:

  volume to be added = diluent volume − displacement volume

Interpretation of drug information

OBJECTIVES

At the end of this chapter, you should be familiar with the following:

- Content of a summary of product characteristics (SPC)
- Content of a product information sheet

Before administering any drug, you should have some idea of how that drug acts, its effect on the body and possible side-effects. This is certainly true when dealing with parenteral products, as they have a more immediate and dramatic effect than oral preparations.

Basic drug information can be found in reference books (such as the *British National Formulary* or BNF) and from information produced or supplied by drug manufacturers. Information is produced in the form of a drug data sheet or summary of product characteristics.

SUMMARY OF PRODUCT CHARACTERISTICS (SPC)

Before a drug is marketed, it is extensively researched and tested over many years. During this time, a great deal of information is gathered about efficacy, side-effects and toxicology.

The most important information regarding the drug is documented in the summary of product characteristics – the SPC, also called the data sheet – which is officially approved when the medicine is licensed for use.

The main purpose of an SPC is to provide essential information to ensure that the drug or medicine is used correctly, effectively and safely.

WHAT AN SPC CONTAINS

All SPCs are presented in the same way, using standard headings. In this section you will find a brief description of these headings.

1 Trade name of the medicinal product

The brand name of the drug or medicine.

2 Qualitative and quantitative composition

The generic or chemical names of the active ingredients and the amount of each active ingredient, e.g. amount per tablet, amount per volume of solution, etc.

3 Pharmaceutical form

The physical form in which the medicine is presented, e.g. tablets, suppositories, ointment, etc.

4 Clinical particulars

Information that is essential for prescribers, to ensure that patients are treated appropriately, taking into account the patient's medical history, any other co-existing diseases or conditions and other current treatments.

4.1 Therapeutic indications

The diseases or conditions that the medicine is licensed to treat.

4.2 Posology and method of administration

Posology refers to the science of dosage, i.e. how much of a medicine should be given to a patient. The dose of the drug is given, including any changes in dose that may be necessary according to age or other disease or condition, such as renal or hepatic impairment. Where relevant, information is also given on the timing of doses in relation to meals.

The maximum single dose, the maximum daily dose and the maximum dose for a course of treatment may also be given.

4.3 Contra-indications

Anything about a patient's condition, medical history or current treatments that may indicate that this medicine should not be given.

4.4 Special warnings and special precautions for use

Any circumstances or condition where the drug should be used with particular care.

4.5 Interactions with other medicaments and other forms of interaction

Any other medicines, or anything else that the patient is likely to take, which may react with the drug, for example, food or alcohol as well as other drugs. These reactions may mean that some precautions should be taken or possibly that the medicine should not be used.

4.6 Pregnancy and lactation

Advice on the risks associated with using the drug at various stages of pregnancy and in fertile women, based upon the results of animal studies and any observations in humans that may have been recorded.

If the drug or any of its metabolites are excreted in breast milk, the probability and nature of any adverse effects on the infant are described, together with advice on whether breast-feeding should continue or not.

4.7 Effects on ability to drive and use machines

Whether or not the medicine is likely to impair a patient's ability to drive or operate machinery and if so, the extent of the effect.

4.8 Undesirable effects

A description of the side-effects that may occur, including how likely they are to happen, how severe they may be and for how long they are likely to last.

4.9 Overdose

A description of the signs and symptoms of overdose, together with advice on how to treat.

5 Pharmacological properties

Information about how the medicine works, how it is handled in the body and how it is excreted, e.g. in the urine or the faeces.

5.1 Pharmacodynamic properties

Pharmacodynamics is the study of the biochemical and physiological effects of drugs and the way in which they work. Information is given as to the time taken for the medicine to have an effect and reach its maximum effect and steady state.

5.2 Pharmacokinetic properties

Pharmacokinetics is the study of how a drug acts on the body over a period of time. It includes information regarding the absorption, distribution within the body, and excretion of the drug concerned.

Where appropriate, additional information may be included as to how the pharmacokinetics may change according to, for example, the patient's age or state of health.

5.3 Preclinical safety data

Describes the effects of the drug that were observed in studies before being used in humans, which could be of relevance to the prescriber in assessing the risks and benefits of treatment.

6 Pharmaceutical particulars

Information about excipients that the medicine contains, important incompatibilities and for how long the medicine may be stored and under what conditions is given. In addition, a description of the packaging and any special instructions for the use or handling of the medicine.

6.1 List of excipients

The contents of the medicine apart from the active ingredients, such as binding agents, solvents and flavourings.

6.2 Incompatibilities

In addition to the information given under 'Interaction with other medicaments and other forms of interaction', any other medicines or materials that interact with the drug and with which it should therefore not be used or mixed.

This information is particularly relevant to parenteral medicines, since they are often mixed or co-administered with other drugs. They may also, in some circumstances, react with the plastics from which syringes and infusion containers are made.

6.3 Shelf life

The maximum length of time for which the medicine may be stored under the specified conditions and after which it should not be used.

6.4 Special precautions for storage

The conditions in which the medicine must be stored to avoid degradation, for example, excessive temperatures or light.

6.5 Nature and contents of container

Description of the packaging and any other materials included in the pack, such as desiccants.

6.6 Instructions for use/handling

Instructions for the preparation or administration of the medicine in addition to those given under 'Posology and method of administration'.

7 Marketing authorization holder

The drug company holding the marketing authorization granted by the licensing authority.

8 Marketing authorization number

The licence number for the marketing authorization granted by the licensing authority.

9 Date of first authorization/renewal of authorization

The date when the marketing authorization was first granted. If the licence has at some time been suspended, the date when the licence was renewed.

10 Date of (partial) revision of the text

The last date on which an alteration to the wording of the SPC was officially made to reflect, for example, the addition of a new therapeutic indication or a change to the pack sizes available.

The following is an example of an SPC, for clarithromycin injection (Klaricid).

Klaricid IV
(Abbott Laboratories Limited)

1. TRADE NAME OF THE MEDICINAL PRODUCT
Klaricid IV

2. QUALITATIVE AND QUANTITATIVE COMPOSITION

Clarithromycin 500mg/vial

3. PHARMACEUTICAL FORM

Lyophilised powder for reconstitution to give a solution for IV administration.

4. CLINICAL PARTICULARS

4.1 Therapeutic Indications
Klaricid IV is indicated whenever parenteral therapy is required for treatment of infections caused by susceptible organisms in the following conditions;
- Lower respiratory tract infections for example, acute and chronic bronchitis, and pneumonia.
- Upper respiratory tract infections for example, sinusitis and pharyngitis.
- Skin and soft tissue infections.

4.2 Posology and Method of Administration
For intravenous administration only. Intravenous therapy may be given for 2 to 5 days and should be changed to oral clarithromycin therapy when appropriate.
Adults: The recommended dosage of Klaricid IV is 1.0 gram daily, divided into two 500mg doses, appropriately diluted as described below.
Children: At present, there are insufficient data to recommend a dosage regimen for routine use in children.
Elderly: As for adults.
Renal Impairment: In patients with renal impairment who have creatinine clearance less than 30ml/min, the dosage of clarithromycin should be reduced to one half of the normal recommended dose.
Recommended administration: Klaricid IV should be administered into one of the larger proximal veins as an IV infusion over 60 minutes, using a solution concentration of about 2mg/ml. Clarithromycin should not be given as a bolus or an intramuscular injection.

4.3 Contra-indications
Klaricid IV is contra-indicated in patients with known hypersensitivity to macrolide antibiotic drugs.
Klaricid and ergot derivatives should not be co-administered. Concomitant administration of

clarithromycin and any of the following drugs is contraindicated: cisapride, pimozide and terfenadine. Elevated cisapride, pimozide and terfenadine levels have been reported in patients receiving either of these drugs and clarithromycin concomitantly. This may result in QT prolongation and cardiac arrhythmias including ventricular tachycardia, ventricular fibrillation and Torsade de Pointes. Similar effects have been observed with concomitant administration of astemizole and other macrolides.

4.4 Special Warnings and Precautions for Use

Clarithromycin is principally excreted by the liver and kidney. Caution should be exercised in administering this antibiotic to patients with impaired hepatic and renal function.

Prolonged or repeated use of clarithromycin may result in an overgrowth of non-susceptible bacteria or fungi. If super-infection occurs, clarithromycin should be discontinued and appropriate therapy instituted.

4.5 Interaction with other medicaments and other forms of Interaction

Clarithromycin has been shown not to interact with oral contraceptives.

As with other macrolide antibiotics the use of clarithromycin in patients concurrently taking drugs metabolised by the cytochrome p450 system (e.g. warfarin, ergot alkaloids, triazolam, midazolam, disopyramide, lovastatin, rifabutin, phenytoin, cyclosporin _and tacrolimus_) may be associated with elevations in serum levels of these other drugs.

Rhabdomyolysis, co-incident with the co-administration of clarithromycin, and HMG-CoA reductase inhibitors, such as lovastatin and simvastatin has been reported.

The administration of Klaricid to patients who are receiving theophylline has been associated with increased serum theophylline levels and potential theophylline toxicity.

The use of Klaricid in patients receiving warfarin may result in a potentiation of the effects of warfarin. Prothrombin time should be frequently monitored in these patients. The effects of digoxin may be potentiated with concomitant administration of Klaricid. Monitoring of serum digoxin levels should be considered.

Klaricid may potentiate the effects of carbamazepine due to a reduction in the rate of excretion. Simultaneous oral administration of clarithromycin tablets and zidovudine to HIV infected adults may result in decreased steady-state zidovudine concentrations. Since this interaction in adults is thought to be due to interference of clarithromycin with simultaneously administered oral zidovudine, this interaction should not be a problem when clarithromycin is administered intravenously. With oral clarithromycin, the interaction can be largely avoided by staggering the doses; see Summary of Product Characteristics for Klaricid tablets for further information. No similar reaction has been reported in children.

Ritonavir increases the area under the curve (AUC), C_{max} and C_{min} of clarithromycin when administered concurrently. Because of the large therapeutic window for clarithromycin, no dosage reduction should be necessary in patients with normal renal function. However, for patients with renal impairment, the following dosage adjustments should be considered: For patients with CL_{CR} 30 to 60ml/min the dose of clarithromycin should be decreased by 50%. For patients with CL_{CR} <30ml/min the dose of clarithromycin should be decreased by 75%. Doses of clarithromycin greater than 1g/day should not be coadministered with ritonavir.

4.6 Pregnancy and Lactation

The safety of Klaricid during pregnancy and breast feeding of infants has not been established. Klaricid should thus not be used during pregnancy or lactation unless the benefit is considered to outweigh the risk. Some animal studies have suggested an embryotoxic effect but only at dose levels which are clearly toxic to mothers. Clarithromycin has been found in the milk of lactating animals and in human breast milk.

4.7 Effects on Ability to Drive and Use Machines

None reported.

4.8 Undesirable Effects

The most frequently reported infusion-related adverse events in clinical studies were injection-site inflammation, tenderness, phlebitis and pain. The most common non-infusion related adverse event reported was taste perversion. During clinical studies with oral Klaricid, the drug was generally well tolerated. Side-effects included nausea, vomiting, diarrhoea, dyspepsia and abdominal pain and paraesthesia. Stomatitis, glossitis and oral monilia have been reported. Other side-effects include headache, tooth and tongue discolouration, arthralgia, myalgia

and allergic reactions ranging from urticaria, mild skin eruptions and angioedema to anaphylaxis and, rarely, Stevens-Johnson syndrome / _toxic epidermal necrolysis_. Reports of alteration of the sense of smell, usually in conjunction with taste perversion have also been received. There have been reports of transient central nervous system side-effects including dizziness, vertigo, anxiety, insomnia, bad dreams, tinnitus, confusion, disorientation, hallucinations, psychosis, and depersonalisation. There have been reports of hearing loss with clarithromycin which is usually reversible upon withdrawal of therapy.

Pseudomembranous colitis has been reported rarely with clarithromycin, and may range in severity from mild to life threatening.

There have been rare reports of hypoglycaemia, some of which have occurred in patients on concomitant oral hypoglycaemic agents or insulin.

Isolated cases of leukopenia and thrombocytopenia have been reported.

As with other macrolides, hepatic dysfunction (which is usually reversible) including altered liver function tests, hepatitis and cholestasis with or without jaundice, has been reported. Dysfunction may be severe and very rarely fatal hepatic failure has been reported.

Cases of increased serum creatinine, interstitial nephritis, renal failure, _pancreatitis and convulsions_ have been reported rarely.

As with other macrolides, QT prolongation, ventricular tachycardia and Torsade de Pointes have been rarely reported with clarithromycin.

4.9 Overdose

There is no experience of overdosage after IV administration of clarithromycin. However, reports indicate that the ingestion of large amounts of clarithromycin orally can be expected to produce gastro-intestinal symptoms. **Adverse** reactions accompanying overdosage should be treated by gastric lavage and supportive measures.

As with other macrolides, clarithromycin serum levels are not expected to be appreciably affected by haemodialysis or peritoneal dialysis.

One patient who had a history of bipolar disorder ingested 8 grams of clarithromycin and showed altered mental status, paranoid behaviour, hypokalaemia and hypoxaemia.

5. PHARMACOLOGICAL PROPERTIES

5.1 Pharmacodynamic Properties

Clarithromycin is a semi-synthetic derivative of erythromycin A. It exerts its antibacterial action by binding to the 50s ribosomal sub-unit of susceptible bacteria and suppresses protein synthesis. Clarithromycin demonstrates excellent *in vitro* activity against standard strains of clinical isolates. It is highly potent against a wide variety of aerobic and anaerobic gram positive and negative organisms. The minimum inhibitory concentrations (MICs) of clarithromycin are generally two-fold lower than the MICs of erythromycin.

The 14-(R)-hydroxy metabolite of clarithromycin, formed in man by first pass metabolism also has anti-microbial activity. The MICs of this metabolite are equal to or two-fold higher than the MICs of the parent compound except for *H. influenzae* where the 14-hydroxy metabolite is two-fold more active than the parent compound.

Klaricid IV is usually active against the following organisms in vitro:

Gram-positive Bacteria: *Staphylococcus aureus* (methicillin susceptible); *Streptococcus pyogenes* (Group A beta-haemolytic streptococci); alpha-haemolytic streptococcus (viridans group); *Streptococcus (Diplococcus) pneumoniae; Streptococcus agalactiae; Listeria monocytogenes.*

Gram-negative Bacteria: *Haemophilus influenzae, Haemophilus parainfluenzae, Moraxella (Branhamella) catarrhalis, Neisseria gonorrhoeae; Legionella pneumophila, Bordetella pertussis, Helicobacter pylori; Campylobacter jejuni.*

Mycoplasma: *Mycoplasma pneumoniae; Ureaplasma urealyticum.*

Other Organisms: *Chlamydia trachomatis; Mycobacterium avium; Mycobacterium leprae; Chlamydia pneumoniae.*

Anaerobes: Macrolide-susceptible *Bacteriodes fragilis; Clostridium perfringens;* Peptococcus species; Peptostreptococcus species; *Propionibacterium acnes.*

Clarithromycin has bactericidal activity against several bacterial strains. These organisms include *H. influenzae, Streptococcus pneumoniae, Streptococcus pyogenes, Streptococcus agalactiae, Morazella (Brahamella) catarrhalis, Neisseria gonorrhoeae, Helicobacter pylori* and Campylobacter spp. The activity of clarithromycin against *H. pylori* is greater at neutral pH than at acid pH.

5.2 Pharmacokinetic Properties

The microbiologically active metabolite 14-hydroxyclarithro-mycin is formed by first pass metabolism as indicated by lower bioavailability of the metabolite following IV administration. Following IV administration the blood levels of clarithromycin achieved are well in excess of the $MIC_{90}s$ for the common pathogens and the levels of 14-hydroxyclarithromycin exceed the necessary concentrations for important pathogens, e.g. *H. influenzae*.

The pharmacokinetics of clarithromycin and the 14-hydroxy metabolite are non-linear; steady state is achieved by day 3 of IV dosing. Following a single 500mg IV dose over 60 minutes, about 33% clarithromycin and 11% 14-hydroxyclarithromycin is excreted in the urine at 24 hours.

Klaricid IV does not contain tartrazine or other azo dyes, lactose or gluten.

5.3 Preclinical Safety Data

There are no pre-clinical data of relevance to the prescriber which are additional to that already included in other sections of the SPC.

6. PHARMACEUTICAL PARTICULARS

6.1 List of Excipients

Lactobionic acid and Sodium Hydroxide EP.

6.2 Incompatibilities

None known. However, Klaricid IV should only be diluted with the diluents recommended.

6.3 Shelf Life

48 months unopened.
24 hours (at 5 °C–25 °C) once reconstituted in 10ml water for injections.

6 hours (at 25 °C) or 24 hours at (5 °C) once diluted in 250ml of appropriate diluent.

6.4 Special Precautions for Storage

Store at up to 30ºC and protect from light.

6.5 Nature and Contents of Container

30ml Ph.Eur. Type I flint glass tubing vial with a 20mm grey halo-butyllyophilisation stopper with flip-off cap. Vials are packed in units of 1,4 and 6. Pack size 500mg.

6.6 Instructions for Use/Handling

Klaricid IV should be administered into one of the larger proximal veins as an IV infusion over 60 minutes, using a solution concentration of about 2mg/ml. Clarithromycin should not be given as a bolus or an intramuscular injection.

7. MARKETING AUTHORIZATION HOLDER

Abbott Laboratories Limited, Queenborough, Kent. ME11 5EL.

8. MARKETING AUTHORIZATION NUMBER

PL 0037 / 0251

9. DATE OF FIRST AUTHORIZATION/RENEWAL OF AUTHORIZATION

22/09/93

10. DATE OF (PARTIAL) REVISION OF THE TEXT

October 2000

PACKAGE INSERT

The information given in the SPC is also summarized in the package insert found inside the box. The package insert is not as detailed as the SPC but contains the basic information necessary for the administration and monitoring of the drug. It is particularly useful when administering parenteral drugs as it gives information on dosing, diluents, rate of administration, etc.

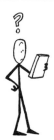

TECHNICAL LEAFLET

KLARICID® I.V.

500 mg clarithromycin

Presentation
Klaricid IV is a sterile freeze-dried powder form of clarithromycin. Each vial is a single dose of clarithromycin and contains: 500 mg Clarithromycin, Lactobionic Acid, Sodium Hydroxide, and Nitrogen.
Details of the preparation of suitable solutions for IV administration are given in the section on Administration.

Actions
Clarithromycin is an anti-bacterial agent. It is a semi-synthetic derivative of erythromycin A.

Uses
For the treatment of infections caused by susceptible organisms, whenever parenteral therapy is required, e.g. upper and lower respiratory tract infections and skin and soft tissue infections.

Contra-indications
Known hypersensitivity to macrolide antibiotic drugs. Concomitant administration of clarithromycin and any of the following drugs is contraindicated: cisapride, pimozide, terfenadine, and ergot derivatives. Similar effects seen with astemizole.

Precautions
Caution in administering to patients with impaired hepatic and renal function. Prolonged or repeated use of clarithromycin may result in an overgrowth of non-susceptible bacteria or fungi. The use of clarithromycin in patients concurrently taking drugs metabolised by the cytochrome p450 system may be associated with elevations in serum levels of these other drugs.

Interactions
No interaction with oral contraceptives.
Drugs metabolised by the cytochrome p450 system (e.g. warfarin, ergot alkaloids, triazolam, midazolam, disopyramide, lovastatin, rifabutin, phenytoin and cyclosporin, and tacrolimus). Rhabdomyolysis co-incident with the co-administration of clarithromycin, and HMG-CoA reductase inhibitors, such as lovastatin and simvastatin has been reported.
Theophylline, warfarin. (Prothrombin time should be frequently monitored in these patients).
Digoxin (Monitoring of serum digoxin levels should be considered.)
Carbamazepine.
Ritonavir, for patients with renal impairment, dosage adjustments should be considered: CL_{CR} 30 to 60 ml/min, reduce dose by 50%, CLCR <30ml/min, reduce dose by 75%.
Doses of clarithromycin greater than 1 g/day should not be coadministered with ritonavir.

Side Effects
Commonest side effects seen at the injection site, e.g. inflammation, tenderness, phlebitis and pain. Others include nausea, vomiting, diarrhoea, paraesthesia, dyspepsia, abdominal pain, headache, tooth and tongue discolouration, arthralgia, myalgia and allergic reactions ranging from urticaria and mild skin eruptions and angioedema to anaphylaxis and, rarely, Stevens-Johnson syndrome/ toxic epidermal necrolysis. Stomatitis, glossitis and oral monilia have been reported. Alteration of the sense of smell, usually in conjunction with taste perversion has also been reported with oral treatment. There have been reports of transient central nervous system side-effects including dizziness, vertigo, anxiety, insomnia, bad dreams, tinnitus, confusion, disorientation, hallucinations, psychosis and depersonalisation. There have been reports of hearing loss with clarithromycin which is usually reversible upon withdrawal of therapy. There have been rare reports of hypoglycaemia, some of which have occurred in patients on concomitant oral hypoglycaemic agents or insulin. Pseudomembranous colitis has been reported rarely with clarithromycin and may range in severity from mild to life threatening. Isolated cases of leukopenia and thrombocytopenia have been reported.
Hepatic dysfunction, including altered liver function tests, cholestasis with or without jaundice and hepatitis has been reported. Cases of increased serum creatinine, interstitial nephritis and renal failure, pancreatitis and convulsions have been reported rarely. As with other macrolides, QT prolongation, ventricular tachycardia and Torsade de Pointes have been rarely reported with clarithromycin.
If any other undesirable effect occurs, which is not mentioned above, the patient should be advised to give details to his/her doctor.

Use In Pregnancy and Lactating Women
Klaricid should not be used during pregnancy or lactation unless the clinical benefit is considered to outweigh the risk. Clarithromycin has been found in the milk of lactating animals and in human breast milk.

Recommended Dosage
Intravenous therapy may be given for 2 to 5 days and should be changed to oral clarithromycin therapy when appropriate.

Adults: The recommended dosage of Klaricid IV is 1.0 gram daily, divided into two 500 mg doses, appropriately diluted as described below.

Children: At present, there are insufficient data to recommend a dosage regime for routine use in child

Elderly: As for adults.

Renal Impairment: In patients with renal impairment who have creatinine clearance less than 30ml/min, the dosage of clarithromycin should be reduced to one half of the normal recommended dose.

Recommended Administration

Clarithromycin should not be given as a bolus or an intramuscular injection.

Klaricid IV should be administered into one of the larger proximal veins as an IV infusion over 60 minutes, using a solution concentration of about 2mg/ml.

STEP 1

Add 10 ml sterilised Water for Injections into the vial and shake
Use within 24 hours
May be stored from 5°C up to room temperature

DO NOT USE
• Diluents containing preservatives • Diluents containing inorganic salts

STEP 2

Add 10ml from Step 1 to 250ml of a suitable diluent (see below)
This provides a 2mg/ml solution
Use within 6 hours (at room temperature) or within 24 hours if stored at 5°C

DO NOT USE
• Solution strengths greater than 2mg/ml (0.2%) • Rapid infusion rates (< 60 minutes) • Failure to observe these precautions may result in pain along the vein

Recommended Diluents

5% dextrose in Lactated Ringer's Solution, 5% dextrose, Lactated Ringer's solution, 5% dextrose in 0.3% sodium chloride, Normosol-M in 5% dextrose, Normosol-R in 5% dextrose, 5% dextrose in 0.45% sodium chloride, or 0.9% sodium chloride. Compatibility with other IV additives has not been established.

Overdosage

There is no experience of overdosage after I.V. administration of clarithromycin. However, reports indicate that the ingestion of large amounts of clarithromycin orally can be expected to produce gastro-intestinal symptoms. Adverse reactions accompanying oral overdosage should be treated by gastric lavage and supportive measures.

As with other macrolides, clarithromycin serum levels are not expected to be appreciably affected by haemodialysis or peritoneal dialysis.

One patient who had a history of bipolar disorder ingested 8 g of clarithromycin and showed altered mental status, paranoid behaviour, hypokalaemia and hypoxaemia.

Storage

Can be stored at up to 30°C. Protect powder from light. See carton and vial for expiry date. The product should not be used after this date.

Product Licence Number
0037/0251

Legal Category
POM

Marketed in the UK by: Abbott Laboratories Ltd., Queenborough, Kent, ME11 5EL

Date of preparation of leaflet: May 1999. Revised: October 2000.   001-897-701

Let's look in more detail at the package insert for clarithromycin injection (Klaricid), as this is the usual form in which you will see drug information.

The important points to note are as follows:

Dosing information

Recommended Dosage
Intravenous therapy may be given for 2 to 5 days and should be changed to oral clarithromycin therapy when appropriate. **Adults:** The recommended dosage of Klaricid IV is 1.0 gram daily, divided into two 500 mg doses, appropriately diluted as described below. **Children:** At present, there are insufficient data to recommend a dosage regime for routine use in childr **Elderly:** As for adults. **Renal Impairment:** In patients with renal impairment who have creatinine clearance less than 30ml/min, the dosage of clarithromycin should be reduced to one half of the normal recommended dose.

- The normal dose for adults (including elderly people) is 500 mg twice a day for 2–5 days.
- In patients with renal impairment, the dose may have to be reduced.
- Clarithromycin is not recommended in children.

Administration information

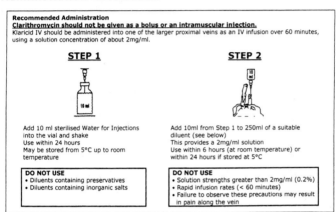

Recommended Administration
Clarithromycin should not be given as a bolus or an intramuscular injection.
Klaricid IV should be administered into one of the larger proximal veins as an IV infusion over 60 minutes, using a solution concentration of about 2mg/ml.

STEP 1

Add 10 ml sterilised Water for Injections into the vial and shake
Use within 24 hours
May be stored from 5°C up to room temperature

DO NOT USE
- Diluents containing preservatives
- Diluents containing inorganic salts

STEP 2

Add 10ml from Step 1 to 250ml of a suitable diluent (see below)
This provides a 2mg/ml solution
Use within 6 hours (at room temperature) or within 24 hours if stored at 5°C

DO NOT USE
- Solution strengths greater than 2mg/ml (0.2%)
- Rapid infusion rates (< 60 minutes)
- Failure to observe these precautions may result in pain along the vein

- Clarithromycin should not be given as a IV bolus or by IM injection – it must be given as an intermittent infusion.
- The infusion must be given over at least 60 minutes.
- The concentration of the infusion should not be greater than 2 mg/mL (0.2%), usually given in 250 mL.

    Let's see how this is calculated. The maximum concentration is 2 mg/mL, which is equal to:

$$1 \text{ mg in } \frac{1}{2} \text{ mL}$$

Therefore for a 500 mg dose:

$$\frac{1}{2} \times 500 = 250 \text{ mL}$$

So the minimum volume for a 500 mg dose would be 250 mL.

- Once added to the infusion bag, it must be used within 6 hours (24 hours if stored in a fridge).

Reconstitution information

- Water for Injection BP must be used.
- The volume for reconstitution is 10 mL.
- Once reconstituted, it must be used within 24 hours.

Recommended diluents

> **Recommended Diluents**
> 5% dextrose in Lactated Ringer's Solution, 5% dextrose, Lactated Ringer's solution, 5% dextrose in 0.3% sodium chloride, Normosol-M in 5% dextrose, Normosol-R in 5% dextrose, 5% dextrose in 0.45% sodium chloride, or 0.9% sodium chloride. Compatibility with other IV additives has not been established.

- Suitable infusion fluids include sodium chloride 0.9% or 5% dextrose.

Other points to note

- Contra-indications: hypersensitivity to clarithromycin, otherwise nothing else of note.
- Precautions: caution in administering to patients with impaired hepatic and renal function.
- Incompatibilities: this information would be useful if several drugs are being given parenterally and going through the same IV line or mixed in the same infusion bag. In this case, nothing is reported.
- Side-effects: the most commonly seen side-effects are those seen at the injection site, e.g. inflammation, tenderness, phlebitis and pain.

SUMMARY OF PRODUCT CHARACTERISTICS (SPC) AND PACKAGE INSERT

The main purpose of an SPC is to provide essential information to ensure that the drug or medicine is used correctly, effectively and safely. The information given in the SPC is also summarized in the package insert found inside the box. All SPCs are presented in the same way, using a standard heading for each section:

1 Trade name of the medicinal product
2 Qualitative and quantitative composition
3 Pharmaceutical form
4 Clinical particulars
    4.1 Therapeutic indications
    4.2 Posology and method of administration
    4.3 Contra-indications
    4.4 Special warnings and special precautions for use
    4.5 Interactions with other medicaments and other forms of interaction
    4.6 Pregnancy and lactation
    4.7 Effects on ability to drive and use machines
    4.8 Undesirable effects
    4.9 Overdose

5 Pharmacological properties
   5.1 Pharmacodynamic properties
   5.2 Pharmacokinetic properties
   5.3 Preclinical safety data
6 Pharmaceutical particulars
   6.1 List of excipients
   6.2 Incompatibilities
   6.3 Shelf life
   6.4 Special precautions for storage
   6.5 Nature and contents of container
   6.6 Instructions for use/handling
7 Marketing authorization holder
8 Marketing authorization number
9 Date of first authorization/renewal of authorization
10 Date of (partial) revision of the text

KEY POINTS

Interpretation of drug information

- Before administering any drug, you should have some idea of how that drug acts, its effect on the body and possible side-effects. This is particularly true for parenteral products as they have a more immediate and dramatic effect than oral preparations.
- Drug information is available in the form of a drug data sheet or summary of product characteristics (SPC).

Revision test

The purpose of this revision test is to test your ability at drug calculations after you have finished the book. You should get most, if not all, of the questions right. If you get the wrong answers for any particular section, then you should go back and re-do that section as it indicates that you have not fully understood that type of calculation.

BASICS

The aim of this section is to see if you have understood basic principles such as fractions, decimals, powers and using calculators.

FRACTIONS

Solve the following, leaving your answer as a fraction.

1 $\dfrac{5}{16} \times \dfrac{5}{7}$

2 $\dfrac{3}{8} \div \dfrac{6}{7}$

Convert to a decimal:

3 $\dfrac{4}{7}$

DECIMALS

Solve the following:

4 2.15×0.64
5 $4.2 \div 0.125$
6 2.6×100
7 $45.67 \div 100$

Convert the following to a fraction:

8 0.4

ROMAN NUMERALS

Write the following as ordinary numbers:

9 III
10 VII

POWERS

Convert the following to a proper number:

11 2.3×10^2

Convert the following number to a power of 10:

12 800,000

UNITS AND EQUIVALENCES

This section is designed to re-test your knowledge in units, and how to convert from one unit to another.

UNITS OF WEIGHT

1 0.125 milligrams = … micrograms
2 0.5 grams = … milligrams
3 0.25 micrograms = … nanograms
4 0.75 kilograms = … grams

UNITS OF VOLUME

5 0.45 litres = … millilitres

UNITS OF AMOUNT OF SUBSTANCE

6 0.15 moles = … millimoles

DOSAGE CALCULATIONS

CALCULATING THE NUMBER OF TABLETS OR CAPSULES REQUIRED

The strength of the tablets or capsules you have available does not always correspond to the dose required. Therefore you have to calculate the number of tablets or capsules needed.

1 Dose prescribed, lisinopril 15 mg. You have 5 mg tablets available. How many tablets do you need?

DRUG DOSAGE

Sometimes the dose is given on a body weight basis or in terms of body surface area. The following tests your ability at calculating doses on these parameters.

Work out the dose required for the following:

2 Dose = 7.5 mg/kg; weight = 78 kg
3 Dose = 4 micrograms/kg/min; weight = 56 g
4 Dose = 4.5 mg/m²; surface area = 1.94 m²

CALCULATING DOSAGES

Calculate how much you need for the following dosages:

5 You have haloperidol injection 5 mg in 1 mL, amount required = 6 mg.
6 You have diazepam suspension 2 mg in 5 mL, amount required = 5 mg.
7 You have codeine phosphate syrup 25 mg in 5 mL, amount required = 30 mg.
8 You have co-trimoxazole injection 480 mg in 5 mL, amount required = 2,040 mg. What volume and how many ampoules do you need?

PERCENT AND PERCENTAGES

This section is designed to see if you understand the concept of percent and percentages.

1 How much is 28% of 250 g?
2 What percentage is 160 g of 400 g?

MOLES AND MILLIMOLES

This section is designed to see if you understood the concept of millimoles.

> **Tip** The following information will be helpful in answering questions in this section.
>
> Molecular weight:
> sodium bicarbonate   84
> sodium chloride   58.5

1 Approximately how many millimoles of sodium are there in a 200 mL infusion of sodium bicarbonate 8.4%.

2 Approximately how many mmol per litre of sodium are there in an infusion containing 4.5 g of sodium chloride per litre?

DRUG STRENGTHS OR CONCENTRATIONS

This section is designed to see if you understood the various ways in which drug strengths can be expressed.

PERCENTAGE CONCENTRATIONS

1 How much glucose (in grams) is there in a 500 mL infusion of glucose 10%?

2 A patient is prescribed 5 mg of salbutamol respiratory solution 0.5% w/v. How much should the patient have?

CONCENTRATIONS IN MG/ML

3 What is the concentration (in mg/mL) of a 30% sodium chloride ampoule?

'1 IN ...' CONCENTRATIONS OR RATIO STRENGTHS

4 You have a 1 mL ampoule of adrenaline (epinephrine) 1 in 1,000. How much adrenaline (epinephrine), in milligrams, does the ampoule contain?

DRUGS EXPRESSED IN UNITS

5 You need to give an infusion of heparin containing 32,000 units over 24 hours. You have ampoules of heparin containing 25,000 units/mL. How much of each ampoule do you need to draw up?

MOLARITY

6 How many grams of sodium chloride is required to make 100 ml of a 0.6 M solution? (The molecular weight of sodium chloride is 58.5).

INFUSION RATE CALCULATIONS

This section tests your knowledge of various infusion rate calculations. It is designed to see if you know the different drop factors for different giving sets and fluids, as well as being able to convert volumes to drops and vice versa.

CALCULATION OF DRIP RATES

1 What is the rate required to give 1 litre of glucose 5% infusion over 6 hours using a standard giving set?
2 What is the rate required to give 1 litre of sodium chloride 0.9% infusion over 8 hours using a standard giving set?
3 What is the rate required to give 1 unit of blood (500 mL) over 6 hours using a standard giving set?

CONVERSION OF INFUSION RATES (ML/HOUR) TO DROPS/MIN

4 You are asked to give a 1 litre infusion of sodium chloride 0.9% at a rate of 100 mL/hour using a standard giving set. What is the rate in drops/min?

CONVERSION OF DOSAGES TO ML/HOUR

5 You have an infusion of dobutamine 250 mg in 250 mL. The dose required is 6 micrograms/kg/min and the patient weighs 77 kg. What is the rate in mL/hour?
6 You are asked to give 500 mL of lidocaine (lignocaine) 0.2% infusion at a rate of 3 mg/min. What is the rate in mL/hour?

CONVERSION OF ML/HOUR TO MICROGRAMS/KG/MIN OR MG/MIN

7 An infusion pump containing 50 mg of glyceryl trinitrate in 100 mL is running at a rate of 8 mL/hour. The dose wanted is 4 mg/hour. Is the pump rate correct?

CALCULATION OF DURATION OF INFUSIONS

8 You have a 500 mL infusion at a rate of 21 drops/min using a standard giving set. Approximately how long will the infusion run?

PAEDIATRIC DOSAGE CALCULATIONS

This section tests your knowledge of paediatric dosage calculations.

1 The dose of morphine for a 6-month-old child (7 kg) is 200 micrograms/kg. How much do you need to draw up if morphine is available as a 10 mg/mL ampoule?
2 You need to give benzylpenicillin at a dose of 25 mg/kg four times a day to a year-old baby weighing 11 kg. How much do you need to

draw up for each dose, assuming each 600 mg vial is to be reconstituted to 5 mL?

ANSWERS

BASICS

Fractions

1 $\frac{5}{28}$

2 $\frac{7}{16}$

3 0.57

Decimals

4 1.376
5 33.6
6 260
7 0.4567
8 $\frac{2}{5}$

Roman numerals

9 3
10 7

Powers

11 230
12 8×10^5

UNITS AND EQUIVALENCES

Units of weight

1 125 micrograms
2 500 mg
3 250 nanograms
4 750 g

Units of volume

5 450 mL

Units of amount of substance

6 150 mmol

DOSAGE CALCULATIONS

Calculating the number of tablets or capsules required

1 3 tablets

Drug dosage

2 585 mg
3 224 micrograms/min
4 87.3 mg

Calculating dosages

5 1.2 mL
6 12.5 mL
7 6 mL
8 21.25 mL; 5 ampoules

PERCENT AND PERCENTAGES

1 332
2 45%

MOLES AND MILLIMOLES

1 200 mmol
2 77 mmol

DRUG STRENGTHS OR CONCENTRATIONS

Percentage concentration

1 50 g
2 1 mL

Concentrations in mg/mL

3 300 mg/mL
4 15 mL

'1 in ...' concentrations or radio strengths

5 1 mg

Drugs expressed in units

6 $1 \times 25,000$ units/mL ampoule **and** $1 \times 5,000$ units/mL ampoule **and** 0.4 mL of a 5,000 units/mL ampoule

INFUSION RATE CALCULATIONS

Calculation of drip rates

1 55.5 drops/min (56 drops/min)
2 41.7 drops/min (42 drops/min)
3 20.8 drops/min (21 drops/min)

Conversion of infusion rates (mL/hour) to drops/min

4 33.3 drops/min (33 drops/min)

Conversion of dosages to drops/min and mL/hour

5 27.72 (28) mL/hour
6 90 mL/hour

Conversion of mL/hour to micrograms/kg per min or mg/min

7 8 mL/hour is equal to 4 mg/hour

Calculation of duration of infusions

8 476 minutes = 7 hours 56 minutes (approximately 8 hours)

PAEDIATRIC DOSAGE CALCULATIONS

1 0.14 mL
2 2.3 mL

Preparations of solutions (dilutions)

It is now rarely necessary to prepare solutions on the ward or even in the pharmacy. Such treatments are no longer used and the calculations are included here for reference only.

PREPARATION OF SIMPLE SOLUTIONS

Most solutions are stored in a concentrated form in order to save storage space. The concentrated or stock solution is then diluted before use. The same stock solution may be used at different concentrations or strengths for different purposes.

WORKED EXAMPLE: PREPARATION OF A SOLUTION FROM A STOCK SOLUTION

What volume of stock solution is needed to give a 45% solution when diluted to 500 mL?

In this case, the original volume of the stock solution does not matter. You are only interested in the final (diluted) solution and how much of the stock solution is needed to make the final solution.

Step 1

Convert the percentage required to the number of mL per 100 mL:

45% v/v = 45 mL in 100 mL

Thus for every 100 mL of your final solution, 45 mL will be the original or stock solution.

Step 2

Work out how much of the stock solution is needed for every 1 mL of the final solution, i.e. divide by 100:

45 mL in 100 mL

1 mL in $\frac{45}{100}$ mL

Step 3

However, you need to prepare 500 mL for your final solution. Calculate the volume of stock solution required by multiplying the volume for 1 mL by the final volume:

1 mL in $\dfrac{45}{100}$ mL

Thus for 500 mL, you will need:

$\dfrac{45}{100} \times 500 = 225$ mL

Step 4

From Step 3, you have just worked out that you need 225 mL of stock solution. Therefore you will need:

500 mL − 225 mL = 275 mL of diluent

Answer: To prepare 500 mL of a 45% solution, you will need 225 mL of stock solution diluted with 275 mL of diluent.

Alternatively, a simple formula can be used:

$$\begin{array}{c} \text{amount of stock} \\ \text{solution required} \\ \text{(in mL)} \end{array} = \dfrac{\begin{array}{c}\text{\% concentration of}\\\text{the final solution}\end{array}}{100} \times \begin{array}{c}\text{final volume of}\\\text{solution required}\\\text{(in mL)}\end{array}$$

where, in this example:

% concentration of the final solution = 45%
final volume required (in mL) = 500 mL

Substitute the figures in the formula:

$\dfrac{45}{100} \times 500 = 225$ mL

Answer: To prepare 500 mL of a 45% solution, you will need 225 mL of stock solution and 275 mL of diluent.

PREPARATION OF SOLUTIONS FOR TOPICAL APPLICATION OR SOAKS

Although solutions for topical application, soaks or disinfectants are not usually made on the ward now, it still may be necessary to prepare potassium permanganate solutions for soaks. These solutions are made from strong or concentrated stock solutions that are diluted to form weaker solutions. The diluted solutions are often expressed in ratio strengths, i.e. '1 in …' concentrations, for example:

- 1 in 10,000 means 1 g dissolved in 10,000 mL
- 1 in 500 means 1 g dissolved in 500 mL

See the chapter on 'Drug strengths or concentrations' for a fuller explanation.

WORKED EXAMPLE: PREPARATION OF A SOAK

A 1 in 10,000 potassium permanganate soak is required. A stock solution of 10 g/litre is available. How much of the stock solution do you need to make a litre of a 1 in 10,000 solution?

When you are trying to solve problems like these, it is much easier to work backwards and convert everything to the number of grams.

Step 1

Write down the final concentration required:

  1 g in 10,000 mL (1 in 10,000)

Step 2

Next calculate how many grams in 1 mL of your final solution by dividing by 10,000:

$$1 \text{ mL} = \frac{1}{10,000} \text{ g}$$

Step 3

Now calculate the total number of grams for the final volume required, i.e. multiply the amount for 1 mL by 1,000 (1 litre = 1,000 mL):

$$1 \text{ mL} = \frac{1}{10,000} \text{ g}$$

For 1,000 mL:

$$\frac{1}{10,000} \times 1,000 \text{ g}$$

You are converting the strength required (1 in 10,000) to the total number of grams or quantity required.

After calculating the number of grams in your final solution, you now need to work out how much of your stock solution is equal to the number of grams needed.

Step 4

Of the stock solution, calculate the volume for 1 g:

  10 g in 1 litre or 10 g in 1,000 mL, so

$$1 \text{ g} = \frac{1,000}{10} \text{ mL}$$

Thus you are converting the strength of the stock solution to a volume containing 1 g.

Step 5

To calculate how much of the stock solution (in mL) is needed, multiply the total number of grams in the final solution (Step 3) by the volume for 1 g of stock solution (Step 4):

$$\frac{1}{10,000} \times 1,000 \times \frac{1,000}{10} = \frac{100}{10} = 10 \text{ mL}$$

Answer: 10 mL of a 10 g/litre stock solution when made up to 1 litre (1,000 mL) will give a 1 in 10,000 solution.

As in earlier dilution problems, a formula can be used to work out the amount of stock solution needed:

$$\begin{array}{c} \text{amount of stock} \\ \text{solution required} \\ \text{(in mL)} \end{array} = \frac{\begin{array}{c}\text{concentration of the} \\ \text{final solution (g/mL)}\end{array}}{\begin{array}{c}\text{concentration of the} \\ \text{stock solution (in g/mL)}\end{array}} \times \begin{array}{c} \text{final volume of} \\ \text{solution required} \\ \text{(in mL)} \end{array}$$

Therefore you have:

concentration of the final solution (g/mL) $= \dfrac{1}{10,000}$

% concentration of the stock solution (g/mL) $= \dfrac{10}{1,000} = \dfrac{1}{100}$

final volume required (in mL) $= 1,000 \text{ mL}$

Substitute the figures in the formula:

$$\frac{\frac{1}{10,000}}{\frac{1}{100}} \times 1,000$$

Because you always invert fractions when dividing, this is rewritten as:

$$\frac{1}{10,000} \times \frac{100}{1} \times 1,000$$

$$\frac{1}{10,000} \times \frac{100}{1} \times 1,000 = 10 \text{ mL}$$

Answer: 10 mL of the stock solution is required.

- As you can see, using the formula can appear a bit complicated. However, if you work slowly and step by step, then you shouldn't have any problems.
- It is usually better to work from first principles.
- If you are using the formula, take care with your calculations.

Preparation of powders

Sometimes the dose required can be extremely small – too small to be given in the form of tablets. If the drug can't be made into a syrup or suspension because they are unstable, the powdered form of the medicine is diluted with an inert substance, such as lactose, and dispensed as individual doses or powders.

This process of dilution is called **trituration**, and several trituations may be required if the dose is very small (e.g. doses for babies or children) or if a potent drug is involved.

There are two methods for preparing powders:

- dilution of the drug as a powder
- weighing and crushing tablets, then diluting with a suitable diluent.

WORKED EXAMPLE

A child needs levothyroxine (thyroxine) at a dose of 35 micrograms. This is too small to be given in the form of a tablet, and a suspension cannot be made, so powders need to be prepared. You need 14 powders.

Method 1: Dilution of the medicine as a powder

To allow for wastage, you usually calculate for an extra two powders. Thus in this case, calculate for 16 powders.

Step 1

Calculate the total amount of drug required for 16 powders. Each powder is to contain 35 micrograms, so for 16 powders you will need:

$16 \times 35 = 560$ micrograms (0.56 mg)

It is impossible to weigh 560 micrograms with the equipment normally available, let alone divide it into 16 equal amounts. Therefore it is necessary to weigh a larger weighable amount and then dilute it by trituration.

Step 2

On a normal dispensing balance (class B balance), it is good dispensing practice never to weigh less than 100 mg. Therefore each final powder must weigh at least 100 mg.

Calculate the total amount for the number of powders required (16):

16 × 100 mg = 1,600 mg

Step 3

You need to dilute the drug until you have a final powder weighing 100 mg that contains 35 micrograms of drug (this may take several dilutions or triturations).

Dilution 1 (1 in 50 dilution):

levothyroxine (thyroxine)	100 mg (minimum weighable amount)
lactose	4,900 mg
	5,000 mg

You have 100 mg levothyroxine (thyroxine) in 5,000 mg, so in each 100 mg of this dilution there are:

$\dfrac{100}{5,000} \times 100 = 2$ mg of levothyroxine (thyroxine)

Step 4

A further dilution is necessary.

Dilution 2 (1 in 20 dilution):

from Dilution 1	100 mg (which contains 2 mg levothyroxine (thyroxine))
lactose	1,900 mg
	2,000 mg

You now have 2 mg levothyroxine (thyroxine) in 2,000 mg, so in each 100 mg there are 0.1 mg (100 micrograms) of levothyroxine (thyroxine):

$\dfrac{2}{2,000} \times 100 = 0.1$ mg (100 micrograms)

Step 5

You have already calculated that you need a final amount of 560 micrograms of levothyroxine (thyroxine) (from Step 1). You know that 100 mg of powder from Dilution 2 contains 100 micrograms of levothyroxine (thyroxine), so for 560 micrograms you will need 560 mg of powder from Dilution 2. The total amount required for 16 powders (Step 2) is 1,600 mg. Therefore, take 560 mg from Dilution 2 and make up to 1,600 mg with lactose.

Dilution 3 (dilution according to the dose required):

```
from Dilution 2    560 mg  (= 560 micrograms of levothyroxine (thyroxine))
lactose          1,040 mg  (1,600 mg − 560 mg)
                 1,600 mg
```

You have 560 micrograms levothyroxine (thyroxine) in 1,600 mg, so each 100 mg of this final dilution will contain 35 micrograms of levothyroxine (thyroxine):

$$\frac{560}{1,600} \times 100 = 35 \text{ micrograms}$$

Therefore you can weigh 16 lots of 100 mg (14 plus 2 backups), as required.

Other 'doses' of varying strengths

If the dose required is in terms of hundreds of micrograms ($\times100$ micrograms) or milligrams' ($\times1$ mg) instead of tens of micrograms ($\times10$ micrograms), then the same methods are used but different dilutions are made:

- Hundreds of micrograms ($\times100$ micrograms)
  Dilution 1: 1 in 20 dilution (100 mg diluted to 2,000 mg)
  Dilution 2: 1 in 5 dilution (100 mg diluted to 500 mg)
  Dilution 3: dilution according to dose required.
- Milligrams ($\times1$ mg)
  Dilution 1: 1 in 10 dilution (100 mg diluted to 1,000 mg)
  Dilution 2: dilution according to dose required.

Example 1: Hundreds of micrograms ($\times100$ micrograms)

The dose required is hyoscine 600 micrograms, and you need 10 powders.

Dilution 1 (1 in 20 dilution):

```
hyoscine   100 mg
lactose  1,900 mg
         2,000 mg
```

You have 100 mg hyoscine in 2,000 mg, so 100 mg of this dilution contains 5 mg of hyoscine:

$$\frac{100}{2,000} \times 100 = 5 \text{ mg}$$

Dilution 2 (1 in 5 dilution):

from Dilution 1	200 mg	(= 10 mg of hyoscine)
lactose	800 mg	
	1,000 mg	

You have 10 mg hyoscine in 1,000 mg, so 100 mg of this dilution contains 1 mg of hyoscine:

$$\frac{10}{1,000} \times 100 = 1 \text{ mg}$$

Dilution 3 (dilution according to the dose required):

You need 10 powders of hyoscine 600 micrograms, so:

total dose required = 600 micrograms × 10 = 6 mg

Take 600 mg from Dilution 2 (= 6 mg of hyoscine) and dilute to 1,000 mg (10 powders of 100 mg = 1,000 mg).

from Dilution 2	600 mg	(= 6 mg of hyoscine)
lactose	400 mg	(1,000 mg − 600 mg)
	1,000 mg	

You have 6 mg hyoscine in 1,000 mg, therefore each 100 mg of this dilution contains 0.6 mg (600 micrograms) of hyoscine:

$$\frac{6}{1,000} \times 100 = 0.6 \text{ mg (600 micrograms)}$$

Example 2: Milligrams (×1 mg)

The dose required is codeine phosphate 1.5 mg, and you need 10 powders.

Dilution 1 (1 in 10 dilution):

codeine phosphate	100 mg
lactose	900 mg
	1,000 mg

You have 100 mg codeine phosphate in 1,000 mg, therefore each 100 mg of this dilution contains 10 mg of codeine phosphate:

$$\frac{100}{1,000} \times 100 = 10 \text{ mg}$$

Dilution 3 (dilution according to the dose required):

You need 10 powders of codeine phosphate 1.5 mg, so:

total dose required = 1.5 mg × 10 = 15 mg

Take 150 mg from Dilution 1 (= 15 mg of codeine phosphate) and dilute to 1,000 mg (10 powders of 100 mg = 1,000 mg).

```
from Dilution 1    150 mg  (= 15 mg of codeine phosphate)
lactose            850 mg  (1,000 mg − 150 mg)
                 1,000 mg
```

You have 15 mg codeine phosphate in 1,000 mg, therefore each 100 mg of this dilution contains 1.5 mg of codeine phosphate:

$$\frac{15}{1,000} \times 100 = 1.5 \text{ mg}$$

Method 2: Crushing tablets

The advantage of this method is that the drug is readily available in a tablet form, whereas it may not be readily available in a powdered form.

We will use the same worked example as before: a dose of 35 micrograms of levothyroxine (thyroxine) is needed for a child. You need to prepare 14 powders, so prepare 2 extra (16 in total) to allow for wastage.

Step 1

First work out the total dose for 16 powders:

$16 \times 35 = 560$ micrograms

Step 2

Levothyroxine (thyroxine) tablets are available in the following strengths: 25 micrograms, 50 micrograms and 100 micrograms.

Obviously, using the above strengths of levothyroxine (thyroxine) tablets, it is impossible to get the required dose of 560 micrograms. The nearest possible dose is either:

550 micrograms = 5 × 100 micrograms + 1 × 50 micrograms
                = 550 micrograms

or

575 micrograms = 5 × 100 micrograms + 1 × 50 micrograms
                        + 1 × 25 micrograms
                = 575 micrograms

If it isn't possible to match the calculated dose exactly, then it is better to go slightly higher, rather than slightly lower.

Step 3

Next work out the number of powders for the nearest (new) total, i.e. divide the new total dose by the dose required:

$$\frac{575}{35} = 16.43 \text{ powders}$$

So 575 micrograms of levothyroxine (thyroxine) is sufficient to provide 16.43 powders.

Step 4

Now work out the total amount required for the final number of powders. Each powder is to weigh 100 mg, so 16.43 powders will equal:

$$16.43 \times 100 = 1{,}643 \text{ mg}$$

Step 5

Weigh the tablets and make up to the final amount required (1,643 mg) with lactose.

$5 \times 100 \text{ micrograms} + 1 \times 50 \text{ micrograms} + 1 \times 25 \text{ micrograms} = 0.7028 \text{ g}$

$= 702.8 \text{ mg} = 703 \text{ mg (rounded up)}$

tablets   703 mg   (contains 575 micrograms of levothyroxine (thyroxine))
lactose   <u>940</u> mg   (1,643 mg − 703 mg)
        1,643 mg

You have 575 micrograms levothyroxine (thyroxine) in 1,643 mg, so each 100 mg of this final dilution will contain 35 micrograms of levothyroxine (thyroxine):

$$\frac{575}{1{,}643} \times 100 = 35 \text{ micrograms}$$

Therefore weigh 16 lots of 100 mg (14 plus 2 backups), as required.

Body surface area estimates

Cancer chemotherapy is usually dosed using body surface area (BSA). BSA has been chosen rather than body weight to calculate doses for two reasons:

- it provides a more accurate estimation of effect and toxicity
- it more closely correlates to blood flow to the liver and kidneys, which are the major organs for drug elimination.

Cancer drugs have a lower therapeutic index (the difference between an effective and a toxic dose) than most other drugs, i.e. the difference between an underdose and an overdose is small and the consequences can be life-threatening. Therefore, cancer chemotherapy needs a precise and reliable method of determining the BSA and dose.

Body surface area is difficult to measure. Several different formulas and nomograms have been derived for predicting surface area from measurements of height and weight. For accuracy, BSA should be calculated to three significant figures. Slide rules and nomograms are incapable of calculating with this degree of accuracy. In addition, they suffer from error associated with their analogue nature and the formulas they are based on.

> Using a recognized formula is a more accurate way to calculate BSA than using a nomogram. Nomograms should only be used as a rough guide or estimate.

FORMULAS FOR CALCULATING BODY SURFACE AREA

There are many formulas for calculating BSA. The formula derived by Mosteller (1987) combines an accurate BSA calculation with ease of use, and has been validated for use in both children and adults.

$$BSA\ (m^2) = \sqrt{\frac{height\ (cm) \times weight\ (kg)}{3600}}$$

This formula can be used on a handheld calculator.

For example, you want to know the body surface area of a child whose weight is 16.4 kg and height 100 cm.

Substitute the figures in the formula:

$$BSA\ (m^2) = \sqrt{\frac{100 \times 16.4}{3600}}$$

$$= \sqrt{\frac{1640}{3600}}$$

$$= \sqrt{0.4555}$$

$$= 0.675$$

Tip First, do the sum in the top line: $100 \times 16.4 = 1640$.
Next, divide by 3600 to give 0.4555.
Finally, find the square root to give an answer of 0.675.

NOMOGRAMS

In 1916, Du Bois and Du Bois derived a formula to estimate BSA on which many nomograms are based. Although they used measurements of only nine individuals, one of whom was a child, and made certain assumptions in developing the formula, this remains the most popular nomogram for calculating BSA.

However, many investigators have since questioned the accuracy of the Du Bois formula. Haycock *et al.* (1978) reported that the formula underestimates surface area by up to 8% in infants, especially as values fell below 0.7 m^2. Nomograms based on the formula derived by Haycock *et al.* are now used in paediatric books, with separate nomograms for infants (Figure A3.1) and for children and adults (Figure A3.2).

Before you can use the nomogram, you have to know the patient's height and weight. Once these have been measured, a straight line edge (e.g. a ruler) is placed from the patient's height in the left column to their weight in the right column, and the intersect on the body surface area column indicates the body surface area.

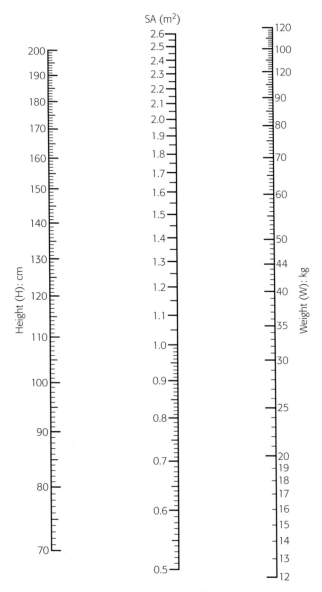

Fig. A3.1 Nomogram for estimating body surface area in infants

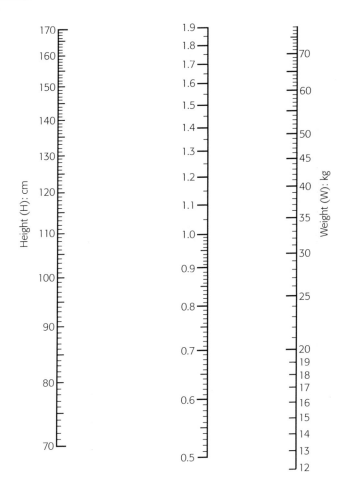

Fig. A3.2 Nomogram for estimating body surface area in children and adults

Example

From our original example (a child weighing 16.4 kg whose height is 100 cm), we can use the nomogram for children and adults.

Align the left-hand side of the ruler against the 100 cm mark on the left-hand column. Next, align the right-hand side of the ruler halfway between 16 and 17 kg on the right-hand column (as close as we can get to 16.4 kg).

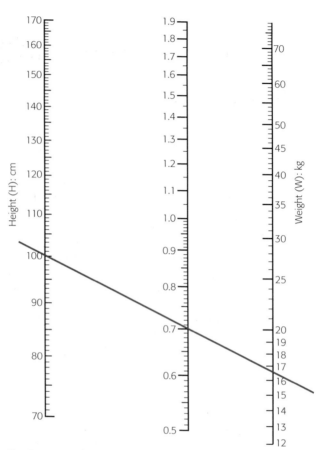

Fig. A3.3 Example of estimating the body surface area for a child

Now read off where the ruler intersects the centre column, which indicates body surface area (Figure A3.3). In this case it is 0.7 m^2.

REFERENCES

Du Bois D, Du Bois EF A formula to estimate the approximate surface area if height and weight be known. *Archives of Internal Medicine* 1916; 17: 863–871.

Haycock GB, Schwartz GJ, Wisotsky DH Geometric method for measuring body surface area: a height-weight formula validated in infants, children and adults. *Journal of Pediatrics* 1978; 93: 62–66.

Mosteller RD Simplified calculation of body-surface area. *New England Journal of Medicine* 1987; 317: 1098.

Body mass index (BMI)

WHAT IS BMI?

Body mass index or BMI (wt/ht^2), based on an individual's height and weight, is a helpful indicator of obesity and underweight in adults.

BMI compares well to body fat, but cannot be interpreted just as a certain percentage of body fat. The relation between fatness and BMI is influenced by age and gender. For example, women are more likely to have a higher percentage of body fat than men for the same BMI. At the same BMI, older people have more body fat than younger adults.

The BMI is used to screen and monitor a population to detect risk of health or nutritional disorders. In an individual, other data must be used to determine if a high BMI is associated with increased risk of disease and death for that person. BMI alone is not diagnostic.

HOW DOES BMI RELATE TO HEALTH AMONG ADULTS?

A healthy BMI for adults is between 18.5 and 24.9. BMI ranges are based on the effect body weight has on disease and death.

A high BMI is predictive of death from cardiovascular disease. Diabetes, cancer, high blood pressure and osteoarthritis are also common consequences of overweight and obesity in adults. Obesity itself is a strong risk factor for premature death.

BMI CUTPOINTS FOR ADULTS

We interpret BMI values for adults with one fixed number, regardless of age or sex, using the following guidelines:

- Underweight   BMI < 20
- Acceptable   BMI 20–25
- Overweight   BMI 25–30
- Obese   BMI 30–40
- Morbidly obese   BMI > 40.

These ranges are indicated in the table.

Table 14 BMI table

Stones	Pounds	Kilograms	5'0" 1.52	5'1" 1.55	5'2" 1.57	5'3" 1.6	5'4" 1.63	5'5" 1.65	5'6" 1.68	5'7" 1.7	5'8" 1.73	5'9" 1.75	5'10" 1.78	5'11" 1.8	6'0" 1.83	6'1" 1.85	6'2" 1.88	6'3" 1.91	6'4" 1.93	6'5" 1.96	6'6" 1.98
6	0	38	16	16	15	15	14	14	13	13	13	12	12	12	11	11	11	10	10	10	10
6	2	39	17	16	16	15	15	14	14	13	13	13	12	12	12	11	11	11	10	10	10
6	4	40	17	17	16	16	15	15	14	14	13	13	13	12	12	12	11	11	11	10	10
6	6	41	18	17	17	16	15	15	15	14	14	13	13	13	12	12	12	11	11	11	10
6	8	42	18	17	17	16	16	15	15	15	14	14	13	13	13	12	12	12	11	11	11
6	10	43	19	18	17	17	16	16	15	15	14	14	14	13	13	13	12	12	12	11	11
6	12	44	19	18	18	17	17	16	16	15	15	14	14	14	13	13	12	12	12	11	11
7	0	44	19	18	18	17	17	16	16	15	15	14	14	14	13	13	12	12	12	11	11
7	2	45	19	19	18	18	17	17	16	16	15	15	14	14	13	13	13	12	12	12	11
7	4	46	20	19	19	18	17	17	16	16	15	15	15	14	14	13	13	13	12	12	12
7	6	47	20	20	19	18	18	17	17	16	16	15	15	15	14	14	13	13	13	12	12
7	8	48	21	20	19	19	18	18	17	17	16	16	15	15	14	14	14	13	13	13	12
7	11	49	21	20	20	19	18	18	17	17	16	16	15	15	15	14	14	13	13	13	13
7	12	50	22	21	20	20	19	18	18	17	17	16	16	15	15	15	14	14	13	13	13
8	0	51	22	21	21	20	19	19	18	18	17	17	16	16	15	15	14	14	14	13	13
8	2	52	23	22	21	20	20	19	18	18	17	17	16	16	16	15	15	14	14	14	13
8	4	53	23	22	22	21	20	19	19	18	18	17	17	16	16	15	15	15	14	14	14
8	6	54	23	22	22	21	20	20	19	19	18	18	17	17	16	16	15	15	15	14	14
8	8	54	23	22	22	21	20	20	19	19	18	18	17	17	16	16	15	15	15	14	14
8	10	55	24	23	22	21	21	20	19	19	18	18	17	17	16	16	16	15	15	14	14
8	12	56	24	23	23	22	21	21	20	19	19	18	18	17	17	16	16	15	15	15	14
9	0	57	25	24	23	22	21	21	20	20	19	19	18	18	17	17	16	16	15	15	15
9	2	58	25	24	24	23	22	21	21	20	19	19	18	18	17	17	16	16	16	15	15

st	lb	kg																		
9	4	59	26	25	25	24	23	22	22	21	20	20	19	19	18	18	17	17	16	15
9	6	60	26	25	25	24	23	23	22	21	20	20	19	19	18	18	17	17	16	16
9	8	61	26	26	25	24	24	23	22	22	21	20	20	19	18	18	17	17	16	16
9	10	62	27	26	26	25	24	23	23	22	21	21	20	20	19	18	18	17	17	16
9	12	63	27	27	26	25	24	24	23	22	22	21	20	20	19	19	18	18	17	16
10	0	64	28	27	27	26	25	24	24	23	22	21	21	20	20	19	18	18	17	17
10	2	64	28	27	27	26	25	25	24	23	22	22	21	20	20	19	19	18	17	17
10	4	65	28	28	27	26	26	25	24	24	23	22	21	21	20	19	19	18	18	17
10	6	66	29	28	28	27	26	25	25	24	23	22	22	21	20	20	19	19	18	18
10	8	67	29	29	28	27	26	26	25	24	24	23	22	21	21	20	20	19	18	18
10	10	68	30	29	29	28	27	26	26	25	24	23	23	22	21	21	20	20	19	19
10	12	69	30	30	29	28	27	27	26	25	25	24	23	22	22	21	21	20	19	19
11	0	70	31	30	30	29	28	27	27	26	25	24	24	23	22	22	21	20	20	19
11	2	71	31	31	30	29	28	28	27	26	26	25	24	23	23	22	21	21	20	20
11	4	72	32	31	31	30	29	28	28	27	26	25	25	24	23	22	22	21	21	20
11	6	73	32	32	31	30	30	29	28	27	27	26	25	24	24	23	22	22	21	20
11	8	74	32	32	32	31	30	29	29	28	27	26	25	25	24	23	23	22	21	21
11	10	74	33	32	32	31	31	30	29	28	28	27	26	25	25	24	23	23	22	21
11	12	75	33	33	32	32	31	30	30	29	28	27	27	26	25	24	24	23	22	22
12	0	76	34	33	33	32	31	31	30	29	29	28	27	26	26	25	24	24	23	22
12	2	77	34	34	33	32	32	31	30	30	29	28	28	27	26	25	25	24	23	23
12	4	78	35	34	34	33	32	32	31	30	30	29	28	28	27	26	25	25	24	23
12	6	79	35	34	34	33	33	32	31	31	30	29	28	28	27	26	26	25	24	24
12	8	80	35	35	34	34	33	32	32	31	30	29	29	28	27	27	26	25	24	24
12	10	81	36	35	35	34	33	33	32	31	31	30	29	28	28	27	26	26	25	24
12	12	82	36	35	35	34	34	33	32	32	31	30	30	29	28	27	26	26	25	25
13	0	83	36	36	35	35	34	33	33	32	31	30	30	29	28	28	27	26	25	25
13	2	83	36	36	35	35	34	34	33	32	32	31	30	29	29	28	27	27	26	25
13	4	84	36	36	35	35	34	34	33	33	32	31	31	30	29	28	28	27	26	26

BMI < 20 = Underweight; BMI 20–25 = Acceptable; BMI 25–30 = Overweight; BMI 30–40 = Obese; BMI >40 = Morbidly obese

Table 14 *continued*

Stones	Pounds	Kilograms	5'0" (1.52)	5'1" (1.55)	5'2" (1.57)	5'3" (1.6)	5'4" (1.63)	5'5" (1.65)	5'6" (1.68)	5'7" (1.7)	5'8" (1.73)	5'9" (1.75)	5'10" (1.78)	5'11" (1.8)	6'0" (1.83)	6'1" (1.85)	6'2" (1.88)	6'3" (1.91)	6'4" (1.93)	6'5" (1.96)	6'6" (1.98)
13	6	85	37	35	34	33	32	31	30	29	28	28	27	26	25	25	24	23	23	22	22
13	8	86	37	36	35	34	32	32	30	30	29	28	27	27	26	25	24	24	23	22	22
13	10	87	38	36	35	34	33	32	31	30	29	28	27	27	26	25	25	24	23	23	22
13	12	88	38	37	36	34	33	32	31	30	29	29	28	27	26	26	25	24	24	23	22
14	0	89	39	37	36	35	33	33	32	31	30	29	28	27	27	26	25	24	24	23	23
14	2	90	39	37	37	35	34	33	32	31	30	29	28	28	27	26	25	25	24	23	23
14	4	91	39	38	37	36	34	33	32	31	30	30	29	28	27	27	25	25	24	24	23
14	6	92	40	38	37	36	35	34	33	32	31	30	29	28	27	27	26	25	25	24	23
14	8	93	40	39	38	36	35	34	33	32	31	30	29	29	28	27	26	25	25	24	24
14	10	93	40	39	38	36	35	34	33	32	31	30	29	29	28	27	26	25	25	24	24
14	12	94	41	39	38	37	35	35	33	33	31	31	30	29	28	27	27	26	25	24	24
15	0	95	41	40	39	37	36	35	34	33	32	31	30	29	28	28	27	26	26	25	24
15	2	96	42	40	39	38	36	35	34	33	32	31	30	30	29	28	27	26	26	25	24
15	4	97	42	40	39	38	37	36	34	34	32	32	31	30	29	28	27	27	26	25	25
15	6	98	42	41	40	38	37	36	35	34	33	32	31	30	29	29	28	27	26	26	25
15	8	99	43	41	40	39	37	36	35	34	33	32	31	31	30	29	28	27	27	26	25
15	10	100	43	42	41	39	38	37	35	35	33	33	32	31	30	29	29	27	27	26	26
15	12	101	44	42	41	39	38	37	36	35	34	33	32	31	30	30	29	28	27	26	26
16	0	102	44	42	41	40	38	37	36	35	34	33	32	31	30	30	29	28	27	27	26
16	2	103	45	43	42	40	39	38	36	36	34	34	33	32	31	30	29	28	28	27	26
16	4	103	45	43	42	40	39	38	36	36	34	34	33	32	31	30	29	28	28	27	27
16	6	104	45	43	42	41	39	39	37	36	35	34	33	32	31	30	30	29	28	27	27
16	8	105	45	44	43	41	40	39	37	36	35	34	33	32	31	31	30	29	28	27	27
16	10	106	46	44	43	41	40	39	38	37	35	35	33	33	32	31	30	29	28	28	27

st–lb	kg																			
16–12	107	46	45	43	42	40	39	38	37	36	35	34	33	32	31	30	29	29	28	27
17–0	108	47	45	44	42	41	40	38	37	36	35	34	33	32	32	31	30	29	28	28
17–2	109	47	45	44	43	41	40	39	38	36	36	34	33	33	32	31	30	29	28	28
17–4	110	48	46	45	43	41	40	39	38	37	36	35	34	33	32	31	30	30	29	28
17–6	111	48	46	45	43	42	41	39	38	37	36	35	34	33	32	31	30	30	29	28
17–8	112	48	47	45	44	42	41	40	39	37	36	35	34	33	33	32	31	30	29	29
17–10	112	48	47	45	44	42	41	40	39	37	37	35	34	33	33	32	31	30	29	29
17–13	114	49	47	46	45	43	41	40	39	38	37	35	35	34	33	32	31	31	30	29
18–0	114	49	47	46	45	43	42	41	39	38	37	36	35	34	33	32	31	31	30	29
18–2	115	50	48	47	45	43	42	41	40	38	37	36	35	34	34	33	31	31	30	29
18–4	116	50	48	47	45	44	42	41	40	39	38	36	36	35	34	33	31	31	30	29
18–6	117	51	49	47	46	44	43	42	41	39	38	37	36	35	34	33	32	31	30	29
18–8	118	51	49	48	46	44	43	42	41	39	38	37	36	35	34	33	32	32	31	30
18–10	119	52	50	48	47	45	44	43	42	40	39	37	37	36	35	34	32	32	31	30
18–12	120	52	50	49	47	45	44	43	42	40	39	37	37	36	35	35	33	32	31	30
19–0	121	52	50	49	48	46	45	43	42	40	39	38	37	36	35	35	33	32	31	30
19–2	122	53	51	49	48	46	45	43	43	41	40	38	37	36	36	36	33	33	31	31
19–4	122	53	51	49	48	46	45	44	43	41	40	38	38	37	36	36	33	33	32	31
19–6	123	53	51	50	48	47	45	44	43	41	40	39	38	37	37	36	33	33	32	31
19–8	124	54	52	50	49	47	46	44	43	42	41	39	38	37	37	36	34	33	32	31
19–10	125	54	52	51	49	47	46	45	44	42	41	39	38	38	37	36	34	34	32	31
19–12	126	55	52	51	50	48	46	45	44	42	41	39	39	38	37	37	34	34	33	31
20–0	127	55	53	52	50	48	47	45	44	43	41	40	39	38	38	37	34	34	33	32
20–2	128	55	53	52	50	49	47	46	45	43	42	40	39	38	38	37	35	35	33	32
20–4	129	56	54	52	51	49	48	46	45	43	42	40	40	39	38	37	35	35	34	32
20–6	130	56	54	53	51	49	48	46	45	44	42	41	40	39	38	37	35	35	34	32
20–8	131	57	55	53	52	50	48	47	46	44	43	41	40	39	39	38	36	35	34	33
20–10	132	57	55	54	52	50	48	47	46	44	43	42	41	39	39	38	36	35	34	34
20–12	132	57	55	54	52	50	48	47	46	44	43	42	41	39	39	38	36	35	34	34

BMI < 20 = Underweight; BMI 20–25 = Acceptable; BMI 25–30 = Overweight; BMI 30–40 = Obese; BMI >40 = Morbidly obese

Estimation of renal function

MEASURING CREATININE CLEARANCE

Creatinine is a muscle breakdown product and the serum concentration of creatinine does not change from day to day because the rate of production is constant and is equal to the rate at which it is eliminated from the body. Thus creatinine clearance (CrCl) is used as a measure of the glomerular filtration rate (GFR) and hence renal function.

The rate of creatinine production is related to the amount of creatinine in the body which, in turn, is related to the lean body mass. This differs between males and females of equal weight and, in addition, the lean body mass decreases with age. Therefore any attempt to correlate serum creatinine to renal function should take into account age, weight and sex of the patient.

Various formulas have been devised and all assume that the patient has normal body mass for their age. However, in cases where this may not be so, e.g. body builders and patients with muscle-wasting disease, errors in estimation can occur.

Cockcroft and Gault (1976) suggested the following formulas, which apply to adults aged 20+:

- Men

$$\text{CrCl (mL/min)} = \frac{1.23 \times (140 - \text{age}) \times \text{weight}}{\text{serum creatinine (micromol/L)}}$$

$$\text{CrCl (mL/min)} = \frac{(140 - \text{age}) \times \text{weight}}{\text{serum creatinine (mg/100 mL)}}$$

- Women

$$\text{CrCl (mL/min)} = \frac{1.04 \times (140 - \text{age}) \times \text{weight}}{\text{serum creatinine (micromol/L)}}$$

$$\text{CrCl (mL/min)} = \frac{(140 - \text{age}) \times \text{weight}}{85 \times \text{serum creatinine (mg/100 mL)}}$$

Ensure that the correct value and units are used for serum
creatinine.

WORKED EXAMPLE

Male patient aged 67 years, weight 72 kg, with a serum creatinine of
125 micromol/L.

As the units of the serum creatinine are given in micromoles, we
must ensure that the right formula is used:

$$\text{CrCl (mL/min)} = \frac{1.23 \times (140 - \text{age}) \times \text{weight}}{\text{serum creatinine (micromol/L)}}$$

where:

age (years) = 67
weight (kg) = 72
serum creatinine (micromol/mL) = 125

Substitute the figures in the formula:

$$\text{CrCl (mL/min)} = \frac{1.23 \times (140 - 67) \times 72}{125 \text{ (micromol /L)}} = 51.7 \text{ mL/min}$$

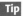 In the top line, the sum within the brackets is done first, i.e.
$(140 - 67) = 73$, then multiply by 1.23 and then by 72, so the
sum is $1.23 \times 73 \times 72 = 6464.88$.

REFERENCE

Cockcroft D, Gault MH. Prediction of creatinine clearance from
serum creatinine. *Nephron* 1976; 16: 31–41.

Abbreviations used in prescriptions

Although directions should preferably be given in English without abbreviation, some Latin abbreviations are still used.

The following is a list of common abbreviations for Latin and other terms that are commonly used. It should be noted that the English version is not an exact translation.

Some of these abbreviations may vary as they depend on local convention.

Table 15 Abbreviations

Abbreviation	Latin derivation	English meaning
a.c.	*ante cibum*	before food
alte die	*alterna die*	alternate days
appli	*applicatio*	an application
aurist.	*auristillae*	ear drops
b.d.	*bis die*	twice daily
b.i.d.	*bis in die*	twice a day
c or c̄	*cum*	with
c.c.	*cum cibum*	with food
		(also: cubic centimetre)
crem	*cremor*	a cream
d	*dies*	daily
elix		elixir
gtt (g)	*guttae*	drops
h	*hors*	hour/at the hour of
h.s.	*hora somni*	at bedtime
		(lit: at the hour of sleep)

Table 15 *continued*

Abbreviation	Latin derivation	English meaning
INH		inhaler/to be inhaled
inj		an injection
IM		intramuscular
irrig	*irrigatio*	an irrigation
IV		intravenously
IU		International Units
m	*mane*	morning
m.d.u	*mor dictus utendus*	to be used or taken as directed
mist	*mistura*	mixture
mitte		please dispense (lit: send)
n	*nocte*	night
NEB		nebules/to be nebulized
o	*omni*	every
oculent (oc)	*oculentum*	eye ointment
o.d. (OD)	*omni die*	every day (daily)
o.m. (OM)	*omni mane*	every morning
o.n. (ON)	*omni nocte*	every night
p.c. (PC)	*post cibum*	after food
p.o. (PO)	*per os*	orally (by mouth)
p.r. (PR)	*per rectum*	rectally
p.r.n. (PRN)	*pro re nata*	occasionally (when required)
p.v. (PV)	*per vagina*	vaginally
q	*quaque*	each/every (e.g. q6h = every 6 hours)
q.i.d. (QID)	*quarter in die*	four times a day
q.d.s. (QDS)	*quater die sumendus*	to be taken four times a day
Rx		'recipe' = take
s̄		without
sig	*signa*	let it be labelled
SC		subcutaneous
SL		sublingual
s.o.s.	*si opus sit*	if required
stat	*statum*	at once
supp *or* suppos	*suppositorium*	a suppository

Table 15 *continued*

Abbreviation	Latin derivation	English meaning
TDD		total daily dose
t.i.d. (TID)	*ter in die*	three times a day
t.d.s. (TDS)	*ter die sumendus*	to be taken three times a day
TOP		topically
U *or* UN		units
ung	*unguentum*	an ointment

Other abbreviations

$\odot$		unit (as in unit of blood)
@		at
1^0		hourly
2^0		2 hourly, etc.
$\frac{2}{7}$		for 2 days, etc.
$\frac{2}{52}$		for 2 weeks, etc.
$\frac{2}{12}$		for 2 months, etc.

Weight and height conversion tables

Patients' weight is often still given in stones and their height in feet and inches. These have to be converted to kilograms and centimetres respectively, especially when working out dosages. A lot of dosages are either calculated on a 'weight basis' (e.g. mg/kg/day) or on a 'surface area basis' (e.g. mg/m², particularly cytotoxic drugs). The following tables show weight and height conversions.

Table 16 Weight conversion table

Stones	Kilograms	Pounds	Kilograms
1	6.4	1	0.5
2	12.7	2	0.9
3	19.1	3	1.4
4	25.4	4	1.8
5	31.8	5	2.3
6	38.1	6	2.7
7	44.5	7	3.2
8	50.8	8	3.6
9	57.2	9	4.1
10	63.5	10	4.5
11	69.9	11	5.0
12	76.2	12	5.4
13	82.6	13	5.9
14	88.9		
15	95.3	Weights correct to 0.1 kg	
16	101.6		
17	108.0	**Weight conversion factors**	
18	114.3	Stones to kilograms: ×6.3503	
19	120.7	Pounds to kilograms: ×0.4536	
20	127.0	Kilograms to stones: ×0.1575	
21	133.4	Kilograms to pounds: ×2.2046	

Table 17 Height conversion table

Feet	Centimetres	Inches	Centimetres
1	30.5	1	2.5
2	61.0	2	5.1
3	91.4	3	7.6
4	121.9	4	10.2
5	152.4	5	12.7
6	182.9	6	15.2
		7	17.8
Heights correct to 0.1 cm		8	20.3
		9	22.9
Height conversion factors		10	25.4
Feet to centimetres: ×30.48		11	27.9
Inches to centimetres: ×2.54			
Centimetres to feet: ×0.328			
Centimetres to inches: ×0.3937			

WORKED EXAMPLE: CONVERTING 14 STONES 4 POUNDS TO THE NEAREST KG

Method 1

Using the conversion table:

$$
\begin{aligned}
14 \text{ stones } &= 88.9 \text{ kg} \\
+ \ 4 \text{ pounds } &= \ \ 1.8 \text{ kg} \\
&= 90.7 \text{ kg}
\end{aligned}
$$

Answer: 91 kg (to nearest kg).

Method 1

Use the conversion factor for stones to kilograms ($\times 6.3503$):

14 stones = $14 \times 6.3503 = 88.9042$ kg

Use the conversion factor for pounds to kilograms ($\times 0.4536$):

4 pounds = $4 \times 0.4536 = 1.8144$ kg

Add the two together:

88.9042 kg + 1.8144 kg = 90.7186 kg

Answer: 91 kg (to nearest kg).

WORKED EXAMPLE: CONVERTING 6 FEET 2 INCHES TO THE NEAREST CM

Method 1

Using the conversion table:

$$
\begin{aligned}
6 \text{ feet } &= 182.9 \text{ cm} \\
+ \ 2 \text{ inches } &= \ \ \ 5.1 \text{ cm} \\
&= 188.0 \text{ cm}
\end{aligned}
$$

Answer: 188 cm (to nearest cm).

Method 2

Using the conversion factors feet to centimetres ($\times 30.48$):

6 feet = $6 \times 30.48 = 182.88$ cm

Use the conversion factor inches to centimetres ($\times 2.54$):

2 inches = $2 \times 2.54 = 5.08$ cm

Add the two together:

182.88 cm + 5.08 cm = 187.96 cm

Answer: 188 cm (to nearest cm).

Index

About the Authors

1 2002 **Janice Maynard** left a career as an primary chool teacher to pursue writing full-time. Her first love creating sexy, character-driven, contemporary omance. She has written for Kensington and NAL, and is very happy to be part of the Mills & Boon family – a ifelong dream. Janice and her husband live in the hadow of the Great Smoky Mountains. They love to hike and travel. Visit her at www.JaniceMaynard.com

SA Today bestselling author **Katherine Garbera** is a wo-time Maggie winner who has written more than inety books. A Florida native who grew up to travel the lobe, Katherine now makes her home in the Midlands f the UK with her husband, two children and a very poiled miniature dachshund. Visit her on the web at tp://www.katherinegarbera.com, connect with her on Facebook and follow her on Twitter @katheringarbera

Andrea Laurence is an award-winning contemporary author who has been a lover of books and writing stories since she learned to read. A dedicated West Coast girl transplanted into the Deep South, she's constantly trying develop a taste for sweet tea and grits while caring for r boyfriend and her old bulldog. You can contact ndrea at her website: http://www.andrealaurence.com

Dynasties

Dynasties: The Montoros

JANICE MAYNARD

KATHERINE GARBERA

ANDREA LAURENCE

MILLS & BOON

First Published in Great Britain 2020
By Mills & Boon, an imprint of HarperCollins*Publishers*
1 London Bridge Street, London, SE1 9GF

DYNASTIES: THE MONTOROS © 2020 Harlequin Books S.A.

Minding Her Boss's Business © 2015 Harlequin Books S.A.
Carrying A King's Child © 2015 Harlequin Books S.A.
Seduced by the Spare Heir © 2015 Harlequin Books S.A.

Special thanks and acknowledgement are given to Janice Maynard,
Katherine Garbera and Andrea Laurence for their contribution to
the *Dynasties: The Montoros* series.

ISBN: 978-0-263-28147-7

This I

Fo

MINDING HER BOSS'S BUSINESS

JANICE MAYNARD

For little girls everywhere who dream of being princesses: This one's for you...

One

Alex Ramon winced as shards of pain lanced his temples. Though the splitting headache was undoubtedly a result of jet lag and too little sleep for the past couple of weeks, it could also be attributed to stress. At the moment, his particular stressor stood on the opposite side of the room…a tall, leggy blonde in a formfitting aquamarine dress and killer heels.

Maria Ferro. Aged twenty-seven. Straight, honey-colored hair that tumbled like a silky waterfall almost to her ass. He probably shouldn't be thinking about her ass. Definitely not. But tonight it was difficult not to notice.

Reluctantly, he dragged his attention from his coworker and surveyed the room. By all accounts, the party was going swimmingly. The delegation of business leaders from the European island nation of Alma mingled with the various members of the Montoro family, everyone chatting with animation and cordiality.

The ballroom was situated on the ground floor of one of Miami's premier hotels. An entire wall of glass showcased the azure ocean. Priceless chandeliers cast sparkles across the polished hardwood floor. The decor was understated, modern and sophisticated. Much like the wealthy Montoro family themselves.

Alex inserted a finger beneath the collar of his tux and tugged. He was more than accustomed to upscale social functions. But in this moment, restlessness plagued him. As Alma's deputy prime minister of commerce, he carried the lion's share of the responsibility for convincing the Montoros to return to their homeland and resume the throne.

A lot was riding on tonight and the days to come.

This evening's soiree was only the beginning…a chance for the delegation to be introduced and to establish personal contact with the family whose ancestors once ruled Alma. Unfortunately, the men and women in the youngest generation, all twenty-somethings, were more interested in hard-driving business deals and hard-partying social lives than in resurrecting any royal roots.

A throaty laugh echoed across the room. Maria was clearly enjoying her handsome companion. Gabriel Montoro, middle child of Rafael III, epitomized the classic bad boy…fun loving, hard to pin down, heedless of anyone's opinion. Alex wanted to dismiss him as a lightweight player, but in fact, Gabriel ran the South American division of Montoro Enterprises with surprising success. He was headquartered in Miami, which meant he would be involved in the upcoming negotiations.

Alex was surprised that the usually sensible Maria didn't see through Gabriel's facade. Perhaps she was blinded by the man's green eyes, tousled hair and golden skin. Alex wasn't jealous. That would be ludicrous. He and Maria were nothing more than business associates. But he was half a dozen years older than she was, and he felt protective of her.

She had worked for his family in London. Then, when political power changed hands in Alma and the Ramons were able to return to their homeland, Maria had come, as well, along with her mother. Alex had watched with satisfaction as Maria's talent and hard work brought opportunities her way. Now, as a marketing and PR expert, she was set to play an integral role in this new venture.

Alex admired and respected Maria. She was too nice a woman to be taken in by a jaded playboy like Gabriel Montoro.

Decades had passed since the last Montoro monarch was deposed by a dictator in the aftermath of the Second World War. Four generations later the family enjoyed the fruits of a shipping and trade empire that spanned half the globe.

The Montoros were happy and successful in Miami… legendary for their wealth and lifestyle. Only time would tell if they could be persuaded by duty and honor to walk a different path.

Alex made his way around the perimeter of the room, stopping to make introductions and to chat with this person and that. In his hotel room he possessed lengthy dossiers on each of the key players in tonight's drama. Though he had glanced over his notes before coming downstairs, the information was stored in his brain.

That was how he worked. Prepare for every eventuality. Plan for any outcome. Make no mistakes.

At last he reached the small alcove where Maria and Gabriel stood. She held a glass of wine in one hand, though Alex hadn't seen her drink more than a few sips. Gabriel

Montoro appeared to be offering her naughty vignettes about their fellow partygoers.

Deliberately, Alex took his place at Maria's side and gave Montoro a steady glance. "Mr. Montoro. I'm Alex Ramon."

Gabriel nodded as the two of them shook hands. "I know. My father speaks highly of you. I have to tell you, though, you may have your work cut out for you. None of us are particularly interested in playing dress up with crowns and thrones and an antiquated system that has seen its day."

Alex rubbed a hand across his chin, hoping to defuse the awkward moment with humor. "Why don't you tell me what you're *really* thinking?" The man's blunt honesty caught him off guard.

Gabriel shrugged. "I'm not sure what all of you hope to gain."

Maria shot Alex a glance as if to caution tact. But Alex was off his game. And irritated. "Alma is in the midst of important changes. Restoring the monarchy in a ceremonial role is a popular idea with the people at large. The offshore oil reserves have made the country wealthy, but we need stability. A royal marriage would ensure that."

Gabriel's smile was mocking. "How very feudal of you, Mr. Ramon."

"This is not something to joke about. The lives and well-being of thousands of people are at stake here. Your family's history is part and parcel of Alma's identity."

Gabriel shook his head. "They threw us out with nothing but the clothes on our backs."

Alex shoved his hands in his pockets. He had the most insane urge to throttle the guy. Wouldn't that be a royal mess… "They didn't throw *you* out," he said, the words even. "You weren't even born. And the people had no say in it. You know what Tantaberra was like. He'd shoot first and ask questions later."

Gabriel shrugged. "Whatever. The point is, if you're trying to make my family and me face up to some kind of obligation, you're way off course. We have a good life here in Miami. Why would we want to return to a tiny backwater collection of islands that time forgot?"

Maria spoke up, her blue-green eyes sparkling with passion. "Alma has changed, Mr. Montoro. We have high-speed broadband internet access, satellite television and radio and a thriving business community. Along with the natural beauty of the land, we have much to offer."

Gabriel wasn't convinced. "I can find all that and more here in the US."

Alex played his trump card. "But think of your aunt… you know what she wants…"

A flicker in the other man's eyes told Alex he'd finally scored a point. Isabella, at seventy-three, was the oldest living Montoro. It was her dearest wish that her grandchildren, grandnieces and grandnephews return to their homeland for the sake of family honor. She was dying… caught up in the advanced stages of Parkinson's disease. Alex had a notion she was hanging on only long enough to see the transfer of power take place.

Gabriel downed the last of his champagne and plucked another crystal flute from the tray offered by a passing waiter. "Aunt Isabella lives in the past. We do not always get what we want."

"I think that's a song," Maria said, smiling. Clearly she was trying to lighten the mood. But Alex was in no frame of mind to be appeased. Gabriel Montoro rubbed him the wrong way. The man had wealth, power, good looks and sex appeal. It was rumored that women besieged him all hours of the night and day. Surely Maria wouldn't be so naive as to be taken in by him.

Gabriel sipped his drink, his gaze stormy. "Lucky for you, my father retains some vestige of the old ways. Perhaps he can be persuaded. Who knows?"

Alex winced, as did Maria. Maria laid a hand on Montoro's arm briefly, as if to placate him. "I think no one has told you," she said softly. "But your father cannot reign."

"Why the hell not?"

It was oddly amusing that even though Gabriel insisted his family had no interest in the monarchy, he was incensed at the notion his father was ineligible.

Alex took a deep breath and exhaled. "Your father is divorced. His marriage was not annulled. Under the tenets of Alma law, that legally disqualifies him."

"Hell of a way to operate a country. You should be damn glad I'm not in the running. If a man of my father's caliber is not on the short list, I'd never make the cut." The sarcasm was laced with disdain.

"This isn't personal, Mr. Montoro. We're merely trying to follow the traditions and expectations of our people."

Maria nodded. "Alex is right, of course. The situation is unprecedented. We are trying our best to make it work."

"But neither of you even lived in Alma until Tantaberra was ousted. Why do you care?"

Alex remained silent, unable to give voice to the emotions roiling inside him. Fortunately, Maria was more vocal. "Alex's family met the same fate as yours long ago, Gabriel. They, however, settled in London and rebuilt their fortunes in oil and gas. When Tantaberra was finally overthrown, Alex's father determined that returning to Alma was the right thing to do."

Gabriel shook his head, draining the second glass of champagne. "I seem to be surrounded by proponents of duty above desire. Thank God, my brother is the one in the hot seat. You'll never find a more honorable man. But whether or not he's interested in a crown remains to be seen."

Alex took Maria's elbow in a loose grip. "If you'll excuse us, Mr. Montoro, Maria and I need to mingle. I'm sure we'll meet again."

Gabriel eyed both of them, his rueful smile half apology, half derision. "I'm sure we will. How long do you anticipate staying in Miami to stir the pot?"

"A month, give or take. We have a great deal of work to do. The official request from Alma to the Montoro family is in the process of being drafted."

Maria spoke up. "And I'll be working on press releases and rollouts to the public. We want everything to be positive and upbeat."

"And if my family refuses?" Gabriel's steely-eyed gaze held not a whit of humor.

It was Alex's turn to shrug. "If your brother agrees, the rest of you will be free to make your own choices. Although, for the sake of a smooth transition, your support will mean a lot to him, I would think."

Maria grimaced. "This is a huge undertaking, Mr. Montoro."

"I asked you to call me Gabriel," he said. "And you, too, Alex. I'm not one to stand on ceremony." If he was making a point, it was subtle.

"Gabriel, then," she said. "We take our charge very seriously. I hope you'll give us a chance to win you over."

He chuckled. "Fair enough."

His relaxed response sent a wave of relief crashing through Alex. It would be bad form to alienate one of the royal family right out of the gate. Gabriel had been pissed a moment ago, but his tone and demeanor were mellower now.

"I appreciate your plain speaking," Alex said, his customary diplomacy back in working order. "I'll look forward to continuing our conversation."

Maria allowed Alex to steer her away from the Montoro bad boy, but for once, she couldn't read her boss. He led her toward the buffet. "Have you eaten anything?" he asked gruffly.

Her stomach rumbled on cue. "No. I was too nervous."

He handed her a plate. "We've both been working nonstop for weeks. I think we deserve a break."

Maria surveyed the bounty with anticipation. Fresh seafood, everything from shrimp cocktail to crab legs to raw oysters, filled silver trays to overflowing. The various salads and breads were no less appealing.

She made her choices and followed Alex to a small table for two. The glass doors were designed to be open for access to the patio, but it was much too hot at the moment for anyone to go outside.

She sat down, tugging the hem of her dress to a decorous level. Alex was in an odd mood. In a tiny pocket she carried a tube of lipstick and a small vial of tablets. Shaking two ibuprofen into her palm, she handed them across the table. "Your head is killing you, I can tell. Take these."

He scowled but didn't argue. She knew that men in general and this one in particular hated showing weakness of any kind. It was a sign of his discomfort that he didn't refuse.

They ate in silence for long minutes. The quiet didn't bother Maria. She'd grown up without brothers or sisters and had often spent time alone at home when her mother was at work.

Tonight, however, she was more aware than usual of her boss. It was no surprise that she'd had a bit of a crush on him over the years. Alex was virile, lean and muscular. Even in the expensive suits he wore, his physical power was evident. Thick black hair, cut conservatively, and deep brown eyes added up to an extremely masculine and sexy man.

In London, she had worked as his secretary. Once they all returned to Alma, however, she had been promoted to her current assignment in media and PR. Her position fell under the auspices of the Ministry of Commerce, but she did not ordinarily answer directly to Alex. For this assignment, however, he was definitely in charge. And that was a problem. Because the longer she knew him, the more she was afraid he would pick up on her reluctant attraction.

She had no illusions on that score. Alex was the eldest son of an aristocratic Alma family. He would marry one day and marry well. But not someone like Maria. Not a woman whose mother had been a laundress in a seedy neighborhood in London to make ends meet.

Maria was practical and ambitious. She would get ahead by virtue of hard work and innate talent. But, once in a while, she let herself fantasize about sharing Alex's bed. All that hard muscle and warm skin at her disposal. A shiver snaked its way from the nape of her neck to a spot low in her belly. Thankfully, Alex was oblivious to her imagination.

He was discreet about his relationships. A very private man with a fine-tuned sense of propriety. She'd seen the hint of disapproval in his gaze tonight as he assessed her party dress. Why, she couldn't say. By Miami standards, her outfit was tame.

Nevertheless, she knew she had blotted her copybook with Alex. Perhaps he thought her décolletage was too

low or her skirt too high. Though the man was incredibly appealing, even she could admit he had a stuffy side.
Perhaps she would have teased him had he not looked so
grim faced. It occurred to her that he took this venture very
personally. As if it was solely up to him to convince the
Montoros to accept the mantle of the monarchy once again.

By the time they'd finished eating, the lines at the corners of Alex's mouth had disappeared. Between the food
and the painkillers, he seemed finally to have relaxed. Still,
she couldn't put a finger on what bothered her about his
interaction with Gabriel Montoro. Instead of being conciliatory and cajoling, he'd been borderline antagonistic.

It made no sense.

She sipped a glass of Chablis and gazed out over the
diverse group of people. The Alma delegation actually
outnumbered the Montoros, but the Montoros had invited
numerous friends and associates.

Rafael Montoro III was the life of the party. His rugged
features belied his age. Though he had already turned fifty,
he could pass for a man a decade younger. Did he harbor
resentment over being bypassed for the throne?

His oldest son, Rafael IV—known as Rafe—was charming and affable and extremely self-possessed, though he
had yet to hit thirty. Except for his age, it was not a stretch
to see him as king of Alma. Rafe's sister, Bella, was much
like her dad, the center of attention and a vivacious extro-
vert. But she was very young, only twenty-three if Maria
remembered correctly.

Then there was Gabriel, who was another story. And
also a close cousin, Juan Carlos, who had been raised with
the Montoro siblings after their parents' deaths. Neither Gabriel nor Juan Carlos would be likely to play much of a
role in the upcoming transition, except for supporting Rafael IV.

The others present were of little interest at this point. It would be Maria's job to craft the image of a royal family that was strong and moral and charismatic. The only person who might make her job difficult was Gabriel. Who knew what skeletons were hidden in *his* closet. It would be up to her to excavate them and make sure they didn't embarrass the Montoro family in the midst of this sea change.

Gabriel, despite his reputation, was not so bad, as far as she could tell. Perhaps a bit cynical, almost definitely a player. Women were always drawn to that kind of fallen-angel mystique.

"I don't know how this is going to go."

She jumped when Alex spoke. She'd been so deep in her thoughts he had startled her. She searched his face. "I've never heard you give voice to the possibility that we might not prevail."

His lips twisted. "Well, look at them. Why do they need Alma or royal titles? The whole family is practically royalty here in the States. If you or I were in their shoes, would we give up all this?"

"Maybe. It's hard to say." Maria pursed her lips. "Everyone likes knowing where he or she comes from. The Montoros' family history goes back hundreds of years. I imagine that once they have some time to think about it they'll be excited about renewing those ties."

"I hope you're right."

At the opposite end of the room, a small orchestra began tuning up. When the musicians launched into their first song, Alex stood and held out his hand. "Do you feel like dancing?"

Her heart fluttered and lifted. "I *always* feel like dancing."

As he led her out onto the floor, she tried not to stiffen up. That would be a dead giveaway that she was nervous.

Alex held her firmly with masculine confidence that was appealing. She was a strong, capable woman, but to move like this… Well, that was another thing entirely. Here she could give in to the mastery of the dance. Alex was in charge, and she was able to let go and let him steer their course.

He smelled of crisp, starched cotton and warm male skin. She was almost certain she caught a whiff of the hotel's signature shower gel. Her heart pounded in her chest, and her knees trembled. This was the first time they had ever been so close.

In Alma, she couldn't think of a single social occasion when she and Alex had interacted so personally. And for such a length of time. Perhaps that was why she felt a change in him.

The first song ended and a second began. Alex made no move to release her. Since she had no real desire to *be* released, she followed where he led. A less pragmatic woman might have called the moment romantic. Maria was neither a romantic nor a wishful thinker. But even a realist could choose to live in the moment once in a while.

Life was serious business most of the time. A woman could be excused for indulging herself on occasion. And Alex Ramon was definitely an indulgence worth savoring.

Two

Alex had made a tactical error. He knew it as soon as he took Maria in his arms. Given the situation, he'd assumed that dancing was a socially acceptable convention…a polite way to pass the time.

He was wrong. Dead wrong. No matter the public venue nor the circumspect way in which he held her, nothing could erase the fact that she was soft and warm in his embrace. The slick fabric of her dress did nothing to disguise the feminine skin beneath.

He found his breath caught in his throat, lodged there by a sharp stab of hunger that caught him off guard. He'd worked so hard these past weeks that he'd let his personal needs slide. Celibacy was neither smart nor sustainable for a man his age. Certainly not when faced with such a deliciously carnal temptation.

How had he never noticed that Maria was such a tall woman…or that her cheek reached his shoulder at exactly the right spot? When he couldn't think of a good reason to let her go, one dance turned into three. Inevitably, his body responded to her nearness.

He was in heaven and hell, shuddering with arousal and unable to do a thing about it.

When Gabriel brushed past them, his petite sister in his arms, Alex remembered what he had meant to say earlier. "Maria…"

"Hmm?"

Her voice had the warm, honeyed sound of a woman pleasured by her lover. Alex cleared his throat. "You need to be careful around Gabriel Montoro."

Maria's reaction was unmistakable. She went rigid in Alex's arms and pulled away. "Excuse me?" Beautiful eyes glared at him.

He tried to continue the dance, but Maria was having none of it. So Alex soldiered on. "He's a mature, experienced man, and you're not accustomed to running in these circles. I'd hate to see him take advantage of you."

Maria went pale but for two spots of hectic color on her cheekbones. "Your concern is duly noted," she said, the words icy. "But you'll have to trust my judgment, I'm afraid. Because I don't plan to avoid him. My job is actually to get close to him, to learn his secrets, to do damage control. And I'm not a child, Alex. I'm insulted by your insinuation."

"I'm not insinuating anything," he said. "But I saw the way he looked at you."

"The man would flirt with a block of wood. I get that. But I certainly don't need you or anyone else to protect me from the big bad wolf."

"You're angry."

"Damn straight, I'm angry." Her eyes snapped with the force of her displeasure. "I was invited to be part of this delegation, and I accepted. I'm here to do a job and to do it to the best of my ability. This assignment means as much to me as it does to you. So I'll thank you to keep your advice to yourself."

"I'm sorry," he said stiffly.

Her posture erect, she gave him a stony stare. "Am I off the clock now, Mr. Ramon? May I go to my room?"

"Don't push me, Maria," he said, his teeth clenched. "It's been a long day, and the ones to come won't be much better."

She wrapped her arms around her waist in a defensive posture. "Maybe it would be best if we avoid each other when we don't have to be working together."

"If that's what you want." How had they gone from dancing to dismay so quickly?

For a brief moment he saw sadness in her gaze. His gut twisted with the sure knowledge that he had put it there.

Her bearing and her expression were dignified. "I'll see you at ten tomorrow," she said.

As he watched her walk away from him, his enjoyment in the evening went flat. He tracked her progress as she spoke to various members of the delegation and said her good-nights. The Montoros were next. Both of the Rafaels. Bella. And of course, Gabriel.

As Alex watched, Gabriel leaned down and whispered something in Maria's ear. Whatever it was, it made her laugh.

Seeing her face light up reminded Alex of how hard she worked. In Alma, he'd never had any problem with their professional relationship. But something about Miami's heat and hedonistic ways blurred the lines between business and pleasure.

Maria was right. Part of her job was to deal with Ga-

briel Montoro so that he didn't embarrass his family and/
or derail the plans to reinstate the monarchy.

Alex understood her priorities. But he didn't have to
like them.

Maria slept poorly and woke early. Her dreams had been
a jumble of Alma and Miami and Alex. Gabriel hadn't
figured in those sequences at all. Which was really no
surprise. Because as handsome and charismatic as the
second-born Montero was, he didn't make her heart beat
faster.

He amused her. He made her laugh. And she liked him
a lot.

But he wasn't Alex.

After fifteen minutes of tossing and turning, it became
clear she wasn't going to be able to go back to sleep. Climbing out of bed, she slipped into her swimsuit, brushed her
teeth and twisted her hair into a messy knot on top of her
head. This was her best chance to get in some sunbathing
before the sun became blistering.

Draped from neck to midcalf in a conservative cover-up
made of ecru lace, she made her way downstairs. Miami
might have different standards, but Maria was a citizen
of Alma and as such, subject to a certain code of dress
and conduct. She would never do anything to embarrass
the delegation.

Other than the occasional hotel employee, she met no
one. These early-morning hours were ones she enjoyed.
Filled with the promise of a new day. Peaceful.

Only when she stepped outside into the heat and humidity did things change. Not because of the weather. But
because she ran headlong into a hard male body.

Catching herself and grabbing for her tote, which threatened to spill everywhere, she looked up in consternation. "Alex."

He wore a gray T-shirt and navy running shorts. With some alarm, she realized that she had never seen his legs bare. If that weren't enough to make her gawk and stutter, she also had to take note of his broad chest and the dark patterns where sweat marked his shirt.

"Hello, Maria. You're up early."

He spoke calmly, as though their last encounter hadn't ended acrimoniously.

She nodded. "I burn easily. I thought it might be nice to spend time at the beach now. I won't be late for our meeting."

He cocked his head. "Am I such an ogre?"

The teasing glint in his eyes made her stomach clench with feelings that were definitely not professional. "Of course not."

"Good."

They both stood there waiting for the other to speak.

"You've been running," she said, as if it weren't obvious.

"Yes." When he removed his aviator sunglasses, his gaze was stormy. "It's a stress reliever."

"You have a lot on your plate."

"The Montoros aren't the only problem I'm juggling at the moment."

"What else is there?" She was genuinely curious.

"This and that." The words were flat. Without inflection. But the dark-eyed gaze held an intensity that made her nipples bead beneath two layers of fabric.

She swallowed hard. "I won't keep you then."

He took a step in her direction but stopped short. "I'd better hit the shower," he muttered. "I'm having breakfast with Rafael Montero."

"Father or son?"

"Father. He's one generation closer to the past. I'm hoping he'll help us sway the younger ones."

"He may be bitter about his own missed opportunity."

"Somehow, I doubt it. He seems to have a very casual approach to life."

"You sound as if you don't approve."

Alex shrugged, the fabric of his T-shirt clinging to a broad, muscular chest. "I'm not sure how the American personality will translate in Alma. The older people still remember days of pomp and circumstance. A laid-back monarchy may be hard to swallow."

"Are you sure we're doing the right thing?"

"No." He grimaced. "But it's the assignment we've been given. If we're in pursuit of the 'good old days,' then the monarchy is necessary for our people to feel as if life has finally returned to normal."

"Better the devil you know?"

Alex chuckled, his face lightening. "Something like that. I'd better get moving. See you at ten."

As he walked away, Maria allowed herself to track his progress. He moved with a rangy masculine gait that encompassed determination and impatience. She wondered if he ever truly relaxed.

Down on the sand, she selected a lounger and spread her towel. At this hour, the sun worshippers were few and far between. A handful of joggers. Several people walking their dogs.

She had just picked up her paperback novel when a shadow fell over her left arm. Shading her eyes with one hand, she looked up. "Gabriel. What are you doing here? I wouldn't have pegged you for an early riser."

He waited for her to move her legs to one side and then

settled on the end of the chaise. "I'm not," he said, yawning. "Just now going to bed."

"Ah."

He shook his head with a wry grin. "Get your mind out of the gutter. I have a weekly poker game with some buddies."

"Did you win?"

"I always win."

Despite his reputation, she couldn't help liking the black sheep Montoro. He seemed very comfortable in his own skin, and that was a trait she admired. "Where do you live?" she asked.

"I have a condo here on the beach. But our family has a compound at Coral Gables. You should let me take you there. It's quite fabulous. You'd like it, I think…"

"I'm here to work," she said, smiling to soften the blow. "But thank you."

"If it's your stick-up-his-butt boss you're worried about, I'll invite him along, as well."

"That's not a very nice thing to say. Alex is a wonderful man. And he cares deeply about his country. I admire him very much."

"Does he know about your…devotion?"

The pause before the last word was pointed. She felt her face flush. "We're colleagues, nothing more."

"And you're okay with that?"

"I'm uncomfortable with this subject," she said, wincing inwardly at how prissy she sounded.

Gabriel waved a hand. "Fine. My apologies." He yawned again. "I need some shut-eye. Don't stay out too long and get burned, pretty Maria."

"Why are people so interested in giving me advice? I'm a grown woman, in case you haven't noticed."

Gabriel stood and stretched, his shoulders blocking out

the sun. "I noticed," he said, the grin turning roguish. "But I know a lost cause when I see one. You're too nice a woman for the likes of me."

"I think I've been insulted."

"Not at all," he protested. "It's just that I don't have a great track record with sweet young things. Someone always gets a heart broken."

"Do you ever take life seriously?"

He glanced back at her as he prepared to walk away. "Not if I can help it, Maria. Not if I can help it."

An hour later she gathered her things and prepared to return to the hotel. She had just enough time to clean up and make it to Alex's suite for their meeting. They were being joined by Jean Claude, the attorney overseeing preparation of the legal documents for the restoration of the constitutional monarchy.

Maria was glad to see the lawyer for more reasons than one. He was good at what he did, but even more importantly, today he was a buffer between Alex and her. The growing awareness she had of Alex's masculinity would have to be stamped out.

For two solid hours the three of them wrangled over language and legal points. Lunch was delivered from the hotel restaurant at noon. In forty-five minutes they were at it again. From the beginning, Maria had been awestruck by the historical importance of the documents they were drafting. Now, though she still recognized the critical nature of the work, being cooped up in a small room for hours on end meant she was more than ready to call it quits when Alex finally indicated they were done.

"We can't finish everything in a day or even this week. But we've made a dent in it."

Jean Claude nodded. "When will we show the Montoros a draft?"

"Not until we have some assurance they plan to accept the offer from Alma," Alex said. "If they turn us down, we'll have to scrap everything and come up with plan B."

Maria groaned. "All this work for nothing? Please don't even hint at it. It's a dreadful thought."

Jean Claude capped his expensive pen and tucked papers into his sleek briefcase. He was in his midthirties, good-looking in a quiet, unflashy way and utterly trustworthy. Which was why he had been chosen for his current position. "I believe we must think positively. The Montoros are surely aware of their family's deep history with the country of their origin. Despite their love of the United States, blood ties will win out."

Alex ran a hand through his hair, ruffling the thick dark strands. "Let's hope you're right."

As the door closed behind Jean Claude, silence fell heavy and awkward. Maria stood, her knee bumping the leg of the table. Wincing, she picked up her things and sidled toward the exit. "Same time in the morning?" she asked, trying for a clean getaway.

Alex stopped her with nothing more than an upraised hand. "Tomorrow is Saturday. The entire delegation has been given instructions to enjoy some time off. We'll reconvene on Monday."

Maria raised an eyebrow. "Can we afford the delay?"

"Any deadlines we come up with are artificial at best. If we're to convince the Montoros of our sincerity and our pragmatism, we can't appear too desperate. It's Miami, Maria. Sun, sand, shopping."

"It's like I don't even recognize you," she teased.

The twist of his lips was self-mocking. "I do understand how to have fun, you know."

"I'll take your word for it."

Suddenly they were back to flirting again.

Alex fiddled with a stack of papers, not looking at her. "Did I ever tell you I had a brother? A twin?"

"No." It wasn't the kind of thing two business associates normally discussed. She wasn't going to ignore the personal overture, though. "But I'd like to hear about him…"

Alex's face was cast in shadow, the sun coming through the window at his back. Suddenly the harsh lighting made him seem a tragic figure. She shivered as if a ghost had walked over her grave.

"He died when we were ten years old," Alex said. "Complications from the flu. My parents were completely crushed."

"And what about you?"

He seemed surprised, as though no one had ever considered the grief of a sibling. "I lost a part of myself," he said slowly. "As if I'd had a limb removed. It was agony."

Maria stood frozen, her belongings clutched to her chest. "Why are you telling me this?" she asked, her voice little more than a whisper.

Alex straightened, his gaze meeting hers without hesitation. "I want us to be friends, Maria…to understand each other. You think of me as a workaholic, don't you?"

She bit her lip, evaluating her answer. "I see you as a very conscientious man."

His brooding expression touched something deep in her heart. "I wasn't always such a stickler for the rules. But after my brother died, I felt as if I had to make up for my brother's loss by being perfect," he said. "That narrow path has become who I am now."

"A difficult way to live."

"Yes. Yes, it is." He stopped, and she saw the muscles

in his throat work. "If I push too hard, call me on it. With you and Jean…with the delegation."

"It's not my place."

"It is. Because that's what I need from you."

They were separated by a space of several feet. Even so, she felt the pull of his magnetic personality. "Is that all you need?"

The words left her mouth as if someone else had spoken them. She saw his eyelashes flicker in shock and was appalled at her impulsive gaffe. "I'm sorry," she said quickly. "I shouldn't have said that."

"Do you not want to hear my answer?"

Every cell in her body trembled with uncertainty. "I think perhaps I should say no."

"I never took you for a coward, Maria."

She shook her head instinctively. "We're away from home…in an unusual environment. We're not ourselves."

"Or maybe we're more ourselves than we're allowed to be in Alma."

His words left her breathless…literally. Until it occurred to her that she had for the moment forgotten how to breathe. Exhaling slowly, she weighed her response. Alex was an attractive, appealing man. Sharing his bed would be memorable. Of that she had no doubt.

But in the end, the two of them came from different classes. The United States might pride itself on the ability of a person with nothing to rise to the top, but Maria knew her limitations. "My mother worked in an industrial laundry ten hours a day in order to put me through school in London. And I had two jobs on top of that."

"I'm familiar with your background."

"The Ramons are aristocracy…on a par with the Montoros as far as Alma is concerned. I don't think it would be wise for you and I to do anything we might regret."

"You're throwing up barriers where none exist. The delegation was handpicked. You're here because of your skills and competence. No one looks down on you for not being a native."

"That's not what I meant and you know it."

"It's the twenty-first century, Maria."

"Maybe so. But Alma values the past. Otherwise, none of us would be here trying to reinstate the monarchy. I am proud of who I am, but I'm a realist. You and I walk different paths. Let's not forget that."

He stared at her long and hard as if he could imprint his will on her by mind control. "You asked me what I need from you."

"I shouldn't have." Her heart fluttered in her throat like a butterfly trapped.

He smiled, a totally unfair act of war. "I'll wait until you ask me again. But next time, I'll answer, Maria."

Three

She fled to her room after that, her legs spaghetti and her mouth dry. It was one thing to know she was attracted to Alex but another entirely to realize that he might be feeling the same pull.

After changing into a set of comfy knit casual wear, she pulled out her phone and initiated a FaceTime call with her mother, who was getting ready for bed. The older woman's image was clear and dear. "Hello, sweetheart. How are things going?"

"Good, Mama. I wish you could be here to see Miami. It's gorgeous."

"I'm so proud of you, Maria."

"None of this would be happening if it weren't for all the sacrifices you've made for me." Her throat was tight suddenly.

Her mother's smile held a quiet joy. "That's a mother's job…and one I did gladly. How is Mr. Ramon?"

"Why would you ask me that?" Did her red cheeks show up on the other end?

"I'm not blind, Maria. I know you have a little crush on him."

She was too startled at her mother's perception to prevaricate. "Well, that's all there is to it. We're business associates, nothing more."

"He could do worse for a wife."

"I think you may be a tiny bit prejudiced."

They talked for five more minutes on less sensitive topics and then Maria said her good-nights. Her body was still on Alma time. The temptation to climb into bed was strong. But she knew she needed to resist if she was going to get past the jet lag.

She wasn't quite brave enough to strike out on her own in a strange city, but she had noticed a charming café in the hotel lobby as well as a series of shops with eye-catching merchandise. That would be exploration enough for one day.

Grabbing her billfold with its modest stash of American dollars, she tucked her room key and cosmetic case in a small tote and went in search of the elevator. She'd feared feeling out of place, but the hotel staff was exceptionally kind and friendly. Because she was on the early end of the dinner hour, she was escorted to a table near the window, perfectly situated to gaze out at the ocean.

After that, it was a toss-up as to whether she enjoyed the food or the view more. Though Alma supported a thriving fishing industry, the variety of seafood here in Miami was out of the ordinary. She ordered baby shrimp in a béchamel sauce with spring vegetables over angel-hair pasta. Every bite was a treat.

Afterward, she browsed the shops, trying not to let her shock show at some of the prices. Clearly the patrons of this hotel were upscale consumers with plenty of disposable income. A designer swimsuit and cover-up for twelve hundred dollars. Seventy-five-dollar rhinestone-studded beach sandals. A rattan tote that cost more that Maria earned in a month.

Fortunately, she had never needed such things to be happy. Her mother had taught her to hunt for bargains and to stretch a euro. Though Maria admired the merchandise, it was more in the nature of appreciating exhibits at a museum. She didn't covet any of it.

When she had worked her way around the main floor of the hotel, it was still too early for bedtime. On a whim, she returned to the restaurant and decided to order dessert. Her table was not as ideally situated this go-round, but the watermelon sorbet and caramel-drizzled shortbread cookie more than made up for it.

She was sipping coffee when a familiar figure surrounded by three or four other men entered the room. Gabriel Montoro stood out no matter where she spotted him. After paying her check, she was preparing to leave when he surprised her by showing up at her table and sitting down in the empty chair.

Lifting an eyebrow, she cocked her head. "I'm on my way out. I recommend the dessert special."

Gabriel picked up an unused table knife and rotated it end over end between his fingers. "If I'd known you were eating solo, I'd have invited you to join me."

"Not necessary. Sometimes it's nice to be alone with my thoughts."

"Ouch," he said, wincing theatrically.

"Oh, for heaven's sake. I didn't mean it that way." She studied his face. For a man who claimed to live life on his own terms, she saw signs of strain. "I appreciate the thought, but I'm fine. Just trying to kill some time before I crash."

He glanced at her empty cup. "Caffeine won't help."

"So I've been told. But the coffee here is amazing."

When she stood, he did, as well. "I'll walk you to the lobby," he said.

"Aren't your friends waiting for you?"

"It's a business thing. And not that urgent."

She was unable to dissuade him. Outside the restaurant, he steered her toward a store she hadn't entered because it was mostly jewelry. "What are you doing?" she asked, frowning.

"I need your advice." He pointed toward a glass case. "Which one is the prettiest? The palm tree? Or the crab…"

She gaped. "Well, uh…" She studied the two pieces. Both were gold with delicate chains. The palm tree had a tiny diamond coconut. The crab sported two emerald eyes. "They're each beautiful."

"But?"

"Well, if I had to pick, I'd go for the crab. He's whimsical."

"Fair enough." He handed the salesclerk a platinum card.

Still baffled, Maria watched him complete the transaction. As they left the shop, Gabriel took her hand and pressed the small, lime-green bag into her palm. "This is my apology," he said. "For being a jerk yesterday. You're doing your best to help my family, and even if we don't really care, it was rude of me to say so."

Maria shoved the bag back at him, appalled. "Oh, no, Mr. Montoro. That's not necessary. Not at all. You don't owe me any apologies."

"I told you to call me Gabriel."

"Gabriel, then. It would be very inappropriate of me to accept such a valuable gift."

"Forgive me for being crass, but this is nothing. Just a way for me to soothe my conscience." He gave her a crooked smile. "I don't want you to judge my family by my behavior. I've gotta run. Sleep well, Maria."

As quickly as he had appeared, he was gone.

Maria stared at the small bag in her hand, feeling a coil of unease settle in her stomach. But what else could she have done? She couldn't afford to offend a member of the royal family.

A masculine voice, cold and clipped, interrupted her reverie. "I think I was wrong about you, Maria. I thought you were too inexperienced and naive to deal with the likes of Gabriel Montoro. But apparently you know *exactly* what you're doing."

She looked up to find Alex regarding her with disdain and patent disapproval. "This isn't what it looks like," she said.

"Cliché, my dear. Cliché. A man gives a woman he barely knows jewelry? I think I'm pretty clear about the facts."

Her temper started to simmer. "First of all, you're way out of line. Second of all, I don't have to explain myself to you. Back off, Alex. You don't know what you're talking about. Gabriel was apologizing for being antagonistic about our efforts yesterday."

"He didn't buy *me* jewelry."

"Oh, for heaven's sake. I'm going up to bed. Good night." His criticism stung, in part because she felt guilty about accepting the bauble.

She didn't make it as far as the elevator before Alex caught up with her. "I called your room, but you didn't answer," he said.

"I've been trying to stay awake a little longer. I ate dinner alone and did some window-shopping. Last time I checked, neither of those was a crime."

Alex's jaw firmed. "I'm sorry if I jumped to conclusions. I was calling to see if you wanted to walk on the beach."

The look in his dark eyes said he was telling the truth. And that his apology was sincere. Late-day stubble shadowed his jawline, giving him a rakish, dangerous air.

Her anger deflated, leaving her dangerously vulnerable to his weary charm. "I appreciate the offer, but I can barely keep my eyes open. Maybe another evening?"

He nodded. "Of course."

"Good night, Alex."

He took her wrist and then released it abruptly when she flinched. "You've made quite an impression on the royal family," he said.

"I don't understand."

"They've invited us to spend tomorrow and Sunday at the family enclave in Coral Gables."

"The whole delegation?"

He shook his head. "Just you and me."

"Oh." Well, shoot. "I can make an excuse. It's more appropriate for you to be there."

He leaned against a marble column, legs crossed at the ankle. "I doubt that would be a popular choice, Maria. And we certainly can't take a chance on insulting them by declining. I told Mr. Montoro we'd be honored to accept. Rafael the third, that is. He seems to be receptive to our cause. Since we need all the help we can get, we're going to be there."

She sighed, feeling exhaustion wash over her. "What time?"

"Someone will pick us up at eleven in the morning.

Bring everything you need for the weekend. We won't check out of our rooms, though."

"That seems extravagant, doesn't it?"

His grin was quick and surprisingly boyish. "Relax, Maria. Your thriftiness is appreciated, but this is the big leagues."

She dreamed about that smile. And other things that left her hot and restless and agitated when she finally awoke. As she showered and dried her hair, she fretted about spending two days in a distinctly *unprofessional* atmosphere with Alex. He continued to keep her off balance. She didn't know if that was deliberate on his part or simply a function of their new circumstances.

At a quarter till eleven, she shouldered her tote and grabbed the handle of her suitcase. No point in summoning a bellman. She was leaving behind her smaller case.

In the lobby, she looked for Alex to no avail. Many people were checking out, and the sizable space was crowded. She found a corner and pulled out her phone to send a text. Before she could do so, a large hand settled on her shoulder.

"Sorry I'm late," Alex said, his expression harried. "I had to deal with a call from Alma. Some members of parliament are expecting news immediately. I tried to explain why that won't be possible."

She followed him outside. "Don't they understand that the royal family is somewhat reluctant?"

Alex donned dark sunglasses, effectively shielding his gaze. "I doubt it has even occurred to them that the Montoros may not be interested in what we have to offer."

A uniformed chauffer held up a sign with their names, and soon they were speeding southwest toward Coral Gables. Maria sat back, content to enjoy the passing view.

Though Alex was dressed casually in khaki pants and a loose ivory cotton shirt in deference to the heat, his posture remained tense as he scrolled through emails on his phone. As deputy prime minister of commerce, he bore an enormous workload, never more so than now in the midst of delicate negotiations.

Maria had done her research before leaving Alma, but at the moment all she could remember about Coral Gables was that it dated back to the 1920s with its origin as a planned community. And that it was home to the University of Miami.

The drive was barely half an hour on a good day, but with traffic could be upward of forty-five minutes. Luck was with them, and the trip was quick. As they passed through a portion of the charming business district and turned into a residential area, Maria's jaw dropped in admiration.

Lush tropical gardens and ornate walls protected private enclaves of the wealthy and oftentimes famous. At the entrance to the Montoros' estate, the chauffeur pressed an intercom button and identified his passengers before the gate rolled back and they were granted admittance.

Even the driveway was beautiful. The ubiquitous palm trees shaded winding paths of crushed shells mixed with white sand. Feral parrots dotted the landscape with pops of intense color.

"It's like something out of a novel," Maria murmured, more to herself than to Alex.

He didn't answer, still engrossed in his work. Biting her lip, she debated how far she dared push him. "Alex."

"Hmm?" He never looked up.

"Alex." This time she put more force behind the word.

He took off his sunglasses and rubbed the heel of his hand across his forehead. "What?"

She forgave him the faint note of irritation in his voice, because she suspected he hadn't slept much last night. Between the stress and the time change, the poor man was in bad shape.

"I think you need to relax," she said. "Look around you. We're in paradise. If nothing else, we've been given an opportunity to make a good impression on the Montoros…to meet them on their turf and show that we understand them."

His chuckle was halfhearted at best. "Do we?" he asked. "Understand them, I mean? Neither you nor I have royal blood. What do we know about the obligations of rank and lineage?"

"That's true," she conceded. "But this is our chance to get beyond the obvious…to see them as they really are. Then maybe we can decide how best to cast the lure."

He put his phone away and lifted an eyebrow, gazing at her with a warm smile that curled her toes. "I'm impressed, Maria. Machiavellian machinations and intrigue. Who knew you had it in you?"

"Don't be so dramatic. All I'm saying is that we should look for their vulnerabilities…their weaknesses. We both know Alma needs the Montoros. What we need to do now is establish exactly why the Montoros need Alma. Once we've done that, the outcome should fall in our favor."

The driver pulled the limo into a circular driveway. Before Alex could respond, Maria had gathered her things and stepped out of the vehicle. A uniformed housekeeper met them and ushered them inside a small guesthouse.

"Welcome," she said in softly accented English. "The Montoros are glad you are here. I have prepared a light meal and afterward you may want to relax for a bit. At four, someone will come to escort you to the main house to join the family."

Alex nodded. "Thank you."

The housekeeper waited patiently as they explored. Maria's wide-eyed expression amused him as she took in the lavish amenities. The villa had two guest rooms, each outfitted with a massive king-size bed and expensive teak furnishings. The chauffeur brought in the luggage, placing Maria's in the dove-gray and shell-pink room, and Alex's in the navy-and-yellow suite.

When the tour was complete, the housekeeper held out a hand. "Would you like to eat in the sunroom?"

Alex looked at Maria and nodded. "Of course."

Soon, they were digging into a light but flavorful luncheon of fish tacos, mango salsa and conch fritters.

Alex took a sip of his really excellent pinot and shook his head. "I think they're trying to impress us."

"Isn't that our role?" Maria had devoured her food every bit as eagerly as he had.

"Maybe they want to make very clear how little they're interested in returning to Alma…in any fashion."

"Oh." Her crestfallen look urged him to comfort her. But the unexpected wave of tenderness made him uneasy. She caused him to feel things that were inappropriate at best and dangerously seductive at worst. How could he fulfill his mission if he were constantly derailed by his baser instincts?

A life of public service meant subverting his own needs for the greater good. For the benefit of his country and for the sake of his pride he would have to ignore the way she made him feel.

She had left her blond hair loose today, confined only by two small tortoiseshell clips, one at either temple. Though he knew she came from a background far less privileged than his, she carried herself with a regal grace and dignity that surpassed her years.

He had suggested her as one of the team for this trip, but ultimately, she had been chosen by the committee. Her talent and hard work impressed everyone who witnessed her in action.

She'd been right to call him on his preoccupation. *Nothing* at the moment was more important than the Montoros.

As they finished their meal, the housekeeper hovered, spiriting away empty plates and keeping their glasses full. At last, she left them alone.

Alex cleared his throat. "Would you like a nap?"

"The answer is yes, but I'm not going to take one. I'm determined to beat this jet lag. How about a walk instead?"

"You do know it's hot as hell out there."

She wrinkled her nose. "Yes. But it's Florida. I've never been here."

He held out his hands. "Far be it from me to stop you. I'll tag along to make sure you don't get lost."

Maria changed clothes so quickly he was stunned. Instead of the subdued navy dress she had worn earlier, she came out of her room wearing white shorts that showcased her long, tanned legs and a raspberry-colored tank top. Her hair was now caught up in a free-falling ponytail. The outfit shaved half a dozen years off her age, reminding him again of how young she was.

He swallowed against a tight throat. "That was fast."

She shrugged. "My mother believes in a woman being herself. Too many lotions and potions breed vanity...or so she claims. I started sneaking mascara and lip gloss when I was fourteen."

"Such a rebel," he teased.

"I tried to behave. I really did, because I adored my mother, even as a bratty teenager. But I wanted to be like all the other girls."

"Not such a terrible failing."

"I suppose not. But she came home from work early one day before I'd had a chance to wash my face, and she was so…"

"Angry?"

"No. Not that. It was worse. I had disappointed her. She told me that it was a mistake for a girl to primp and paint herself to attract a boy. That I should be proud of who I was inside. That the exterior didn't matter."

"Wise words."

"Yes. But they came from a place of pain. I never knew the details, though it was no secret that my father abandoned her before I was born. When it came to love, she had chosen poorly, and she paid for it the rest of her life. My goal has been to earn enough money to set her up in a little retirement flat. I owe her so much. And I want to give her a chance to enjoy life while she is still strong and healthy."

"You're a good daughter."

For a fleeting second he witnessed a surprising vulnerability in her aquamarine eyes. "I hope so."

Four

As they exited the small house, Alex pondered Maria's words. He knew she was ambitious. Unlike some people, he didn't see that as a negative in a woman. He'd like to think he was more of an enlightened male than some of his contemporaries.

But what if Maria's ambitions had more to do with securing a future for her mother and herself than for simply rising in the ranks of government service? Did she want a husband and children? Or had her mother's experience made Maria reluctant to entrust a man with her future? The more he thought about it, the less he was sure of anything.

What bothered him the most was the faint but insistent notion that she might be setting herself up to land in a Montoro's bed. Gabriel's to be exact. Did Maria have fantasies of becoming a princess?

Almost instantly, Alex was ashamed of his doubts. He had no basis at all for such a supposition. Merely his own jealousy. Though he knew a relationship with Maria was not likely to be good for either of them, he winced at the thought of her being with another man. Surely it was a dog-in-the-manger attitude.

As they wandered the grounds, he tried to keep his mind on the flora and fauna and not on the long-legged grace of the beauty in front of him. The more time he spent in Maria's company, the less control he had over his fantasy life. Already, he'd been awakened twice on this trip by intensely erotic dreams.

Now, with her three feet ahead, his hands itched to feel the silky hair that tumbled down her back. It bounced and swung as she walked. In his imagination he could see that same hair spread out across his pillow, those wide-set eyes, drowsy with passion, staring up at him.

Damn it. He was hard and hot and horny, none of which were appropriate conditions for the man who was supposed to be orchestrating a diplomatic dance that could affect thousands of lives.

Clenching his jaw, he concentrated on naming the flowering shrubs they passed. Anything to keep from staring at a heart-shaped butt and narrow waist made for the grasp of a man's hands.

Despite her claim of jet lag, Maria seemed indefatigable. The various pathways were clearly marked, so it was easy to circle back around in the direction of their accommodations. At the very last turn, they lingered beside a small lagoon, taking advantage of a patch of shade.

A pair of peacocks strutted on the far bank. Birdsong echoed from every direction. Maria leaned against a tree trunk, propping one foot behind her. "I like the wildness," she said, smiling dreamily. "The landscape is passionate and alive."

"If it were you, would you go back to a country where

you had never lived? Simply to fulfill a destiny you didn't choose?"

She gazed toward the water, her profile as familiar to him now as his own face in the mirror. "I honestly don't know. My life is so different. Once my mother is gone, I'll never have a chance to press the issue of my father's identity. And she won't even discuss her own family, because they threw her out when she ended up pregnant and unmarried. So the idea of having a family tree that can be traced back almost two thousand years is hard for me to grasp. My past is a blank slate."

"I'm sorry," he said.

"It is what it is."

She wasn't trying to elicit his sympathy. Her words were matter-of-fact. He wondered, though, if she recognized the vein of wistful sadness he heard in them.

Her skin glowed with heat and perspiration. It occurred to him in that quiet moment that her beauty was intrinsic, not dependent at all on the paints and potions she had so whimsically described. She might look much like this after a bout of energetic lovemaking.

Shifting restlessly from one foot to the other, he fought the urge to take her in his arms. Clearing his throat, he glanced at his watch. "We should get back and clean up."

She nodded, smiling at him with such sweet openness that his heart clenched in his chest. "I'm glad I was able to come on this trip. I know you put in a good word for me, and I'm grateful."

He stared at her, his body rigid with desire. "I don't want your gratitude, Maria."

Hurt flickered in her eyes, only to be replaced by dawning surprise as she realized what he wasn't saying. "I asked you before what you needed from me. And you wouldn't answer."

"Correction. I *didn't* answer because you weren't willing to listen."

She straightened from her relaxed pose against the tree and took a step in his direction. "And if I'm ready now?"

He shuddered, no longer able to hide the hunger that rode him hard. "Come here," he said, tugging her by the hand until she landed against his chest. He linked his hands at the small of her back, allowing himself one tiny nibble of a shell-like ear.

She looked up at him, her eyes huge. "Men are strange creatures."

He choked out a laugh. "What does that mean?"

"I'm all sweaty and icky."

Inhaling sharply, he shook his head. "Definitely not icky. Trust me on that one." He found her mouth with his, going in for a quick pass and then lingering to taste every nuance of warm, willing woman.

Maria was not shy, but there was a certain hesitance in her response, a tiny awkwardness that perhaps signified a lack of experience. That same pesky tenderness surfaced, making him want to protect her from himself. And wasn't that a conundrum…

Finally, her arms went around his neck. Now they were pressed chest-to-chest, hip-to-hip. There was no way she could miss the state of his body. He was hard everywhere.

Though it took everything he had, he kept the kiss gentle, the embrace circumspect. They were standing where anyone could see them. And they had a very critical appointment in less than an hour.

One more minute. That's all he needed. His tongue stroked hers. "Hell, Maria. You make me forget my name."

"Alex," she whispered, straining against him, standing on tiptoe. "Smart, sexy, adorable Alex."

"Adorable?" He frowned, trying to focus as she sucked on his bottom lip.

"Adorable," she said firmly. "You're so serious and dedicated and straight-arrow. It's lovable and charming."

He forced himself to release her, though when she clung to him in protest, his resolve weakened. His heart slamming in his chest like a pile driver, he took her wrists in his hands and dragged them away from his neck. "I'm not feeling at all dedicated right now, Maria. If it weren't for the possibility of alligators in that lagoon, I'd be tempted to pull you down on the ground and have my adorable wicked way with you."

"Alligators?" Her shriek sent a flock of birds skyward.

If he'd hoped to derail the possibility of sex, he'd succeeded beyond his wildest dreams. His companion looked scared to death.

He shook his head in bemusement. "You do know where we are, right? Alligator alley?"

"I didn't think they were everywhere." She clung to his arm as he led her back toward their quarters.

Alex ushered her inside the villa and shut the door. "I didn't mean to frighten you. Gators aren't aggressive as a rule. Though they might grab the occasional cat or dog."

"Oh, Lord." When she went white, he realized his assurances weren't helping.

"Go take your shower," he said. "As long as you stay out of unknown pools and ponds, you've got nothing to worry about, I swear." He leaned down for one last kiss. "I'll protect you."

Maria turned the water as hot as she could bear it, stepping into the shower and trying to stop shaking. Maybe her fear was irrational, but while she could handle the occasional mouse or nasty spider, alligators were beyond her experience. Maybe this was what people meant when they said every Eden has its serpent.

Miami and Coral Gables were beautiful beyond belief. Lush…tropical…a garden paradise. She'd never anticipated a dark side.

As she dried off and re-dressed in the outfit she'd worn earlier, she hoped she had chosen appropriate attire for the weekend. Unfortunately, there was no manual for how to hobnob with royalty in America.

Her navy linen sheath dress was very plain, its only adornment a trio of quirky wooden buttons on either shoulder. Her shoes were low-heeled strappy sandals in a neutral shade with cork soles. She stared in the mirror. Too casual? Not casual enough?

The decision was moot now, because she didn't have enough clothing with her for endless choices. Truthfully, it probably didn't matter. She was not a key player in this drama. Alex was the one in the hot seat. The Montoros would be grilling him, not Maria. Poor Alex.

She finished drying her hair and brushed it out, leaving it as it had been when she arrived. The clips kept it off her face. Presumably this afternoon's gathering would be inside an air-conditioned space. One thing she had already learned about Florida was that even if the outside temperatures were sweltering, inside most buildings, it was cold enough to hang meat.

Alex was waiting in the living room when she went in search of him. His smile was automatic and held no hint that only minutes earlier they had been passionately entwined in a kiss that had made her weak with longing.

She decided to match his air of calm. "Are we ready?"

He nodded. At that same moment the doorbell chimed. A young man, probably Maria's age, stood waiting with a polite posture. His grin was quick and easy. A navy knit polo shirt, stretched across his broad shoulders, identified him as an employee of Montoro Enterprises.

"I'm here to take you to the main house," he said. "The Jeep's right outside."

The vehicle was spotless, though perhaps not designed for women wearing dresses. Maria's cheeks flamed when she was forced to accept Alex's help climbing into the rear seat. The two men sat up front.

It dawned on her that this compound must be even larger than she had imagined, because it took five minutes to drive to their destination. All the buildings, large or small, had been designed in the same vein, with whitewashed stucco walls and blue tile roofs.

Most of the places they passed she couldn't identify, but she did see a gardening shed and a transportation corral that housed multiple golf carts. When they arrived at the Montoros' residence, she was not surprised to find that it was the largest building on the property.

It was a work of art…two stories, with wraparound porches, ceiling fans and rattan furnishings. And there were windows…lots of windows. The glass was probably tinted, because otherwise, the sun would bake the inhabitants.

Their escort parked at the base of a shallow set of steps and abandoned them. "Just knock," he said, whistling as he wandered away.

Maria looked at Alex askance. "I guess we're on our own."

He shaded his eyes and looked around with curiosity. "I guess we are." He didn't seem a fraction as nervous as she felt. But then again, his family was every bit as prestigious as the Montoros, though not royal. If Alex so desired, he could probably be elected to lead the country when the current prime minister's term was over.

Together, she and Alex ascended the stairs. Moments after Alex rang the buzzer, a honey-skinned gray-haired man answered the door. He was dressed much like Alex in clothes that gave deference to the climate, though his manner was anything but relaxed. An English butler couldn't have been more dignified.

"Welcome to Casa Montoro," he said. "The family awaits you in the salon."

The house reminded Maria of a spread she'd once envied in *Architectural Digest*. Every detail was harmonious perfection. Polished hardwood floors, colorful rag rugs. And views. Wow. One entire wall of glass framed the ocean in the distance.

When she and Alex entered the large room, Rafael III jumped to his feet. "You're here at last. We're honored to welcome you to our home." He shook Alex's hand and kissed Maria on both cheeks.

One glance around the assemblage told Maria that the key players in this drama were present. Rafael's three children—Gabriel, Bella and Rafael IV. Juan Carlos II, the cousin. And, last but not least, the frail but indomitable Isabella Salazar.

At seventy-three, she should still have a number of good years ahead of her, but her body had been ravaged with Parkinson's. Though bound to a wheelchair when she was able to get out of bed, she was an imposing figure. Grandmother to Juan Carlos and great-aunt to his cousins, Isabella wielded considerable influence. *And* she was a proponent of the old ways. Which made her automatically an ally.

With the exception of Isabella, Maria and Alex had met everyone the night of the reception. Knowing that, and as a matter of courtesy, Rafael took them immediately to sit with his aunt.

The old woman might have been trapped in a broken body, but her mind was sharp and her eyesight keen. "Do you know why we invited the two of you today?" she asked, the words abrupt.

Maria gulped inwardly and saw by Alex's reaction that he was as taken aback as she was. Alex recovered first. "Not exactly, ma'am."

"You're wondering why we didn't bring the entire delegation out here."

Alex was brave enough to give her the truth. "The thought crossed our minds."

"It's simple, boy. Your people are supposed to have the weekend free to relax and enjoy Miami. Correct?"

"Yes."

"So we left them alone. But the two of you are here because Gabriel over there owned up to being a bit of an ass when he first met you. He's hotheaded, but he's a good boy, and he thought better of his actions. On behalf of our extended family, we want to apologize for any ill manners on the part of the Montoros, and I assure you, you'll find us receptive to your proposal when it is ready."

Maria glanced around the room, not at all convinced. Gabriel and Bella wore identical mulish expressions. Rafael, the father, was sober. Rafael, the son, appeared uncomfortable. Only Juan Carlos, who was not a key player in all of this, seemed calm.

Alex, ever the politician, spoke carefully. "Maria and I are very appreciative of the invitation to be here with you today. But apologies are unnecessary. This is a difficult time for everyone involved. I'd expect there to be certain tensions along the way. Hopefully, in the end we'll be able to work out solutions beneficial to Alma and to your family, as well."

Rafael III nodded. He had allowed his aunt the courtesy of speaking due to her age and position, but now he took control. "Mr. Ramon, my elder son and I would like to sit down with you in my office and go over our business situation so you have a clear idea of our responsibilities. I've asked Bella and Gabriel to entertain Ms. Ferro."

Juan Carlos, the tall young man with the reserved manner, spoke up. "My grandmother has a social engagement this afternoon, and I have promised to escort her. But we will rejoin you for dinner later this evening. Please excuse us."

When those two left the room, Maria saw Alex glance at Gabriel with an inscrutable expression. Was he unhappy that Maria was to spend time with the Montoro bad boy... even with Bella as chaperone? If he was, it was too bad. Maria couldn't refuse without insulting her hosts, and besides, she didn't want to refuse. Gabriel was an interesting man whose company she enjoyed, and this would also be an opportune moment to get acquainted with the very young and very pretty Bella.

As Rafael escorted his son and Alex out a door on the opposite side of the salon, Bella clapped her hands softly. "Alone at last. I'm so tired of all this Alma talk. No offense, Miss Ferro."

"None taken. But please call me Maria."

Gabriel squeezed his sibling's shoulders. "My baby sister thought you might enjoy the pool. She has enough bikinis to outfit every woman in a twenty-mile radius. But if you're not a sun worshipper, Maria, we can go out on the boat instead."

"The pool sounds delightful, actually. And I did bring a suit. As long as you have sunscreen, I'd love a swim."

Bella wrinkled her nose. "I'll let you two be energetic. I had a late night last night, so I may snooze behind my sunglasses."

Gabriel chuckled. "Maria, it's no secret that my Bella is a party girl. She knows every hot spot in Miami. But somehow she manages to stay out of trouble."

"Which is more than *you* ever did at my age," Bella shot back with a fond smile that told Maria these two were close, indeed.

Seeing Bella in a bikini made Maria very glad she had brought her own swimsuit. The younger woman's style and body were flawless. Maria had a decent self-image, but she was more than happy to don the conservative navy maillot she'd brought along.

When she and Bella exited the changing cabana, Gabriel was already in the pool, his broad shoulders gleaming wet and golden in the blistering sun. The man was incredibly handsome, but oddly, he didn't increase her heart rate one bit. Apparently she had a thing for focused, überconscientious oil barons with black hair and deep brown eyes.

Determined to forget about work and Alex and Alma for a while, she stepped up onto the diving board, walked to the end and executed a simple dive into the aquamarine water.

Five

When she surfaced, she laughed out loud, exhilarated by the feel of the silky cool water against her overheated skin. "This is amazing," she said. "It was raining when we left home…in fact, it had been raining for a week. I could get used to perpetual sunshine."

Bella adjusted the back of her lounge chair and smoothed her beach towel before stretching out with an audible sigh. "Perfection gets boring after a while, Maria. Ask our older brother."

Gabriel slicked a hand through his hair, sending droplets of water flying, his green eyes gleaming. "You're not being fair to Rafe, Bella. You try being CEO of Montoro Enterprises and see how you like it."

Bella donned dark glasses, shuddering. "No thank you. My job is to spend money, not make it."

When his sister subsided in a somnolent pose, Gabriel swam to where Maria paddled lazily in the deep end.

"She's putting on a show for you," he said in a low whisper. "Bella gets tagged as flighty and shallow, but my sister is a good actress. Few outside the family know about her charity work and her passion for preserving the environment."

"Why the charade?"

"I think people made assumptions about her as a teenager, and at that vulnerable age, the criticism hurt. Now she goes out of her way to appear as a wealthy diva without a care in the world."

"How does she feel about the possibility of becoming a royal and living in Alma?"

He shrugged. "I don't really know. I'm the only one who has been clear from the beginning about my feelings. The rest of them are playing their cards close to the chest. Maybe Bella likes the idea of starting over somewhere new, who knows? But we're still being premature…right?"

Maria sighed. "What's so terrible about reclaiming a throne and a legacy that are your birthright? The history of the Montoro family is inextricably interwoven with Alma's past."

"You're talking about tearing my family apart. If Rafe agrees to this madness, he'll move across the ocean."

"You've heard of jets, haven't you?"

Gabriel flicked water at her. "It's not the same. My family is exceedingly close. If we agree to accept this offer from Alma, someone will have to stay here to run the business. Decades of work have gone into making our company a player on two continents."

"I don't know what to tell you, Gabriel. This proposal from Alma to your family has taken on a life of its own. I sympathize with your position, but I have to move ahead with my responsibilities until someone tells me differently."

"You think our family is going to accept, don't you?"

She weighed her answer. "I hope so. Alma has suffered through years of deprivation and corruption and abuse. Now, finally, good things are beginning to happen. Having a Montoro on the throne again would be a huge boost to morale and for the identity of the people. Can you blame me for wanting to see that come to pass?"

For once, there wasn't a hint of humor or teasing on his face. "No. I suppose not."

"Let's wait and see what happens. A lot of the outcome hinges on your brother. It's a shame your father isn't eligible to ascend the throne, though. He's a very young fifty, and so exuberant and gregarious. I think he would have made an impressive king."

"My brother will, as well…if it comes to that."

"You're very protective of your family, aren't you? And very proud."

"Any one of them is worth three dozen of me. I'm a cynic, Maria…and I don't trust easily. This whole monarchy thing stinks of self-serving on the part of your chosen country. It's insulting for my family to be trotted out as puppet royalty so the merchants of Alma can sell postcards and T-shirts."

She studied his Greek god features, seeing the restless agitation and his genuine dismay. "Give us a chance," she said quietly. "I think you'll be pleasantly surprised when you see the actual proposal. No one wants to diminish the stature of the Montoros. In fact, quite the opposite. You have royal blood. That means something."

His expression lightened, but she sensed he wasn't convinced. They both clung to opposite sides of the ladder, their legs moving lazily in deep water. For a brief moment, she considered the odd situation. Perhaps this was the equivalent of doing business on the golf course.

Although Gabriel was a big flirt, he had neither said nor done anything to make her feel uncomfortable at being so close to him and wearing such skimpy clothing. They had spoken of deep, important matters. If anything, being in the water had kept their conversation from overheating.

It was difficult to fly off the handle when in the midst of such sybaritic surroundings. Truthfully, she felt sorry for Gabriel. It must be difficult to see the people he loved struggling with such gargantuan changes.

"You'll be royalty, too," she said quietly. "If this plays out like I think it will."

"No way," he said firmly. "If my brother decides he has to fall on the sword, I'll support him in every way I know how. But I'm not going to be a damned royal. Bella tried to make me play Prince Eric to her Ariel doll when we were little kids. I didn't like it then, and I haven't changed in that regard. I know who I am and who I'm not."

She didn't waste her breath explaining the role he would play in his brother's coronation…or in describing the richly ornamental robes and jewels of state that had been hidden away for decades. Time enough for him to get used to all that later. Right now, she had two jobs. One—impress upon him the importance of the Montoros to Alma's rebirth. And two—determine what, if any, of his bad-boy past might pop up and cause damage to the royal family's reputation.

"You can fight it all you want," she said earnestly, "but blood will tell, as they say."

"You're wrong," he said firmly. "If I were to cut your arm or you mine, our blood would look the same. I'm an American. We built this country on principles of equality."

"That may be so, but you can't rewrite history."

Bella lifted her head, sliding her sunglasses to the top of her head to glare at them. "Oh, for God's sake. Give it a rest. Can't we talk about books or movies or baseball? The two of you are giving me a headache."

Gabriel touched Maria's shoulder briefly. "Though I hate to admit it, my sister is right. This is a day for relaxing."

Alex stepped outside just in time to see Gabriel caress Maria's bare arm. The surge of primitive fury that racked him found no outlet. He was forced to clench his jaw and walk forward as if nothing was wrong.

Maria's face lit up when she saw him, appeasing his displeasure somewhat. "Alex…did you bring something to change into?"

Gabriel shaded his eyes. "Plenty of swim trunks in the cabana."

Alex debated his options. What he would *like* to do was spirit Maria back to their villa and make love to her until the sun came up. But since that wasn't an option, he might as well make the best of things.

By the time he had stripped down, changed and made it back to the pool, his feet were uncomfortably warm from the hot concrete. Even Bella had given up on sunbathing and was now frolicking in the water. Someone had set up a net midway across the pool, and brother and sister had apparently formed a team.

Maria beckoned him. "Hurry. They think they're champions, but I told them you were a big athlete at university."

"Not in volleyball," he said mildly, sliding into the cool water with an inward sigh of bliss.

"Doesn't matter," Maria declared. "I think we can take them."

Maria's scantily clad body was a definite handicap to his concentration. But when Gabriel scored two points right off the bat, Alex dragged his attention from her rounded breasts and sexy wet hair to the competition at hand. With Maria gazing at him in supplication, he brought his A game. The adrenaline rush of competition was a great stress reliever. And it was damn fun.

Maria and Bella were both nimble and coordinated. They set up shots and the two men took turns smashing points over the net. Time and again Maria dove for saves, her face dripping water and her eyes lit up with laughter.

He was, at some level, struck dumb by her beauty. She was so alive, so eager, so joyful. He felt the pull in his gut and wanted badly to kiss her. Because of Alex's addled state, Gabriel was able to spike the ball for yet another point. The smug smile on the other man's face told Alex that his opponent might have put Maria on Alex's team on purpose.

Of course, watching her across the net with Gabriel would have been just as bad.

After each team won two games apiece, it was mutually decided to play best three out of five. All four competitors were out of breath from battling the water to reach the ball.

Alex shot Maria a glance, trying not to notice the way her nipples beaded against the thin fabric of her suit. "You okay?"

"Of course." She moved closer and lowered her voice. "And I want to win."

He grinned, for the moment forgetting his responsibilities and his governmental role. "Then let's do it."

The game was fierce and quick, each side battling for supremacy. The Montoro team edged ahead by two or three only to be matched by Alex and Maria in the next few minutes.

Bella was short, but she was a master at setting up the ball. It was clear that she and her brother had teamed up before. Maria was taller and could occasionally punch a shot over the net, but mostly she fed the ball to Alex.

They had made it to game point a half-dozen times when the older Rafael appeared poolside and signaled their attention with a broad smile. "Dinner in half an hour. Don't make me come after you."

Alex grinned at his partner. Her cheeks were pink from the sun or from exertion or both. Her eyes sparkled amid spiky lashes. "We've come too far to lose," he said.

"My feelings exactly."

In that moment, he knew that they could have as easily been talking about their mission as the game.

Alex turned back to the net. "We're ready."

Bella pumped a perfect serve deep into her opponent's watery court. Maria fielded it, set it up for Alex, and he shot it over the net. Back and forth, back and forth.

Finally, Maria began to tire. But she still made her play and got the ball to Alex. He jumped, ready to spike a point, when he lost his balance and fell into the net. Gabriel seized the moment and hammered the ball into enemy territory.

Unfortunately, the driving slam struck Maria in the face, and down she went.

"Good God." Alex's heart stopped. Vaguely he was aware of shouts from Bella and Gabriel, but he got to Maria first and dragged her up out of the water. Her eyes were closed, her face contorted in pain. Already a large knot had formed over her left eye.

Gabriel shoved his way close. "Let me see her."

Alex glared at him. "You could have knocked her out."

Gabriel touched her hair. "Damn, I'm sorry. Stupid competitive urges. I should be shot."

Maria tried to stand up. "I'm fine. No permanent damage."

Alex tightened his arms around her. "Don't move. I've got you." He strode toward the ladder, Gabriel at his elbow. Gabriel nudged him. "Give her to me and hop out. I'll hand her up to you."

Alex bristled. "No. I can handle this." Awkwardly, he tried to reach the first step.

Bella got between him and the ladder, her expression combative. "You two boneheads are acting like Neanderthals. Back off. Maria can get up the ladder on her own." She bit her lip. "Can't you, honey?"

Maria nodded. "Of course."

Reluctantly, Alex allowed Maria to wriggle out of his embrace. He steadied her when she was on her feet. "Are you sure?"

"Yes." Her face was pale, but she managed the three steps and made it up onto the side of the pool.

Alex sprinted behind her and picked her up again.

Gabriel and Bella followed him. "There's a sofa in the cabana," Bella said.

As Alex deposited his precious cargo on the comfy couch, Gabriel frowned. "I'll call 9-1-1."

"No, no, no." Maria sat up despite their protests. "It's a bump on the head. That's all. Give me some aspirin and I'll be fine."

Maria was embarrassed and mortified. Her three companions hovered like broody hens. And despite her wishes, the Montoros' private physician was summoned. The speed at which he arrived startled her.

Everyone was sent out of the cabana while the doctor did his exam. He was kind and gentle and thorough. At last he gave her the all clear. No concussion, but plenty of headaches on the way.

When the other three were allowed to return, Maria

struggled to sit up. "We have to change. Dinner is already late because of me."

Gabriel crouched beside her. "Let Alex take you back to the villa. You're in no shape to suffer through a formal meal. My family will understand, of course. If you feel better in the morning, you're welcome to join us for breakfast."

Bella nodded. "My bull-in-the-china-shop brother is right. I'll have dinner sent down to you. Take the evening to recover." She gathered up Maria's things, as well as Alex's, and tucked them in a large canvas tote.

Gabriel handed Alex a set of keys. "Take the golf cart that's outside. Call the main house if you need anything or if she gets worse."

"I'm sitting right here," Maria said, exasperated. What was it about powerful men that made them feel as if they had to control the world?

Alex steadied her as she stood. "Take it slow."

Outside, Bella gave her a hug. "I'm so sorry about this."

Gabriel said nothing, his expression frustrated and guilty.

"It's nothing," Maria insisted. "I'll be fine."

At last she and Alex were allowed to escape. He drove the cart expertly, of course. And though she couldn't remember for sure where all the turns were, Alex tracked the route without error.

Back at their lodging, she held him off with an upraised hand. "I can walk inside." Still wearing a damp swimsuit, she felt distinctly at a disadvantage, even though Alex was half-naked, as well. Perhaps *because* Alex was half-naked. Despite her pounding headache, she wasn't immune to his overt masculinity.

She was accustomed to seeing him dressed to the nines,

sartorial perfection from head to toe. And *that* man was wildly attractive.

But something about all the bare skin between them sent a pulse thrumming low in her belly. Alex's lightly hair dusted chest and powerful thighs said louder than words that he was a virile man in his prime. If she hadn't been indisposed, she'd have been hard-pressed not to jump his bones. As it was, she had to admire him with a modicum of restraint.

Though she would die before admitting it, she was woozy by the time they made it inside and to her room. Alex allowed her to move at her own pace, but he stayed close. At last, she faced him with a wry smile. "I'm going to take a shower. I'll be careful, I promise."

"Is that wise?" She could see that he didn't like her choice. But short of tying her to a chair, he had no recourse but to step back and close the bedroom door.

When he was gone, her legs gave out and she sat down on the side of the bed. Her head hurt like crazy. When she chanced a peek in the mirror over the dresser, she groaned. Her eye and part of her cheek were swollen, giving her face an odd, lopsided look.

Well, if she'd ever had any hope of luring Alex into her bed, all bets were off. He might be willing to kiss hot-and-sweaty Maria, but what guy would be attracted to a woman who looked like she'd gone three rounds with a boxing champ?

Dispirited and hurting, she gathered her clean undies and her short gown and robe. Their deep plum color should have boosted her spirits, but all she could think about was how her eye was probably going to be a perfect match.

It actually hurt for the water in the shower to hit her face, so she turned the faucet away and managed to wash the chlorine out of her hair without too much discomfort.

After drying off and donning her sleepwear, she sat and dried her hair.

There were times—now being one of them—that she debated cutting her hair. Its length was pure vanity. But the thought of chopping it off made her wince. So she put up with the time it took to wash and dry it.

When she was done, her aches and pains had begun to make themselves felt in earnest. The doctor had left some painkillers. But she needed to take them with food. And, besides, she was starving.

Barefoot, she padded into the living room. Her robe was thigh length, but perfectly respectable, especially given the climate. She found Alex sprawled on the sofa, flipping channels. He was dressed in the casual shirt and slacks he had worn on arrival.

He jumped to his feet. "The food's in the kitchen. Are you interested in eating?"

She nodded, a lump in her throat. The genuine concern on his face and in his dark eyes made her feel cared for and protected. It was a warm, fuzzy sensation. "I'm really hungry," she said softly.

He insisted on seating her at the table and serving her plate from the variety of dishes on the counter.

Maria was barely conscious of what she ate. The food was hot and delicious, but she tasted little of it. She was far too aware of the tension in the room. She remembered their kiss earlier in the day, and it was a good bet Alex did, too.

Six

Alex tried not to let Maria see how worried he was about her. Fatigue was visible in the curve of her shoulders and the pale cast of her skin. She seemed to be holding herself upright by sheer stubbornness.

The knot where the volleyball had made contact with her eye socket had already gone down some, but the bruise was blooming rapidly.

He joined her at the table to eat, though he had no real interest in food. "I was going to offer you a glass of wine," he said. "But I thought better of it. Didn't seem like a good idea if you're taking pain pills."

She pulled a prescription bottle from the pocket of her robe. "The doctor said I can take two at a time, but I'm going to start with one and see how I do."

As he watched, she shook one tablet into her hand and washed it down with water. When her head tilted back, the silky fabric of her nightwear shifted and pulled, making it clear that she was bare underneath. Which made perfect sense, of course. But it also played havoc with his physical state.

He cleared his throat. "It's not late, but you may want to go on to bed."

She shook her head. "I've only now adjusted to the time change. I don't want to start over again. Do you think we could watch a movie?"

He would have done anything she asked in that moment. "Of course," he said, the words gruff.

When they finished their meal, he gathered the dishes and put them in the sink. Maria sat staring at him. "This is weird," she said.

He turned to look at her. "What do you mean?"

"We have a working relationship. And a very important job to do. But suddenly you're having to play nurse. I'm sorry."

He couldn't help himself. Wiping his hands on a dry cloth, he went to her and gathered her hair gently, tucking it over her shoulder so it covered one breast. "Nothing is weird unless we let it be. I kissed you today, Maria. And you kissed me back. Your bump on the head is unfortunate, but I don't regret this time together."

Taking her hand in his, he slowly pulled her to her feet.

When he scooped her into his arms, she protested as she had earlier. "I can walk into the living room."

His arms tightened a fraction. He was a bit drunk on the smell and feel of her. "Humor me. I happen to like having you in my arms."

When he set her gently on the sofa, she stared up at him, wide-eyed. "Are you sure about this?"

She wasn't referring to the movie, of course. "I'm not sure about anything here in Florida," he joked. "Least of all this. But I plan to go with the flow."

He felt her gaze boring into his back as he selected a disc and inserted it into the Blu-ray player and muted the volume. The movie didn't really matter. He had other plans.

When he joined her, she wrapped her arms around her waist and tugged at the hem of her robe. "I've known you for a very long time, Alex…and even on your wildest days, I'd never call you a go-with-the-flow kind of guy."

Her lips quirked, her teasing smile softening what might have been a criticism. But the gentle light in her eyes told him she understood what he was saying.

An attack of conscience struck him as he settled into the soft, plump couch cushions. "If you'd rather watch this alone, I'll leave you. I've plenty of work to do in my room."

One small hand landed on his thigh…not moving…just searing him with heat. "I want you to stay."

He swallowed, for one brief second questioning his sanity. There was a better than even chance that Gabriel Montoro had plans for Maria. Could Alex risk offending a member of the royal family in the midst of delicate negotiations?

But when his hand closed over Maria's, their fingers twining together, he sucked in a deep breath as he realized that for once in his life he was prepared to put his personal wishes and feelings before his obligations.

Gently, giving her every chance to protest, he scooped her into his lap. Her head settled against his collarbone as if he had been holding her like this for a lifetime. "How do you feel?" he asked.

She stroked his jaw with a single finger. "Well enough for whatever you have in mind."

"I seriously doubt that." If she knew what he was thinking, what he wanted, she might run for the hills. "We'll take this slow," he promised. "Tonight and always. I don't want to hurt you."

"I'm a grown woman, Alex. You may have a lot of responsibilities, but I'm not one of them."

The spark of temper reminded him that his Maria was a female of strength and purpose. "I can't apologize for wanting to take care of you. You bring out the gentleman in me."

She curled a hand behind his neck, dragging his head lower to press her lips to his. "Maybe I don't want the gentleman," she muttered. "Kiss me, Alex."

Whatever measure of control he'd maintained up until that second finally snapped. Easing her down onto her back, he parted the lapels of her robe. Lust was a kick to his chest. But it was wrapped in wonder and tenderness. He touched a tight, rosy nipple. "You're so damned beautiful." The words stuck in his throat. He felt he could barely breathe.

"I look like a clown."

He heard the feminine pique in her words and had to smile. "You may be a trifle the worse for wear, dear Maria, but it only makes me want you more."

She rolled her eyes at him. "Is that how you win over your conquests? With outright lies?"

He put his hand, palm flat over her heart, cupping the curves of her breast. "I work too hard to have much of a personal life," he said, willing to be brutally honest if it meant relieving her misgivings. "And when I do spend time with a woman, I am always honest."

"Somehow, I believe you." Her chest rose and fell with her quickened breathing. Despite her poor face, all he could see was the arousal darkening her gaze.

The sofa was oversize and perfectly designed for the things he had in mind. Easing down beside her on one elbow, he separated the robe completely, taking in the minuscule pair of satiny black undies she wore. He traced the tiny elastic edging, feeling the soft skin of her flat stomach.

Reluctantly, he gave her the truth he had promised. "We're not going to be reckless, Maria. I draw the line at making love to an injured woman."

"That's not fair. I get a vote, don't I?"

He shook his head. "Not tonight." Though it would cost him dearly, he decided he could play with fire. Moving carefully so as not to cause her any distress, he sucked in a sharp breath when touching her hardened his sex to the point of pain. "God, you make me crazy," he groaned.

Kissing her was like diving into a pool of quicksand. But aligning their bodies so that warm, feminine flesh nestled against him was far worse. Shaking, he slid a hand between her legs, noting the warmth and dampness that told him she was ready for his possession.

The foreplay tormented them both. Though he would have liked to pleasure her until she came apart in his arms, he feared her poor head would suffer for the orgasm. Reluctantly, he moved his fingers to less volatile territory.

She smelled of exotic shower gel and honeysuckle shampoo. Unable to resist a taste, he caught one nipple between his teeth and tugged gently. Maria cried out, her face now flushed with wild color. "Alex, please," she begged, panting.

Temptation beckoned. The prospect of burying himself inside her and satisfying the craving that had built for weeks was almost irresistible. He could almost feel the warm clasp of her sex on his.

But when her fingers went to the buttons of his shirt, he stopped her, shuddering and dragging in great lungfuls of air as he struggled for control. "We can't. We can't. Not tonight."

Had she been a hundred percent, she would have done

everything in her power to change his mind. He knew that. But she was weak and hurting, her energy at a low ebb.

Tears glistened on her eyelashes, making him feel like the world's biggest cad. "Go away," she cried.

That was one request he couldn't honor. He sat up, moving so that she rested her full length on her side with her head in his lap, her cheek on his thigh. Reaching for the remote, he backed to the opening scene and raised the volume. The film was a black-and-white classic.

He touched her forehead. "Rest, sweetheart. Please."

Though her eyes were open, he couldn't see her expression. For a little while, her body was tense, but gradually he felt her relax. When he thought she was half-asleep, he began to stroke her hair.

The experience changed him. He recognized the seismic shift and marveled at it. Work and pleasing his father had driven his life for so long he scarcely remembered any other way. But tonight…with Maria…he found himself yearning for something he couldn't even identify.

He had never considered himself a jealous man. The truth was, he had never cared enough before for such an emotion to be an issue.

Maria responded to him physically. There was no question of that. But she guarded her feelings and emotions. Did she want anything more from him than physical release?

The thing that bothered him the most was the notion that she might be eventually won over by the bad-boy prince, Gabriel. The other man was apparently irresistible to women. His exploits were the fodder of international gossip rags, even without a royal role.

Worse still was the inescapable truth that Gabriel liked and admired Maria, and vice versa. If such a relationship softened Gabriel to the notion of the Montoros reclaiming the monarchy, could Alex in all good conscience stand in the way? He had devoted weeks and months of his life and his career to affecting this change for the good of Alma.

If a match between Gabriel and Maria made the Montoros more receptive to the proposal, the smartest thing for Alex to do was step aside. But every cell in his body rejected the idea. He'd perfected the art of being a politician first and a man second. Now, integrity be damned, the idea was repugnant to him.

He was not here in Florida, however, to pursue his own agenda. He had been sent as deputy prime minister of commerce to solidify an ancient bond that would take Alma with confidence into the twenty-first century as a world player.

How could he betray the trust of his people for his own selfish ends?

At last, Maria's steady breathing told him she was asleep. Her eyelashes, a shade darker than her hair, fanned out on her cheeks. He knew he probably should have made sure she iced her face, but in his urge to find intimacy with her, the thought had escaped him.

Now, he couldn't bear to wake her.

The medicine had done its work. When he eased out from under her and stood, she barely stirred. Unfortunately, her robe was still unbelted, her breasts bared to his hungry gaze.

Looking at her without her knowledge seemed wrong. Carefully, he tucked the garment around her and knotted the sash. Leaving her for a moment, he went into her bedroom and turned down the covers of her bed. He flipped on a small light in the bathroom and closed the door except for a narrow crack. She might awaken confused in the night.

When he returned to the living room, his heart contracted in his chest. She was smiling in her sleep. He would give a hell of a lot to know if he figured in that pleasant dream.

Gritting his teeth against the rush of need that assaulted him, he bent and lifted her carefully into his arms. Though her robe sheltered her now, he had a very good memory.

Maria was limp in his arms. He worried about that, but he had to trust that the doctor knew his business. Tucking her into bed, he adjusted the sheet and the light, summer-weight comforter. He doubted he would sleep much. Unappeased sexual arousal and a very real concern about Maria's injury guaranteed a wakeful night.

Pulling his phone from his pocket, he set the alarm. He would check on her every hour. She would never know, but it would give him peace of mind.

Maria stretched and winced as her head throbbed. Oh, Lordy. All of the events of yesterday came flooding back in living color…including the memory of Alex's big warm hands on her body.

She flushed from head to toe. And as she did, she grimaced when she realized she had no clue how she had made it from the sofa to the bed. Alex seemed to have a thing for carrying her, so that was a good guess.

Somehow, the thought of him looking after her when she was asleep made her uneasy. Vulnerability was dangerous. She needed to be on her guard, because it would be a mistake to let Alex get too close until she knew what he had in mind.

A business-trip fling was one thing. His position was secure. She had the most to lose.

But what if he wanted more? Back in Alma life would revert to the status quo. Alex would continue to be wealthy and powerful and influential while Maria would go back to being the bastard daughter of a laundress.

That wasn't self-pity talking. It was simply the cold, hard truth.

When she climbed out of bed and stood upright, her head throbbed, but not too badly. The worst part was looking in the bathroom mirror. Holy cow. It was a good thing she had makeup with her. It was going to take a deft hand to ensure her face was presentable for a day with the Montoros.

A day with the Montoros. She chuckled out loud. That sounded like a television series. The trouble was, Maria didn't have the luxury of changing the channel. She had to dress and play her part. Even if today's agenda was ostensibly relaxation and recreation, she and Alex were still officially on the clock. Everything they said or did could have implications for the new regime. That responsibility was never far from her mind.

It took her a half hour to dress and cover up the worst of the bruising around her eye socket. By parting her hair differently and leaving one side loose to fall across her cheek, she managed to improve her appearance significantly.

The headache was bearable this morning, so she decided to skip the prescription stuff in favor of simple ibuprofen. Only then did she notice the small folded slip of paper on the bedside table.

Picking up the note with fingers that trembled, she opened it and studied the bold, masculine scrawl…

Gone up for breakfast at the main house. We all thought you needed to sleep more than eat. When you're hungry, the housekeeper has something fixed for you in the kitchen.
A

If she'd been expecting a tender missive, she was way off base. Not by any stretch of the imagination could the words be construed as personal. And the "we all" was probably only Alex making his usual sweeping judgments, thinking he knew what was best.

Well, darn him, in this case he was right. It was almost ten-thirty and she was only now feeling halfway human and presentable. Given the late hour and the fact that lunch was not far off, she only nibbled at the beautifully prepared tray of food set out in the kitchen beneath a layer of thin linen napkins.

The kiwi and grapefruit and mangoes tempted her the most. And the pitcher of freshly squeezed juice. She did allow herself one of the small perfect cinnamon rolls, as well.

By the time she had eaten and brushed her teeth, there was still no sign of anyone coming to fetch her. Not willing to sit cooling her heels, she went outside and found that a golf cart sat waiting, key in the ignition. Mindful of Alex's alligator warnings, she eyed the open side of the low-slung vehicle with reservation.

But boredom and curiosity won out. She only took one wrong turn and recognized it immediately, so she was justifiably proud when she made it to the Montoro house without incident. The same dignified man from yesterday answered the door when she rang the bell.

Feeling unaccountably nervous, she followed him down the hall to the salon where she and Alex had met the family. Gabriel was the first to spot her hovering in the doorway. He jumped to his feet and met her halfway as she entered the room.

His hands on her shoulders, he cocked his head and studied her face, his own gaze anxious. "How do you feel, Maria?" Gently, he brushed aside a swath of hair to see the bruises she had tried so hard to disguise.

Even his gentle fingertip on her brow made her wince. "Much better," she said. "It's not so bad…honestly."

He kissed her on both cheeks in the European way and released her. "I believe you are a really bad liar."

Bella hovered, as well, surprising Maria with a quick hug. "I worried about you last night. I know the doctor said you didn't have a concussion, but they do make mistakes sometimes."

Being the center of attention was not a comfortable position, particularly with the entire Montoro clan in attendance. "I'm fine, really. But I appreciate your concern."

Rafael Montoro, the older, offered her a seat at his side. "We've been talking business. Alex wanted more information about our company's plans for expansion."

She glanced at Alex, perturbed to find his expression curiously blank. "I thought this was a social visit," she said, smiling.

Rafael nodded. "Bella just called us out on that very subject right before you arrived. I promised her no more boring talk today. I believe you young people are in for a treat. Gabriel has arranged for an airboat tour of the Everglades."

Maria clenched the arm of the love seat. "That's very kind, but I'm sure all of you have been there often. No need to play tourist for us."

Alex raised an eyebrow. He was standing near the window, one hand in his pocket. His posture was relaxed, but she knew him well enough to see the traces of tension in the way he held his mouth. "What Maria isn't saying," he drawled, "is that she is not fond of alligators."

Everyone looked at her, including Isabella. The older woman seemed taken aback. "It's entirely safe," she said in her quavering voice. "I used to love those trips when I was younger."

Even Rafe, Gabriel's brother, nodded. "It's a gorgeous day. You'll love it. I promise."

Juan Carlos chimed in. "Ordinarily, I'd be joining you, too, Miss Ferro. The trip will be delightful. Unfortunately, I have another commitment today. But you really have nothing to worry about."

Maria swallowed her misgivings, realizing she had no choice in the matter. "Sounds like fun."

Seven

Two hours later, after a sumptuous lunch of roasted pork and summer squash, Maria found herself with Bella in the backseat of a large, luxuriously outfitted van. Up front, Gabriel sat at the wheel with his brother in the passenger seat. Alex occupied the middle row, flanked by two large coolers filled with beverages and snacks.

Maria eyed the coolers with misgivings. Exactly how long *was* this trip? Eventually, they pulled into a nondescript gas station and met up with their guide, who then led them in his ancient pickup truck out to the docks where the boats were tethered.

On the upside, the airboats appeared to be modern and well maintained. The padded seats, three and three, were elevated to provide the best vantage point for viewing wildlife. But there was no railing of any kind.

Bella took her arm. "We'll give you the seat in the middle."

That was some small comfort. Maria had assumed Alex might want to sit beside her, but he joined Rafael in the other row. Leaving Gabriel to flank her opposite Bella.

When the guide handed out headphones to block the noise of the motor, Maria eyed her set askance, deciding that she'd rather be deaf than have that thing pressing on her injured head. Gabriel fished out a plastic-wrapped pair of earbuds from his pocket. "You may not need any of this. It's up to you. But I brought you these, just in case."

"That was sweet of you."

He shook his head ruefully. "Merely my guilty conscience at work."

As it turned out, the airboat was noisy, but not incredibly so. The pilot scudded rapidly through the waterways until they reached the Everglades proper. Now he slowed the pace, sliding over the surface of the water as they entered the grasslands. Birds flew everywhere. One of the first varieties of wildlife they spotted in the water was not an alligator at all, but actually a banded snake that turned out to be very rare.

In the midst of the beauty and wonder of it all, Maria forgot to be afraid. Almost. The vegetation was lush and the heat oppressive. Before starting out, she had pulled her hair into a high ponytail and donned a hat and dark sunglasses. Even so, the saunalike atmosphere was sweltering. Soon they were deep in a mangrove swamp. The creek they traversed narrowed in spots until there was barely room for the boat.

All the while she was conscious of Alex sitting behind her. What was he thinking? Maybe not about her at all. Perhaps last night meant nothing more to him than a bit of fooling around. The thought left a sick feeling in the pit of her stomach. And the taste of shame.

It was one thing to initiate something that might be serious, but another entirely to think that Alex saw her as an easy mark.

When Gabriel touched her arm, pointing out a bald eagle, she forced herself to ignore Alex completely. The Everglades were fascinating, 4,300 square miles, a river of grass...unlike anything she had ever seen.

Again, she asked herself why the Montoros would choose to go home to Alma. For the generation sitting in the boat today, Alma was no more home than it was to Maria. She had chosen to move there so she could keep her job when the Ramons relocated their oil business. But for Bella and Rafael and Gabriel, there was nothing but the history in dry books to tie them to the island nation. Who could expect them to tear up roots and make a new home four thousand miles away?

After they had been touring for an hour and a half, the captain steered the boat to a halt and tied it to an outcropping of bushes. Maria looked around with a frown. "Why are we stopping?"

Rafael spoke up. "We like to explore the island. You can get a feel for what it was like before humans came."

"Um, no thanks. I'll wait for you here."

The other four and the grizzled captain stared at her.

She shrugged. "I looked up fatal alligator attacks on humans on the internet yesterday afternoon. I'll be fine right here. I promise."

The captain chewed a toothpick in the side of his mouth. "Reckon you'll be safer on land. No gator's gonna go after six adults together. But one might take a notion to climb into an empty airboat."

Maria scrambled onto shore without another word, enduring the laughter that followed her. The men set up a folding table and some deck chairs. Their guide started opening the coolers and pulling out packets of boiled shrimp and French bread.

The meal had a surreal feel to it. Though Alex still avoided her, she found a quiet pleasure in the day. This trip to the States might be her last chance to travel for many years. Her position paid well as such jobs went, but if she planned to help her mother retire early, there would be little extra money, certainly not for worldwide jaunts.

The negatives facing her had piled up; the negotiations in particular were not going well. Alex was giving her the cold shoulder. She had a bruise the size of a small country around her eye, with a headache to match. But even so, she couldn't be sorry about today. The Montoros were fun and interesting people. She was seeing an ecosystem that was both fragile and starkly beautiful.

When the meal was finished, the Montoro siblings squabbled about how to pack up the leftovers. The guide headed back to the boat. For a moment, Maria and Alex were isolated in a bubble of silence a few yards away from the others. She summoned her courage and spoke her mind. "Are you angry with me, Alex?"

She saw a muscle in his throat work. "No. Of course not."

"You've barely looked at me all day. I can't help thinking the change in you is about last night."

Beneath his tan he was pale. He glanced around, perhaps hoping for rescue, but the Montoros were oblivious. "I don't know what you mean," he said.

Her temper flared. "Oh, please, Alex. Don't lie to me. Surely I deserve better than that."

He clenched his jaw, perspiration beading on his forehead from the thick, heavy air. "It isn't the time or place to talk about this."

"This what?" she asked, her gaze curious, though she knew exactly what he meant.

"We made a mistake," he said through clenched teeth. His voice was low, barely audible. "We're here in Miami to do a job. We have to finish writing the proposal and we have to convince them to sign it. We don't have the luxury of…" He trailed off, but his meaning was clear.

"I see." Hurt made her breathless. Emotion stung the backs of her eyes, but she wouldn't cry. Her injury and her restless night had left her defenses at low ebb. "I won't mention it again. It was nothing anyway."

Alex watched her walk away from him and wanted to curse long and loud. The very thing he'd hoped to avoid had happened. He had hurt Maria, and all because he hadn't been able to resist touching her.

She joined the Montoro siblings, pitching in to clean up the last of the picnic debris. When Gabriel suggested a short walk, Maria nodded. That told Alex more than anything about the state of her mind. She would rather venture into a cypress swamp rife with alligators than remain in his presence one second longer.

He let them go, unable to stomach the sight of Maria's arm tucked in Gabriel's. As the foursome wandered off, Rafael and Bella joked about "*lions and tigers and bears, oh my.*" Gabriel merely kept Maria close to his side, promising to defend her to the death. His dramatic vow made Maria laugh. Alex kicked a root at the happy sound, his thoughts grim.

It was becoming clearer every day that Gabriel Montoro liked Maria. A lot. In a romantic way? Who knew…? But Alex needed to back off or risk damaging the relationships that were integral to the success of his mission for Alma.

As he sat on the airboat and listened to the old captain

tell stories of the Florida that existed before Disney and the interstate highway system, only half of Alex's attention was engaged. He was debating his options. He could send Maria back to Alma on some pretext. That would put an end to his temptation, and she would also be out of Gabriel's reach.

But the idea lasted only a nanosecond. Maria was a gifted, hardworking member of the delegation, and she deserved this chance to shine. Alex had no right to kick her off the team; nor did he have the moral imperative to step in between her and Gabriel.

His conclusions were sound. But he didn't have to like them.

In another twenty minutes, the explorers returned to the boat, all in one piece as Gabriel pointed out, poking Maria in the ribs with a sly smile.

"No thanks to you," she said, settling into her original seat and sparing no glance for Alex.

The captain started up the boat, and the rest of the afternoon passed without incident. To Alex's critical eye, Maria seemed to flag by the end of the day, but he had abdicated any right to check on her well-being. When the Montoros dropped off Alex and Maria at the guesthouse, Maria disappeared into her bedroom without so much as a word.

Though they later rode in a golf cart together up to the main house, the journey was silent.

Dinner that night was both pleasant and awkward if such a thing was possible. Isabella was in attendance, her wheelchair pulled to the edge of the table at Rafael III's right hand. Her nephew encouraged her to tell stories of the old times, and the elderly woman did so with enthusiasm.

She'd had one of her rare good spells today. Though her body trembled and her voice was weak, it was clear to everyone present that her spirit was unquenched. Isabella had been a very young child when the royal family was overthrown. In all likelihood, she didn't actually remember any of the details. But the tales of the traumatic events had been repeated often as she grew up, and to her, the end of the Montoro reign was still vivid.

Alex knew—as did her family, he supposed—that Isabella would not be happy until another Montoro ascended the throne that was rightfully theirs. She was in a fragile state. The span of her life was uncertain. What would happen if she died before a decision had been reached? Would the Montoro family choose to stay in Miami?

Alex had plenty of questions and not enough answers.

Gabriel asked Maria to stay for coffee after dinner adjourned. He glanced at Alex. "I'll bring her home before curfew, I promise."

Alex managed a smile, but his gut churned. Walking out of that house and leaving Maria with Gabriel was one of the hardest things he had ever had to do. The hollow feeling in his chest told him he was in deep trouble. He had been lying to himself about the intensity of his feelings for Maria.

With that knowledge came stinging regret. Had he crushed something new and beautiful beneath the heel of his duty and ambition?

He should have been proud of his dedication and resolve.

But it wasn't pride that kept him awake until three in the morning, when he heard the front door of the villa open and shut...

By Monday morning, Maria was able to conceal most of the vestiges of her contact with Gabriel's spiked volleyball. The swelling around her eye had gone down, and, with artful concealer, her appearance was close to normal.

She had never been more thankful for the presence of the lawyer, Jean Claude. Having a buffer meant that she and Alex were able to work side by side on the draft of the official proposition without acknowledging the events of the weekend. By noon, they were so deeply involved in the knotty questions of language and ceremony that personal situations were pushed aside.

The document was shaping up nicely. Alex and Maria were composing the actual words. Jean Claude was guiding them with the necessary legal language. The collaborative effort flowed well, though as Maria worked feverishly at her laptop, transcribing the conversations, she couldn't help but wonder if all of this would be in vain.

That night she ordered room service for dinner and fell into bed soon after, too tired from the intensity of the day's efforts to do more than dream of Alex. The same pattern repeated itself for the following three days. On Friday morning, the rough draft of the document was complete. Though satisfying, it was only the first step. It would have to be faxed to the prime minister back in Alma. In addition, the entire delegation was to meet the following week to pick it apart and look for weaknesses.

Unfortunately, Jean Claude received a phone call midday summoning him back to Alma for a family funeral. Harried and sad, he offered Alex a bulging folder. "You and Maria can handle editing and polishing over the weekend. Here are all my notes. I'll check in with you before Monday to see if you have any questions."

When he was gone, the silence in the room became oppressive. Maria swallowed hard. She and Alex had shared barely half a dozen personal words since the day of the airboat ride. She hated the rift between them. For years they had worked together in harmony.

Even when she was promoted to a new position and no

longer reported directly to Alex, they still had frequent
contact in the Department of Commerce. And of course,
here in Miami, he *was* her boss. She had been thrilled to
be picked for the delegation, especially knowing it would
be a chance to work with Alex again.

Since coming to Miami, she'd seen him in a new light—
in all honesty, as a potential lover. And it had seemed to her
as if Alex was experiencing the same shift in dynamics.
There was awareness between them. An unspoken bond
that had bloomed out in the open in Miami's atmosphere
of hedonism and fun.

Their first kiss had rocked her…had forced her to be
honest with herself about the fact that her admiration for
Alex had segued into something much deeper and more
volatile. She wanted him.

When she was injured and he cared for her with such
wildly intimate results, she'd been sure he was feeling the
same desperate, crazy passion that she was. But almost in
the next instant, he had shut her down. Which said that his
emotions were unengaged.

He might have a physical response to her as a woman.
But she needed and wanted far more. So much more.

"Shall we continue?" she asked. "With the editing, I
mean."

His face was hard to read. "I think not. We've worked
incredibly hard this week. Why don't we take the rest of
the day for ourselves? Call a truce. Play tourist."

Her heart sank. He was offering an olive branch at the
worst possible time. "That's very kind of you, Alex. And
very tempting. But I'm meeting Bella and Gabriel and
Rafe for an early dinner."

His dark eyes flashed fire for a brief second before his
expression shuttered. "I see."

She shoved her hands through her hair. "No. I don't

think you do. They're concerned about the future. And they know I'm not a native of Alma, so they think I can be objective."

"And can you?"

The derision in his voice hurt. "I've given a hundred percent to the work of the delegation. And I'll do everything in my power to convince them the monarchy is important for everyone."

"Anything else?"

The sarcasm was overt, but she was angry enough now not to be affected by his scorn. "If you must know, I'm trying to get closer to Gabriel."

"I'll bet you are."

"Oh, grow up," she said. "Somebody has to ferret out his bad-boy secrets, not to mention defusing anything that might embarrass the Montoros once they return to Alma."

"And that has to be you?"

"Do you have a better idea? He likes me. I think he trusts me. So I'm going to use that connection to do my job."

Alex's glare could have melted a Titanic-sized iceberg. He held up his hands, his cheekbones streaked with color. "Don't let me stand in your way, Ms. Ferro. Good luck."

Fury sent her across the room to go toe-to-toe with the irritating man. "I can't believe I ever thought you were a nice guy. You're overbearing, hostile, argumentative—"

He shut her up abruptly by the simple expedient of slamming his mouth down on hers. Neither suave nor sophisticated, the move reeked of desperation.

Shock held her immobile for two seconds before she put her hands on his shoulders in a token attempt to shove him away. "I won't let you kiss me," she muttered. But her arms curled around his neck and her lips parted to allow his tongue entrance.

She was so damned mad at him, but somehow all that feeling transmuted into hunger that consumed her from the inside out.

He wedged a leg between hers. "I don't know what to do about you, Maria. God help me, I don't."

With some last vestige of self-respect, she jerked out of his embrace. Her knees trembled, and she could barely breathe. But she wouldn't let him toy with her emotions. Not like this.

She wiped the back of her hand across her mouth, trying to eradicate the taste of him. "You need to make up your mind, Alex," she whispered raggedly. "Either I'm a valued employee or a prospective lover or a gold digger looking to marry into the royal family. When you figure out the answer, be sure to let me know."

Walking toward the door, she stopped abruptly and gave him one last withering glance. "I'll see you here Monday morning at nine o'clock sharp. If you need any edits on the document over the weekend, email them to me. I think it would be better for everyone concerned if you and I stay away from each other."

Eight

By the time dinner rolled around Maria had run the gamut of emotions. She had burned with anger, cried with regret and at last found a certain measure of peace by reminding herself that she was only a small part of a much larger purpose. Her relationship with Alex, or lack thereof, was secondary to the job she had been engaged to do.

Alma, as a nation, faced a critical juncture. At such points in history, personal agendas often took a backseat to working for the greater good. This wasn't wartime, but in a sense, she and Alex were living in the midst of a volatile shift in national identity.

Reminding herself of what was at stake helped put her own troubles in perspective. Broken hearts were a dime a dozen. She'd get over hers. Besides, it was probably only bruised. She'd had a crush. That was all…

Meeting Bella, Rafe and Gabriel in the hotel lobby was interesting to say the least. Paparazzi were not as ubiquitous in Miami as they were in some parts of the world. But the Montoros were both famous and flamboyant. The public enjoyed their antics...even more so now that gossip had begun to circulate about a possible tie to Alma.

Though Maria found it disconcerting when a camera flash went off in her face, the Montoro trio seemed to take it in stride. They had planned to walk the block and a half to their favorite seafood place. When it became clear to the guy carrying the camera that nothing too dramatic was afoot, he slunk away without further incident.

The restaurant overlooked the water and was crowded even at this early hour. Reservations required. When the Montoro party was granted a premium table near the window, Maria began to see that this branch of modern royalty was comfortable with the trappings of wealth and privilege. They might have to adapt to a new country and new titles, but theirs was no rags-to-riches story.

Over a meal that was exquisite in every way, her dinner companions grilled her about Alma and its current state.

She grimaced as she dabbed her lips with a linen napkin. "Where do I start? You'll be happy to know that the government has made technology a priority, both for education and in the private sector. Certain books and movies were banned under the old regime, but now information and entertainment flow freely."

Bella wanted to know about the palace. "Is it habitable?"

"Oh, yes. Tantaberra, and later his son and grandson, made themselves very comfortable over the years. Even during the revolt, little was damaged. Efforts are already underway to update the furnishings and to clean and remodel. I think you'll be pleasantly surprised when you see it."

Rafe frowned. "*If*, not when."

She felt her face heat. "Sorry. Didn't mean to get ahead of myself."

Gabriel appeared far more serious than she had seen him on other occasions. "Are the people really in favor of this move, or is it the brainchild of a favored few?"

"The press has done good job of advancing the idea. In a recent poll, seventy-two percent favored a return of the traditional monarchy."

Bella grimaced. "And what about the other twenty-eight percent?"

"Some of those are young people who are suspicious of anything that reeks of being told what to do and how to act. They want assurances of freedom and personal choice. Once they see that Alma functions well with the constitutional monarchy, I think the poll numbers will be even higher."

Rafe was still the quietest of the three. She couldn't quite tell if it was because of the situation or because his personality was more measured than his younger siblings. He lifted a shoulder, as if to say he was taking a fatalistic view. "In the end, what difference will it make if I say yes or say no?"

Maria started to respond with the official line but then pulled back and spoke from the heart. "I grew up in London. My mother and I had nothing. Every day was a struggle for her. But she adored the royal family. It was as if they represented something special about England that was a part of her, as well, though she was never likely to meet a royal or see one in person. I watched her swell with pride when good things happened to them and shake her head in grief when tragedies happened."

"Then why did you move away from England?" Gabriel asked.

"I had been working for Alex's family for several years

when things changed in Alma and the Ramons decided to return to their homeland. My job paid well, far more than my mother was making. And in Alma I would have opportunities for advancement. So together, we made the decision to leave England. I can tell you, though, that she will be one to cheer the loudest if the Montoros return. She understands what the monarchy means to the common people."

The table fell silent. Maria hadn't spoken with the intent of making anyone feel sorry for her or her mother. But there could no longer be any doubt that the social chasm between the two Ferro women and the Montoros—or the Ramons, for that matter—was vast.

She couldn't decide if she had done more harm than good when her companions consumed their desserts in silence. Had she been too frank? Did they think she was too pushy? Should she have let more senior members of the team do the persuading?

At last, she pushed her plate aside, her lemon meringue pie only half-eaten. "One more thing, and then we can abandon this topic."

Gabriel shook his head. "Why stop now? You're on a roll."

"Very funny." She clasped her hands in her lap, feeling the damp palms that signaled her nervousness. More than anything, she wished Alex were here beside her. For more reasons than one. "Your family is very well-known in Florida, probably across the States, too. But the publicity storm that will be unleashed if you agree to reclaim your positions as royal family will be unprecedented. You think Prince William and Kate and baby George have been photographed continually? That will be nothing compared to your return."

Bella wrinkled her nose. "Surely you're exaggerating."

"I don't think so. We're talking about a throne that has been empty for seven decades. And a new king who is handsome and charismatic and single. Your whole family will be in the public eye."

Gabriel slumped back in his chair. "Oh, goody."

Rafe lapsed into silence. Bella excused herself to go to the ladies' room. Maria fixed Gabriel with a half-apologetic stare. "Part of my job is going to be media spin and public relations. Since you seem to carry the black sheep reputation, I have to ask…are there are any situations we will need to know about?"

His chuckle was dry. "To the best of my knowledge, I have no secret offspring hidden about the state. And no outstanding warrants. The worst of my sins are more gray than black. Wouldn't you agree, Rafe?"

His older brother grinned widely, for once looking almost carefree. "Far be it from me to weigh in on your confessional. But I promise, Maria, Gabriel won't embarrass us. He's too smooth and charming. If critics pop up, he'll simply woo them or schmooze them. They'll never know what hit them."

Rafe's assurances removed most of her concerns. Maybe Gabriel wasn't quite the loose cannon she had expected. Which was a good thing for everyone involved.

When Bella returned to the table, the group rose to leave. Bella and Rafael were headed out to a party. Gabriel offered to walk Maria back to her hotel. Along the way, she was startled when he opened up to her in a very serious voice. "I'm worried about my brother," he said, his voice flat. "I don't want him to give up his life."

"Has he said much to you?"

"Not really. But I found out today that he and my father have known about this monarchy thing for at least a couple of months."

"And you didn't?"

"No. Apparently the prime minister of Alma contacted our father and told him what was brewing…along with pointing out that Dad was not going to be king."

"That must have been an uncomfortable conversation."

"Indeed. Anyway, Rafael was sworn to secrecy until the delegation arrived. But it explains a lot."

"What do you mean?"

"Well, a few weeks ago, Rafe took off to Key West for an unexpected trip. I offered to go with him…we often fish and snorkel there together. But he told me no…that he needed some time alone to clear his head. At the moment, I had no idea what he was talking about."

"But now you do."

Gabriel paused in front of Maria's hotel. "Yes. Now I do."

She touched his arm. "You'll be a big help to him. Whichever way the decision goes. I can tell he thinks a lot of you."

"I appreciate the pep talk, Maria. It's no wonder Alex is madly in love with you."

"Excuse me?" She took a step backward in shock.

"Oh, come on. Surely you've noticed. Every time I get close to you, he practically bares his teeth at me."

Her head pounded and her chest tightened with anxiety. "You're mistaken. We're colleagues. That's all."

"Trust me on this one. I'm a guy. I know how guys think."

"He accused me of trying to cozy up to you so I could be a princess."

Gabriel laughed out loud. "And do you want to be a princess?"

"Not particularly," she said, truthful but wry.

He gave her an oddly sweet smile. "I think you and I

will turn out to be good friends by the time this is all over. And I could use a friend right about now."

"You have a reputation for being a party lover. I find it hard to believe you don't have a confidante on every street corner."

"Plenty of women in my life. I'll admit to that. But they all want something. You're an open book, Maria. I like you a lot, even if we aren't romantically inclined."

"And Alex?"

He grimaced. "I don't have the same warm, fuzzy feelings about your boss. My family will tell you that I get a kick out of stirring up trouble. I could help you make him jealous."

"No, thank you." Imagining Alex's glacial expression if he thought Maria was encouraging Gabriel's interest made her cringe. "Besides, I told him there was nothing between us but friendship."

"And did he believe you?"

"I don't know what he believes," she said, realizing that this was a highly inappropriate conversation to be having with a member of Alma's prospective royal family. "I should go now," she said quietly.

"I've embarrassed you. I'm sorry."

"No. I'm fine. But I shouldn't overstep my bounds. You and your family are very important to the future of Alma. I don't want you to think I take that lightly."

"No one thinks that, Maria. Believe it or not, none of us gives a damn about Alma's class hierarchy."

"You may not, but others do. I appreciate your taking the time tonight to let me talk to you. Please reiterate my thanks to your brother and sister."

"So formal. So serious."

She knew he was teasing her, but she was suddenly desperate to regain some sense of formality between them...as if Alex could see the fact that she and Gabriel were comfortable with each other. "Good night, Gabriel," she said.

He watched her walk up the steps. "It will all work out, Maria. Things always do."

"I hope you're right."

Alex paced the confines of his hotel room, feeling the walls close in around him. It had been eight hours, give or take, since he last saw Maria. If she had her way, the two of them wouldn't meet again until Monday morning when they were surrounded by the Alma delegation.

He had handled things with her poorly from the beginning…probably, because for once in his life, he didn't have a clear idea of how to proceed. Not in regard to the proposal and the Montoros. That path was well defined. It was his personal life that seemed out of control. Hell, up until the past few weeks, he hadn't even allowed himself to imagine a personal life that included any woman on a permanent basis.

But with Maria at his side and under his nose day in and day out, it was becoming increasingly difficult to convince himself that he was a patriot first and a man second.

He glanced at his watch. It was late, but not too late. He wasn't going to be able to sleep unless he saw her. That in itself was disturbing. They had known each other for a long time now. Had worked together in a number of settings. When had things started to change? When had he begun to notice the way her smile hit him in the gut? Or been stricken with the need to touch her? To make her laugh?

Grabbing up his key and his phone, he strode across the room. But when he jerked open the door in preparation for leaving, Maria stood in the hallway, her hand raised to knock.

Her arm dropped, and her eyes widened. "Alex."

He pulled up short, his adrenaline-fueled momentum stymied by the fact that she had come to him. "Maria."

To an outsider, the tableau would have seemed comical. Maria recovered first, already backing away. "You were going out," she said. "I can talk to you later."

He grabbed her arm and dragged her inside, closing the door firmly. "No. We'll talk now."

"But—"

He put a hand over her mouth. "I was coming to find you," he said gruffly.

Maria freed herself from his loose hold and moved to stand beside the window. "If you're going to yell at me again, I'd just as soon pass."

He shook his head. "I didn't yell."

"What would you call it?"

"Mutual aggravation?"

That coaxed a smile from her. "Fair enough."

"Why did you come to find me?" he asked.

"I wanted to let you know how the dinner went."

His chest tightened with disappointment. So much for the personal agenda. "Okay. Let's hear it."

"May I have a seat?"

"Of course."

They moved to the nearby grouping of sofas and chairs. The room was extremely large. Though Alex hadn't asked for it, he presumed that his position as head of the delegation had warranted the generous quarters.

Maria was dressed casually in a soft multicolored skirt that touched her knees and a thin, sleeveless top of ivory silk. The barely there sandals she wore showcased pink toenails.

Although she sat on the love seat, he was too antsy to join her at the moment. He ran a hand through his hair. "So tell me. How did it go?"

She shrugged, her expression pensive. "It's hard to say. They asked a million questions. Good questions. Rafe, as always, was reserved."

"Do they seem at all receptive to the proposal?"

"They're guarding their options. We have to remember that they haven't even seen a copy of it yet."

"True. If the rough draft gets an okay next week, the plan was to go ahead and let the Montoros take a look."

"Does that mean they get a chance to approve or disapprove?"

"I don't think the delegation will like that idea. Unless we have a solid commitment first."

"In other words, two stubborn entities in a standoff."

"No one wants to lose face or operate from a position of weakness."

"I think the key to winning them over is going to be the personal touch. If they trust you and the delegation, they're going to be much more likely to agree to our proposal."

"Well, they trust *you*. That's a start."

She crossed her arms and thrust out her chin. "There you go again. Flinging insults."

He held out his hands. "I certainly did not. It was a compliment."

Her expression was skeptical. "Didn't sound like one."

Judging himself sufficiently in control of his emotions to get closer, he sat down beside her and touched her arm. "I'm glad they feel comfortable talking to you. Really I am. You're an incredible asset to the team."

She stared at him, vulnerability in the depths of her gaze. At times he forgot about her humble beginnings and that her maturity belied her years. "I'm serious," he said softly. "I admire you, Maria. You're smart and quick-thinking and you have a better grasp of human emotions than I do. Thank you for meeting with Rafe and Bella and Gabriel tonight."

"You're welcome," she said, her words barely audible.

She no longer met his gaze, so he had to lift her chin with his finger. "I don't like it when we fight," he muttered.

Maria didn't reply, but her hand came up to cover his. He thought she meant to push him away, but instead, she twined her fingers with his. "I don't like it, either."

Ten seconds passed. Or maybe a hundred. Awareness quivered in the air. He could hear the thump of his own heartbeat in his ears. Maria's cheeks flushed, her eyes starry with something he dared not put a name to. Later, he couldn't remember which of them moved first.

Their lips met softly…tentatively. He slid a hand beneath her hair to cup the back of her neck. The top of her spine was fragile, the curve of her nape feminine. "I want you," he said. He had an advanced degree in diplomacy and a reputation as a persuasive leader. But in that moment he felt as awkward as a high school kid on his first date.

Maria leaned into him, her posture both eager and trusting. He should try to be worthy of that trust, but if such a thing meant sending her away, then he was doomed.

She put a hand against his cheek, stroking the stubble that appeared if he didn't shave twice a day. Her gaze clashed with his, her eyes deep enough to drown in. "I want you, too, Alex. But without regrets. If this time in Miami is all we have, let it be enough."

Nine

The wording made him frown. What she was offering would be the perfect scenario for most men. A temporary liaison. No strings attached. Yet, oddly, her plea unsettled him.

Because he didn't want to answer, he let his actions tell her what he couldn't yet say. The silk shell she wore came off easily over her head. He caught a ragged breath at the sight of her breasts barely covered in smooth, ivory satin. When he tossed the top aside, he realized that his hands were shaking.

Maria had gone still, her wary gaze alert, like a doe in the forest scenting danger. But she didn't stop him when he drew her to her feet. "I need you naked," he groaned, unzipping her skirt and drawing it down and off. Her French-cut undies matched the bra. Plain…unadorned…but sexy as hell. "Ah, Maria."

She hadn't said a word since he began unwrapping the

most wonderful present he'd ever been offered. Was it shyness that kept her silent?

"I don't know what you're thinking," he muttered. The bra fell away. He steadied her as she stepped out of the sandals. Tracing the elastic band of her only remaining item of clothing, he sighed. "Please say something."

Her smile was tremulous. "I haven't done this very often."

"I don't need an accounting." In fact, he'd rather not know. The thought of his Maria with other men made him a little crazy.

"That's not what I mean." She started in on his shirt buttons. "I want to please you. But my experience is—"

He put a hand over her mouth for the second time that night. "Your experience is irrelevant. That's what it is... irrelevant. Neither of us has ever been here before. Everything we say and do in this room is brand-new." He tucked her hair aside and kissed the soft skin beneath her ear. "Brand-new, Maria."

It took a great deal of fortitude to allow her to unclothe him. But she was so sweetly intent on her task he clenched his fists at his hips and let her take the lead. When her fingers touched his belt buckle, he inhaled sharply, the sound a quick hiss of startled shock.

Since when had a woman ever been able to arouse him with such innocent motions? Stretched on a rack of unfilled desire, he braced himself as she slid his shirt from his shoulders and then tugged his trousers to his knees. When she paused, he kicked off his socks and shoes and pants in one ungainly dance.

His navy boxers did little to hide how much he wanted her.

And still his would-be lover was mute. "I think we could

adjourn to the bed," he said, smiling with a grimace that was supposed to be reassuring.

Maria nodded, allowing him to take her hand and draw her toward the king-size mattress that could sleep half a dozen men. The coverlet was navy damask, the contrasting pillows and trim taupe. Against the heavy, ornate fabric, Maria's skin would glow.

At the last instant, he picked her up in his arms and used one hand to fling back the covers. Maria looked up at him, her eyelashes at half-mast, her throat and chest flushed with color. "I'm on the pill," she said.

All members of the delegation had undergone fairly stringent physicals before leaving for the States. Though he had condoms with him, he found himself fiercely glad that they would be unnecessary.

"Are you sure?" he asked hoarsely. "I don't want you to think I'm coercing you."

For the first time since she entered his suite, her face lightened, and she laughed out loud. "I'm pretty sure you're not. It's a little insulting that I had to work so hard to get your attention."

He deposited her on the soft sheets and followed her down. "Are you kidding? I noticed you the first day you came to work for our company in London. But you were way too young and I was way too busy."

"And later?" Her arms remained at her sides, as if she were afraid to move.

He traced a fingertip from the center of her forehead, down her nose, between her breasts, all the way to her navel, where he stopped to let both of them catch their breath. "In Alma I watched you bloom from a pretty young girl to a mature, fascinating woman. But we were both consumed with the work at hand—steering Alma's fate."

"Did you have this in mind when you suggested me to be on the delegation?"

Her quiet question caught him off guard. He was the one to flush this time. Had he envisioned this moment? Really? It troubled him that he couldn't give her an unequivocal answer.

She stroked his collarbone with both hands, moving down his chest as he leaned over her on one elbow. "It doesn't matter," she said. "Because even if you didn't, I did. I've had the worst crush on you. Then somehow, when we got to Florida, everything got worse."

"Worse? Or better?" He lightly rubbed her nipples one after the other, breathing harder when she arched off the bed and called his name.

This time...this precious first time. He knew he wanted it to be special for her, but lust rode him like a wild animal, consuming everything in its path. Honor...tenderness...gentle care.

Maria trembled against him, as nervous as a wide-eyed cat. "Relax," he muttered. "I won't do anything you don't like." But when he buried his face between her thighs and feasted on the taste of her, nothing short of cataclysm could have made him stop before he pushed her off the edge of a choked climax.

"More," he groaned. "We'll do more later. But I can't wait."

He felt the last flutters of her climax against his shaft as he pushed his way inside her. The tight fit...the heat... all of it overwhelmed him. Because in the midst of intense physical euphoria he felt something else. A notion that terrified him and made him weak.

He might be in love with her.

Maria still reeled in the aftermath of what had been an unprecedented orgasm. She'd been sure such things were the stuff of movies and books. Who could believe that the earth actually rocked on its axis when the right man staked a claim?

Alex filled her completely, in a way she barely understood. He was a man with all the usual equipment, but even in her limited experience, she recognized that this was something far beyond a casual hookup. Maybe not for him, but certainly for her.

And because she had courted this moment, watched for it, waited for it to happen, she would be the one with the most to lose. Alex Ramon was not available for everlasting love. He was smart and wonderful and passionate, but he was not hers.

That dreadful reality refused to take root in light of the fact that he was thrusting inside her wildly, rolling to his back and encouraging her own acrobatics. "Take what you want, Maria. Take it all."

His breathless grin encompassed a masculine satisfaction that should have made her want to smack him for his impudence…if she hadn't been trembling on the brink of yet another exquisite climax. "Who's taking whom?" she asked primly, stingingly aware that he felt larger and more determined from this angle.

"Doesn't matter." He groaned when she dared to reach behind and touch the base of his erection.

Where his fingers gripped her buttocks, she would likely have bruises tomorrow. She looked down at him, seeing the power in his broad shoulders, the pleasing symmetry of his pectoral muscles, the sleek delineation of his rib cage.

"You are a beautiful man," she breathed, squeezing inwardly as he dragged her down onto his hard flesh again and again. "I never knew what you were hiding beneath all those hand-tailored suits."

His head pressed into the pillow as he gasped. "Well, we're even then, because I may never let you get dressed again."

With one last twist of his hips, he took them both into the deep end. As the wave crashed over her, violent and deeply satisfying, she slumped onto his chest and counted the beats of his heart.

Alex couldn't feel his legs. Paralysis was, as a rule, a frightening state. But at this particular juncture in his life, he couldn't bring himself to care.

Maria slept like the dead, her limp body draped over him as the softest, sweetest of blankets. Her hair was in his mouth and his nose, and one of her knees threatened his male anatomy. But all he could do was smile and thank his guardian angel for arranging this tryst.

Did angels even know about sex? Well, of course they did, because it was pretty clear that he'd just caught a glimpse of heaven.

His feelings were all over the map. Since he was not a man to even recognize the fact that he *had* emotions, the sharp shift in outlook was both alarming and bemusing.

Maria. It was all about Maria. Offstage, problems loitered, ready to shatter his giddy, postcoital bliss. But he refused to countenance them. One night. One mad, insanely wonderful night. That's all he wanted, all he asked for. When the sun rose, he would pick up the reins of civic obligation once again.

But tonight was his. His and Maria's.

He woke her with a kiss. A kiss that started with a quick nibble on a tender earlobe and ended up with her stretched out on her back, his teeth raking the spot where neck and shoulder met.

"What are you doing?" she mumbled, refusing to open her eyes.

"If you have to ask, I must be doing it wrong."

"Alexxx..." Two syllables stretched to the breaking point.

Her shoulder was particularly sexy. How had he never noticed that? "You're sweet and soft and I want you more now than I did a half hour ago."

"Is that even possible?"

He choked out a laugh, trying to decide what he should taste next. "Look at me and tell me you feel it, too."

Long lashes tipped in gold lifted. Her irises were more blue than green right now. Her pupils were dilated. She was sated and drowsy and completely irresistible.

When she licked her lips, he could swear it was unconscious...that she had no clue what that little movement did to him.

"I should go to my room, Alex."

He frowned. "Why?"

"We have to be circumspect. You're a very important man. Gossip could be detrimental to your career."

"Screw my career." How could she even think like that? They were naked and wrapped in each other's arms. It pissed him off that she had the presence of mind to be concerned about propriety.

She feathered the fingers of both hands through his hair, sending a shiver down his spine. "Be sensible, Alex. Please."

"I'm *always* sensible," he said through clenched teeth. "I'm sick of being sensible. As far as I'm concerned, you're not leaving this room until Monday morning."

"What about the editing and revising?"

Bless her wonderful, conscientious, puritanical heart. She was trying to save him from himself. "We both have laptops. No one expects to hear from us tomorrow or Sunday. It's the perfect scenario. I'll make love to you until neither of us can breathe, then we'll order room service, work on the document a bit and go back to bed."

"You're serious…" Her gaze searched his face, looking for God knows what.

Even he could see that his behavior was an anomaly. His father would be horrified. But his father was far, far away, and Alex was in the midst of a sexual awakening of unprecedented proportions.

What if sex with Maria was more than scratching an itch? What if this was what he'd been missing his entire adult life?

She exhaled, perhaps signaling capitulation. "I'd still have to go to my room and get a few things. What if someone sees me?"

"We're on the same floor. Opposite halls, granted…but it will be a quick trip. Quit worrying."

At long last she nodded slightly. "Okay."

When she climbed out of bed and began to search for her clothes, he was stricken with the notion that she might not return. He took her chin in his hand and stared into her eyes. "You won't change your mind?"

He'd meant the words to sound like a command, but they came out closer to a plea than he would have liked.

Both of them were naked. Upright. He could lift her and take her again right now. The image made him breathless.

"I'll come back," she said.

As a bit of insurance, he confiscated her bra and undies and stuffed them in a dresser drawer. "I want you to think of me when you're walking half-naked down the hall."

"I can't do that," she said, her expression aghast. "What if someone sees?"

"I suppose you'd better hurry."

* * *

Maria scuttled down the carpeted hallway, her arms wrapped around her waist. The building was air-conditioned to arctic levels, and she knew her bare breasts were noticeable beneath her thin top. The knowledge made her face hot, but not as much as reliving what had just transpired in Alex's suite.

If she had not promised to return, there was a good chance she would have avoided him until Monday. Could he read her that well?

Once safely inside her own room, she rested her back against the door, breathing rapidly. She was not the kind of woman who had affairs right under the noses of people who knew her...who expected her to be hardworking and ethical and dedicated to Alma's cause.

Were all those expectations in her head? Maybe people were just people...fallible, unable to predict, good and bad.

Wanting Alex as a lover didn't negate her contributions to the work of the delegation. As a group, the delegation had been sent to Miami with express instructions to take the weekends off. Healthy, productive humans knew how to relax. So why was Maria freaked out about the notion of being spontaneous and irresponsible with Alex Ramon?

Avoiding her own question, she found a straw tote that looked more like a purse than a suitcase and began stuffing it with essentials: toiletries, clean undies, her billfold, a comfy pair of yoga pants and a loose cotton top. The paperback novel she was in the midst of.

On second thought, she took the book out of the bag. Chances were, Alex didn't plan to give her much opportunity for reading.

When she had rounded up everything she thought she might need for the weekend, she stared at the perfectly made bed. *Damn.* She wasn't cut out for a life of deception and hanky-panky. Placing the tote beside the door, she set to work making the room look lived-in.

She tossed the covers until the bed was a tumbled mess. Then she went into the bathroom, dampened a towel and washcloth and crumpled them on the floor. Finally, she opened a packet of soap and wet it before placing it in the shower.

Feeling more than a little ridiculous, she examined her quarters with an eagle eye. The delegation was well-known already, at least within the hotel. Service workers noticed all sorts of intimate details. Maria wanted to make it perfectly clear to anyone who might be paying attention that she had definitely slept in her own room, tonight...*not* in room 1724.

Grimacing at the realization that she would likely have to repeat this same charade tomorrow afternoon, she shook her head at her own foolishness and decided she had kept Alex waiting long enough.

Opening the door to the hallway a crack, she gazed left and right. No one in sight. Though she managed to hold up her head and walk with confidence down the corridor, around the atrium and back to the far wing, her heart was beating so rapidly she felt dizzy.

When she knocked on Alex's door, and he opened it immediately, she practically fell into his arms. "No one saw me," she whispered.

Alex was dressed again...in the same clothes he had worn earlier, minus the shoes and socks. His bare feet were long and sexy.

He took her shoulders in his hands, looking at her with alarm. "You're shaking, Maria."

"Adrenaline," she said on a sigh, thrusting her bag into his arms and dropping into an armchair. "I think I need a drink."

He poured her a glass of white wine and crouched at her side, his warm, dark eyes dancing with amusement. "If I had known it was such a big deal, I would have gone to your room myself."

She raised an eyebrow. "And let you riffle through my unmentionables? I don't think so. We don't know each other that well."

He stroked a finger down her arm, making her shiver. "I've seen you naked," he said solemnly. "I think I'm allowed to touch your underwear."

"It's a slippery slope. First it's the underwear and next thing you know you'll be asking me to spend the night."

His chiseled, masculine lips quirked. "I think I already did."

She stared at him moodily. They were so close at this angle all she had to do was lean forward three or four inches and she could touch her mouth to his. "Do you really think we can concentrate on work in between…um…you know?"

His breath was warm on her cheek. "I have no idea. But I'm willing to find out. Besides, we're supposed to be taking the weekend off."

"Doesn't matter. You and I both know that we have to make sure the proposal is ready for the briefing."

"We'll get it done, I promise. I work best under pressure."

"And what if we can't stop having sex? What if we ravage each other 24/7 until we barely know if it's day or night?"

Ten

Alex's erection had abated during Maria's absence. But if she planned to say things like that to him, how was he supposed to keep his head? His imagination exhibited a sudden astounding propensity for cinematic sexual fantasy. Clearing his throat, he rose to his feet and put some distance between them. "I suppose that's a risk we'll have to take."

The chair was oversize. Maria had curled her legs beneath her and huddled into the depths of the cushions until it seemed as if she were trying to become invisible.

Small, perfect white teeth mauled her bottom lip. "You're not taking me seriously."

His hoarse chuckle was strained. "I've never been *more* serious. But I'd feel a whole lot better if you weren't regarding spending two days and nights with me as the equivalent of going in for a root canal. Sex is fun, Maria."

"Not with you."

She'd spoken rapidly and with conviction. Without the hint of a smile on her face. "I'm almost afraid to ask you to elaborate," he muttered, telling himself grown men didn't get their feelings hurt.

Maria's hands gripped the arms of the chair, her knuckles white. "It wasn't fun earlier. Earth-shattering, maybe. Mind-blowing. Unequivocally wonderful. But not *fun*. That's a word for carnival rides and animated movies and walking barefoot in the rain."

Her earnest speech might have been good for his ego if she didn't seemed so distressed.

He scooped her out of the chair and sat back down with her in his lap. "You're overthinking this, Maria." He nuzzled her ear. "Maybe we didn't start with fun. I'll give you that one. But we'll get there. Eventually. Good sex, I think, hits all the positive adjectives eventually."

She sighed, resting her cheek against his heart. "Have you had *bad* sex?"

"Enough to know the difference." He stroked her hair. "Trust me, sweetheart. Trust *us*."

"You make it sound so easy."

"And you're making it far too complicated. We're here in this room. A man and a woman. Attracted to each other. Unattached. With time on our hands. What makes you think something bad is going to happen?"

"Superstition?"

He laughed ruefully. It was hard to argue the point that the old ways in Alma were laden with superstition. Legends. Folk tales. Fables delineating the fates of those who tempted the gods. Alma's was a culture steeped in centuries of oral tradition.

"You're a thoroughly modern woman. We're here representing the best and brightest of a country eager to make its mark on a new millennium. Relax. There's nothing to worry about."

"I think it's all those years of my mother warning me that misbehavior on my part would have drastic consequences. It was a very effective deterrent."

"I'll protect you if the sky starts to fall."

"Not funny."

He tickled her rib. "A little bit funny. Admit it."

Her body relaxed in his embrace. They had broken some awkward barrier and made it safely through to the other side.

She put her hand on his thigh. "Did you mention room service?"

Alex watched Maria eat a strawberry and was forced to lean forward to lick juice from the slope of her breast. "I'll order more of those," he promised.

They were both naked. It was three in the morning, and they had chosen to shore up their energy with a snack of fresh fruit and champagne.

Maria's hair tumbled around her shoulders. Dark smudges beneath her eyes attested to the fact that so far he hadn't managed to let her sleep for more than thirty minutes at a stretch.

How could he? When she nestled close to him, her bottom cradled against his groin, he wanted her again and again.

More juice dribbled onto her cleavage. "You're doing that on purpose," he accused.

She eyed him innocently, her lips closing on a bite of red berry. "Are you complaining?"

"Hell, no." This time when he licked her velvety soft skin, he shuddered. "We need to sleep." His hands were at her hips, tugging her down onto the mattress. He had no intention at all of closing his eyes.

"We can sleep when we're dead," she said, the words slurred with exhaustion. She was so beautiful in her sensual abandon that it hurt to look at her.

Those six words were all the invitation he needed. He eased her onto her side facing away from him. Lifting her leg over his thigh, he entered her from behind, joining their bodies with an ease that made his head swim. This was so perfect...so right.

Maria's head rested on her arm.

"Are you asleep?" he asked, smiling though she couldn't see him.

"Just catnapping. Keep up the good work."

"I never knew you were such a smart-ass," he teased. He withdrew and thrust firmly, burying himself all the way to the hilt and making each of them gasp in unison.

"I've been on my best behavior at work."

"Will you be insulted if I say I like this version of you even more?"

He curled an arm around her hip and reached for the spot that controlled her pleasure. Toying gently with the small nub, he slowed his penetration to enjoy her restless arousal.

"Not insulted," she moaned. "Don't stop."

He felt his climax bearing down on him and willed it back. "What will you do for me if I let you come?" he asked, the words ragged.

"Anything, everything. Damn you, Alex. Please..."

She tried to twist in his embrace so she could face him, but he held her firmly. Already he felt small contractions in her sex that told him she was close, so close. "I like it when you beg." He bit the back of her neck. "Will you let me kiss you in public?"

He didn't even know where the question came from...
hadn't realized he was about to ask it.

Maria stiffened, the small shake of her head unmistakable. "Not that. Nothing out in the open. I'm offering you
this room, this weekend, these two nights. Anything and
everything. No holds barred."

Though her words promised a sexual carte blanche, he
was pissed at her refusal to have a real relationship with
him in the light of day. Really pissed...but not enough to
let her go. "Fine." He forced the word past clenched teeth.
"But I'll make you pay for that."

He couldn't wait any longer. Cursing softly, he released
the tight control he'd maintained and plunged wildly, taking her again and again with a force and fury that rocked
the bed and sent them both into a fiery crash with orgas-
mic pleasure so intense they collapsed instantly into a
deep, sated sleep.

Maria awoke completely disoriented. For a split second she thought she was in her small apartment in Alma.
Then gradually, everything came back to her, including
the fact that a large, naked man held her tightly with both
arms locked around her even as he slept.

For a moment, she remained still, struggling to assimilate everything that had happened. Fragments of memories...pieces of the night before, sent hot color to her face
and made her wonder how much was dream and how much
reality.

But when Alex murmured in his sleep, his face buried in her hair, she couldn't pretend any longer. She and
Alex had made love...repeatedly. And the experience had
changed her forever. She had given him a part of her soul
and it wasn't something she could or would take back.

Panic rose in her chest. She had done the one thing she

knew was dangerous. She had let Alex get too close. It wasn't just the sex, though that was bad enough. But even worse, she had let down her guard with him...let him see who she really was.

Whatever professional distance had existed between them had been obliterated in one unprecedented night. Alex clearly wasn't alarmed by that. He seemed to have some notion that it was no big deal.

But Maria knew the truth. Soon they would return to Alma, and there it would be impossible to continue whatever this was between them. Alma was struggling to assimilate the fast-moving future with their traditional past, but it was a struggle that would take more than a week or a month or even a year. In the meantime, the old lines of class and social standing would remain mostly intact.

Not only was Maria not a native of Alma, she was a woman with no past. No father, no relatives, no lineage. Only a hardworking mother who had done her best to keep food on the table.

Oh, what the hell. Just because heartbreak lurked around the corner, it didn't negate the benefits of a weekend in bed with the man she lo—

She pulled herself up short. *Love* was an inappropriate word in this context. She wasn't in love with Alex. In lust maybe. But who could blame her? He was smart and sexy, and underneath that oh-so-serious exterior, he was an animal.

Even so, one of them had to show some sense. Carefully, over the space of at least a minute and a half, she stealthily eased out of his embrace and off the bed. Poor man never even moved. He had expended an impressive amount of energy in the past twelve hours.

Maria's insides clenched in helpless longing as she remembered the crazed fervor of his lovemaking. He'd been like a man possessed, as if trying to make up for lost time. Or maybe, deep down, he knew as she did that their time together was limited.

In the bathroom with the door closed, she showered, dried her hair and secured it at the back of her neck. The comfy clothes she'd grabbed while in her room last night would be perfect for an informal workday.

She'd expected to find Alex awake by the time she finished. Opening the door to the bedroom stealthily, she saw that he still slept. Only now, he was facedown on his stomach. His broad, muscular shoulders and smoothly tanned back narrowed to a taut waist and buttocks that were… well…it was a good thing the sheet hadn't slid any lower.

She jumped when low, amused words startled her. "Are you going to stand there staring or are you going to come back to bed?" He reared up on one elbow and turned to look at her. His voice sounded as if he had swallowed sand.

"It's nine o'clock. We need to order breakfast and get to work on the proposal."

He sat up and scrubbed his hands through his hair, yawning. "Are you always so perky at this hour?"

"If you're trying to make me mad, it won't work. Tell me what you want to eat and I'll have it waiting when you get out of the shower."

When he swung his legs over the side of the bed, she held up a hand. "Wrap the sheet around you, for heaven's sake."

He stretched, the muscles in his broad chest doing some kind of mesmerizing flex and ripple. "Are we shy this morning?"

"Not at all," she said primly. "But we don't need to get sidetracked. There's work to do."

He stood up, sans sheet, and crossed the room in three long strides. Putting a finger beneath her chin, he tilted her face up to his, searching her eyes. "You okay, sweet thing? We got a little crazy last night."

She couldn't do a thing about her blush, aggravating as it was. "I'm fine. Better than fine. But seriously, Alex. It's late. One of us has to remember why we're here."

He kissed her long and slow, telling her in no uncertain terms what he thought of her work ethic. Her arms went around his neck and clung. Every inch of his big, honed body pressed against hers, stealing the oxygen from her lungs.

When he finally released her, she had to grab hold of him for a few seconds until her world settled back on its axis. "Stop that," she whispered, going up on tiptoe to kiss him again.

His low, triumphant laugh was masculine arrogance personified, but she couldn't fault his confidence since she was clearly besotted. Did anyone even use that word anymore? If not, they should. It was a perfect description of her current state. Intoxicated. Infatuated. As if all her good sense had flown out the window, and she didn't even care.

But she could pretend. Releasing him reluctantly, she took a deep breath. "More kissing later. Go, Alex. Now."

He bowed, managing despite his nudity to look perfectly relaxed. "Far be it from me to argue with a lady."

When he disappeared into the bathroom, she exhaled, not realizing she had been holding her breath. Dealing with Alex in his current mood was like trying to tame a big, determined tiger.

While he was gone, she escaped to the living room. After a moment's consideration, she moved the vase of fresh flowers from the cherry writing desk. Opening the drapes that framed a stunning view of the Atlantic, she dragged the ornate table in front of the window. Next, she located both laptops, plugged them in behind the new workspace, booted her computer and opened up the rough draft of the Alma proposal to the Montoros.

Once that was done, she called in two orders of scrambled eggs, bacon and black coffee. Room service at this hotel was extremely efficient. She didn't want the food to get cold.

She would have liked to sit down and start working to show Alex that she was taking their new relationship in stride, but it was impossible. She paced the room. Today was a watershed moment for her and Alex. She recognized the importance of what would happen in the next few hours. So she felt a certain amount of pressure to guard her emotions.

Alex was a guy. He was going to have one thing on his mind. Despite his position as deputy prime minister of commerce, he would be able to compartmentalize. Sex wouldn't interfere with his position or his responsibilities.

But for Maria, life wasn't so clear-cut and simple. Could she have an intimate physical relationship with him and still be able to carry on with business as usual when they were with other members of the delegation?

She was so deep in thought that she never heard his footsteps on the plush carpet. When his hand landed on her shoulder, she spun around. "You scared me," she said, not quite able to meet his gaze.

"Who were you expecting, Maria?"

A knock at the door saved her from answering. "I'm going in the bedroom," she whispered. "I don't want anyone to know I'm here."

Alex shook his head with a wry smile but let her go.

When he gave her the all clear, she returned to a beautifully laid out breakfast. Linen napkins, real silver utensils, crystal stemware and delicate china. "That smells wonderful," she said as her stomach growled audibly.

He held out her chair, leaning down to kiss her cheek. "Looks pretty damn good, too."

Fortunately for her peace of mind, Alex was content to eat in silence. They were both starving. He caught her eye at one point and grinned, as if to say he knew exactly what she was thinking. She hid behind a cup of hot tea and wondered how long it would be before they ended up back in bed. *Bad Maria*, her conscience chastised.

But apparently, she had convinced Alex of her dedication to the project at hand. Once they were done with their meal, he carried his coffee to the desk where she had placed two chairs side by side.

"How do you think we should approach this?" he asked, waking his own laptop and clicking on a file.

His matter-of-fact attitude took her aback. She'd been prepared to convince him, to deflect amorous advances. Was he genuinely so cavalier about working with her?

When he burst out laughing, she stiffened. "What's so funny?" she demanded, finishing her tea and standing up. She couldn't quite make her feet move in his direction.

"You," he said, his smile gentle. "You told me we had to be all business this morning. But when I took you at your word, you were disappointed."

"No, I wasn't," she said. The rebuttal wasn't convincing, even to her.

"Well, I am," he said firmly. "We're going to get this done as quickly as possible so I can get you back in bed."

Her spirits lightened. "You must think me awfully naive, Alex. I'm not accustomed to combining business with pleasure. This is new territory to me."

He frowned, leaning a hip against the desk. "What do you think it is to me? I don't make a habit of sleeping with coworkers. In fact, you're the first."

"Why me?"

"I could ask you the same thing," he said, watching her with a hooded gaze. "If you want explanations, I'm fresh out."

"So where and how do we go from here?"

"Does everything in life have to be explained? Let's file this thing between us under the same category as raindrops trapped in cobwebs or the color of the sky at dawn."

Her eyes widened. "Why, Alex, I never knew you were a poet."

His expression was impassive, not a trace of humor in sight. "There's a lot you don't know about me, Maria. So how about giving both of us a chance to learn something and possibly to be surprised?"

There was an odd tone in his voice, some tiny indication that he was not as certain as she thought he was about what had happened between them last night.

It was then she realized she wasn't being fair. Either she was in this, or she wasn't.

It took courage, but she walked to where he stood and slid her arms around his waist. "I've been second-guessing myself, Alex. But that's over. I'm content to take things one day at a time. I can't guarantee I'll be able to work with you and not want to jump your bones, but I'll try."

He hugged her so tightly she thought her ribs would crack. "God, Maria." He pulled back and rubbed his thumb over her cheekbone. "I thought I might have scared you off."

Eleven

"I don't scare that easily, Mr. Ramon."

"Thank God." Her cheeky grin was adorable. Alex felt as if he had dodged a bullet. There had been women in his life who had walked away. At least one or two. But none whose defection had given him heartburn.

This morning when he woke up alone, his heart had gone cold until he heard faint sounds from the bathroom. In those moments when he thought she had fled to her room, he'd felt a little sick. Not for anything in the world would he have her feel uneasy about what had happened between them. He decided then and there that if she wasn't a hundred percent on board with this new slant to their relationship, he wasn't going to chase after her. Not because of any pride on his part, but because Maria was too nice a woman to have to fend off unwanted advances from a coworker.

He wrapped a hand in her silky hair, wishing he could take her hard and fast, but they had reached a tentative accord.

Maybe he should show some restraint. "I suppose we need to work," he said, finding little enthusiasm for the prospect.

"Definitely," she said. "And if we get a lot done, we might have time for some recreation later."

Alex replayed that promise repeatedly over the next three hours. It wasn't easy to stay focused, but he tried. Fortunately, once they delved into the draft of the proposal, he was able to keep his attention mostly on the words they were shaping rather than the scent of Maria's hair.

It touched him that she was so sweetly intent on their task. Though not a native of Alma, she took her responsibilities very seriously. The powers that be had been right to include her in the delegation.

The opening language of the proposal was flowery and formal, based mostly on historic documents. From there, Alex and Maria struggled with the order of points relating to the royal family's return. Should the legalities of power and function be first, or was it more politically correct to mention the palace and what was left of the Montoro fortune from before Tantaberra's regime?

At least they had Jean Claude's extensive notes when it came to lawyer-speak. Neither Alex nor Maria was trained in such areas. But they were both good editors, Alex catching the occasional typo and Maria smoothing out style and syntax.

At one in the afternoon, he called a halt. Standing behind her chair, he put his hand on her shoulders. "My eyes are crossing. We've done enough for now. I need food, woman."

"But we only have—"

He put his hand over her mouth. "It's for your own good, Miss Ferro. I'm seeing symptoms of workaholic-itis. It's a terrible disease and one that has to be nipped in the bud."

She stood up and stretched. "You're so full of it. But yeah…I guess we should stop. What do you want for lunch?"

He took her hand and reeled her in, tucking her against his chest and resting his forehead against hers. "You," he muttered. "Only you."

They eventually got around to ordering pizza. Alex threw on some pants to answer the door and tip the delivery guy, but undressed again quickly so he could eat naked in bed with Maria.

"This is really a smart idea," she said, rescuing a blob of tomato sauce from her bare arm. "I don't have to worry about spilling anything on my clothes."

Alex nodded solemnly. "All part of my plan to keep you here indefinitely as my sexual plaything."

"Plaything?"

"What?" he asked. "You don't like the word?"

She pursed her lips, curling her tongue to rescue a string of cheese. "I was thinking more along the lines of erotic goddess."

He reclined on both elbows, suddenly uninterested in pizza. "I stand corrected," he said huskily.

Maria dabbed her lips with a napkin and frowned at him. "Stop that."

"Stop what?"

"Undressing me with your eyes."

"Um…I'm pretty sure that's not a fair rap. You're buck naked, my sweet. Or hadn't you noticed?"

She crossed her arms over her chest. "A gentleman wouldn't say things like that."

He grabbed her ankle and pulled, laughing when she pretended to struggle. "Then I guess I'm no gentleman."

Maria felt as if another woman had possessed her body. A female who was sexy and fun and carefree. Maybe she was channeling a 1940s film star. Glamorous. Mysterious. Living on the edge.

Alex's head rested on her bare belly, his hair tickling her leg. She stroked the outside of his ear. "You amaze me," she whispered. Her back rested against the headboard. As she cast her gaze over the bed, the view almost made her laugh. All the covers were on the floor. She and Alex lay sprawled on top of the fitted sheet.

She might have been cold if the man's body hadn't radiated heat like a furnace.

He yawned. "Amaze you how?"

"The whole Clark Kent/Superman thing. I've worked *for* you and *with* you for years and only this weekend have I discovered all your superpowers."

"Maybe not all," he said, his smug, masculine grin rekindling a slow burn in her secret feminine places. "I just might have a few more surprises up my sleeve."

"Bragging isn't attractive, Alex." She squeezed his bicep. "And I might point out that you don't have any sleeves."

He pretended to frown as his hand roved her bare thigh, sending gooseflesh all over her body. "Details, woman. Details. You need to look at the big picture."

She brushed his erection with a fingertip. "Oh, I'm looking," she said.

When he laughed, she felt a jolt of pure happiness. Alone in this room, he had shown her a glimpse of the kind of relationship she had always wanted. But the Alex with her now didn't often come out to play.

He was dedicated to his country and to his responsibilities and to his role as deputy prime minister of commerce. The livelihoods of common people rested in his hands. He wielded tremendous talent and carried a tremendous load.

Alex sat up and hooked a hand behind her neck to kiss her. "Pepperoni," he muttered. "My favorite."

Suddenly, she was painfully aware of the ticking of the clock...of the invisible hourglass whose sand was draining away at an alarming pace. "Make love to me, Alex. I need you."

Neither of them noticed or cared when the pizza box fell to the floor. Alex's warm hands on her body caressed and petted and stroked and generally drove her insane. He liked to torment them both, to reduce each of them to desperation before finally moving over and into her with a slow, firm thrust that forged a connection she'd never known or understood.

Her body seemed already to recognize his...

The weight of him pinned her down. Her fingers clenched on his back, searching for purchase in the gathering storm. With her legs wrapped around his waist, she canted her hips, trying to force him deeper.

Alex gasped, his skin damp, his gaze unfocused. "I can't get enough. It's never enough..."

She knew what he meant. In the breathless moments after climax, she was as eager for him as she had been before he first touched her. Clinging to him as if he might be wrenched from her arms, she relished his hard frame, his hair-roughened arms, his male scent.

Everything about him was so different from her body. She was tall and strong, but in his embrace she felt the sweet vulnerability of a woman whose man wants her beyond all reason.

When they both crested at almost the same moment, a rush of moisture in her eyes caught her by surprise. There was nothing to cry about...nothing at all. She would carry the memories of this weekend with her for the rest of her life.

They dozed again for maybe an hour and then rose to

finish their work on the draft. Finally, when they were both satisfied, Alex emailed the document to Jean Claude for his perusal. If everything passed muster, Alex and Maria would meet with the delegation on Monday morning to go over the proposal step by step.

After that, it would be up to the Montoros...

Alex stretched, his face shadowed by a day's growth of beard. "How about a walk on the beach? As much as I love hiding out in this room with you, I could use some fresh air."

"Definitely." They both slipped on the clothes they had worn Friday evening. Spending a naked weekend had definite pluses...less laundry to worry about.

She lobbied for leaving the room separately, but Alex put his foot down. "You're being silly. I'll check the hall if it will make you feel better, but we're not going to skulk around like we're doing something wrong."

Nevertheless, Maria was relieved when they took the back staircase and made it outside unobserved. They traversed the path to the sand in single file. When they reached the beach, Alex took her hand.

Her fingers linked with his as they meandered down toward the firmer sand revealed by low tide. They were not the only night owls out and about, but there was plenty of privacy for a pleasant stroll.

The moon hung low on the horizon, casting a silvery path across the sea. Maria wanted to capture the moment somehow. A photograph wouldn't do it justice. And she was no good as an artist. The fragrance of night-blooming jasmine scented the air. She would have to rely on imagination and sensory recall to hold on to this memory.

Alex adjusted his stride to hers, keeping the pace relaxed.

She felt her muscles relax, her misgivings washing away

in the waves that curled onto the shore. "Have you ever wanted to buy a boat and sail toward the unknown?" she asked, not pausing to consider whether he would think her question a bit odd.

"Every boy dreams of that, I think…at least the ones who have seen the ocean. What did you want to be when you were a kid?"

"Oh, that's easy…a Disney princess."

"Which one?"

"Ariel and Snow White were my favorites, but the hair color was all wrong. My mother bought me a very beautiful Cinderella doll the Christmas I was six years old, and after that, Cinderella was the one I wanted. I carried her everywhere and decided I could be just like her when I grew up. Little girls' dreams are silly, I guess."

"No sillier than boys who want to be soldiers and firemen and police officers."

"But those are attainable goals. A girl can't actually grow up to be a princess. Unless, of course, you're Kate Middleton or someone like that."

Alex told himself not to read too much into her innocent confession. There were a million little girls around the world who wore princess outfits for Halloween costumes and considered sparkly tiaras a vital accessory. It didn't mean a thing.

Still, the evening lost some of its bloom.

They walked for half an hour and then retraced their steps. Afterward, Alex hailed a cab out at the street, despite Maria's insistence that they were far too messy to go anywhere.

But when she saw the all-night diner, her protests died. They binged on chicken-fried steak and homemade mashed potatoes. Alex tried to coax her into apple pie, but she shook her head.

"I'm stuffed," she said. "But you go for it."

When the dessert arrived, Alex forked up a generous bite and held it out to her. "At least taste it."

Staring at him with a small smile that made his skin tighten on the back of his neck, she leaned forward and opened her mouth, allowing him to feed her the rich mix of fruit and spices and crumbly crust.

After she swallowed, a look of bliss crossed her face. "Oh, my gosh. That's amazing."

"More?" Her sensual enjoyment made him shift restlessly in his seat. He did a quick calculation of how long it would take to get back to the hotel.

Maria leaned away and shook her hand. "I can't. We've eaten like kings since we've been in Miami. I don't want to go home with an extra five pounds."

He finished the pie rapidly and lifted a hand for the check. Outside, he pushed her against the side of the building and kissed her wildly, his breathing ragged. "You're perfect the way you are," he muttered. "And I want you… now."

Fortunately, good sense prevailed and he managed to make it back to his suite before getting Maria naked. Little bits of sand showered down onto the carpet. "We should take a shower," she said. "So we won't get sand in the bed."

Nodding jerkily, unable to speak, he dragged her toward the bathroom, aware all the while that Maria was laughing at him. He undressed her in record time and adjusted the water temperature before ripping off all his clothes. Even now, he could see that she was a little shy.

"Look at me, Maria." He took her hand and pulled her beneath the spray. The water darkened her hair immediately and dripped from the tips of her breasts. It was always a toss-up as to whether her eyes were going to be more green than blue. In the tiled shower stall with cavorting dolphins and wave motifs, her irises gleamed pale emerald.

She cast her gaze downward. "I'm looking, Alex. Believe me, I am."

When she wrapped one hand around his aching shaft, his head dropped back against the wall of the shower. *Holy hell.* Her fingers explored him above and below, making sweat break out on his forehead. His knees quivered embarrassingly. "Enough," he croaked.

When she tried to soap him up, he had to intervene. A man could only stand so much torture. "You first." Gliding his hands over slick female flesh made him shake again. He took care of his own ablutions and then hustled them both out of the shower, handing Maria a big fluffy towel.

Perhaps she'd been expecting him to suggest shower sex standing up, but he wanted her to be comfortable with him. Baby steps. Build her trust and her comfort level. Sooner or later she would feel at home in his arms and in his bed. He was counting on it.

By the time they dried off, he had convinced himself not to pounce on her. While he and Maria had walked the beach earlier, housekeeping had been in to service the room. The bed looked inviting, the covers pristine.

Maria, with the towel wrapped sarong-style around her torso, cocked her head. "Almost seems a shame to mess it up."

"What did you have in mind?" he asked, his hands fisting at his sides.

She pointed. At the foot of the bed stood a narrow cushioned bench. Instantly, he saw the possibilities. "I like the way you think." He dragged it away from the footboard and tested the springiness of the navy padding with two fingers. "Bottom or top?" he asked with a straight face.

Maria turned cherry red from the edge of the towel to her hairline. "I'll leave that up to you."

It was so much fun to tease her. She did her best to be nonchalant about what they were doing, but that shy reserve was never far below the surface. He ditched his towel and stretched out on his back, his feet on the floor. The height was perfect. His arousal was out in the open, his shaft full and heavy as it bobbed against his abdomen.

He held out a hand. "Come and get me," he said.

She kept a death grip on the towel, though she did walk a few steps in his direction. Her attention focused on his eager sex, but her expression was hard to read.

"I may have been too hasty. I like having covers to hide beneath."

"You're exquisite," he answered, dead serious. "It would be a crime to cover that gorgeous body. Drop the towel, sweetheart."

For a moment he thought she was going to refuse. But gradually, she unclenched her fingers and lifted her arms until the large, damp rectangle fell to her feet.

Alex sucked in a sharp breath, feeling the last bit of blood in his head rush south. "I'm cold. Come warm me up."

At last, a small smile. "You're never cold. And besides, I'm not exactly sure how to go about this."

"I'll help. It's like riding a bike. You never really forget."

"You're a riot," she said, biting her lip.

In the end, she started at his knees, straddling him with ladylike grace and *walking* up his body until his erection and her soft, damp sex were aligned. He grabbed her hips. "See…that wasn't so difficult."

Leaning forward, she put her hands on his shoulders and lowered herself onto him. They both made a noise halfway between a curse and a sigh. Her silky wet hair fell around them. He was conditioned by now to the smell of her shampoo. It made him want to gobble her up.

He didn't move for a few moments, giving her a chance to adjust to this new position. "You okay?" he asked. Her silence always bothered him. He never knew what she was thinking.

Maria did a little bump and grind with her hips that made him catch his breath. "I don't know," she muttered. "You tell me."

Twelve

Maria had taken a gymnastics class in college to satisfy a PE requirement. Nothing she learned during that semester prepared her for this current experience. Technically, she was in the dominant position. But in reality, Alex called the shots.

She had no objection to that at all. For one thing, she didn't have the sexual confidence yet to orchestrate their coupling. And for another, he was so damned good at sex. Feeling like a rank novice, she squeezed her inner muscles. When he gasped, she smiled.

"I like having you at my mercy," she said, her words little more than a whisper. She kissed him teasingly, nipping his bottom lip with her teeth. His response was to thrust upward…hard.

His hands tangled in her hair, anchoring her head so he could drag her mouth to his and hold her captive. In between kisses, his ragged, breathless praise seduced her. "You wanted to be an erotic goddess, right?"

She barely had the oxygen to answer. "Not really. That was just me being silly."

"Too bad," he groaned. "'Cause you're already there. Sit up," he said urgently.

When she did as he asked, the feel of him inside her was indescribable. Now she could see his face. His cheekbones were ruddy with color, his thick, inky-black hair mussed. He stared at her in return, capturing her attention with nothing more than the hungry look in his eyes.

"Lean back," he demanded. "Put your hands behind you on my thighs."

She obeyed, feeling intensely vulnerable and wildly excited at the same time. He cupped her breasts in his hands, teasing her nipples with his thumbs until the pink rosebuds puckered tightly.

Unable to bear the intense tableau, she closed her eyes.

"Look at me, Maria." The note of authority brooked no opposition. "Do you like what I'm doing to you?"

She tried to swallow. But her throat was dry. "Yes."

He plucked at her sensitive flesh, sending dual arrows of fire arcing to the spot where their bodies were joined. "Alex…" Her sharp cry echoed in the silent room.

His laugh encompassed masculine triumph and sexual intent. "Don't close your eyes. Keep watching."

He found her pleasure center and stroked the tiny bud carefully. When she jerked away instinctively his hands clamped on her hips. "Ride me, Maria. Make me come. I dare you."

The game was on, but she was so lost to reason she barely had the presence of mind to understand what he was saying. Bracing her feet, she pushed off from the floor, and came down hard. Her climax hit with the force of a tidal wave, tumbling her in a maelstrom of confusion and sharp physical pleasure.

Alex went wild beneath her, ramming into her repeatedly, then shouting as he exploded inside her, filling her with his release.

She slumped on top of him, her heart beating loudly in her ears. Beneath her cheek, his chest was damp and *his* heart sounded as if it might leap out of his body.

"Are you good at *everything*?" she muttered, still half dazed.

Long seconds passed when she wondered if he was going to answer. Finally, he stroked her back, his words gruff. "It's you, Maria. You inspire me."

Afterward, she was never sure how long they lay there recovering. But her butt was chilled and her legs ached by the time Alex finally stirred. "Sleep," he said groggily. "We have to sleep."

They stumbled into the bathroom for a quick, strictly platonic shower. Then, with a nod to brushing teeth and a halfhearted attempt by the both of them to tame her hair, they finally gave up and went to bed. The sheets were cool and crisp and heavenly soft.

Alex wrapped an arm around her and tucked her against his side. She thought he was already asleep, so it startled her when he whispered something in her hair.

"I want to keep seeing you when we go home," he said.

She froze, resenting him for introducing conflict in the midst of their wonderful aftermath. "You'll see me every day," she said. "We work in the same office."

"That's not what I mean and you know it."

"Don't ruin what we have," she pleaded. "We can talk about it later."

Alex felt the rejection and marveled that something could be so painful. Was this all a game to Maria? Was he entertaining her while she waited for her chance with

Gabriel? Had the little girl who wanted to grow up to be a Disney princess suddenly realized she had a shot at the real thing?

He didn't want to believe it. But he had no idea what it meant to come from nothing, to struggle financially, to feel the constant ache of uncertainty in every aspect of life. How could he fault her for seeking out financial security and a fairy-tale ending?

Or maybe it was Gabriel. Maybe Gabriel was pursuing her so convincingly that she had to consider what it might mean to be a princess in real life. Alex had money to burn, but he was never going to be a prince. And because of the delicate state of the negotiations, he couldn't stand in the way if Gabriel wanted Maria.

She seemed naive sexually, as if there had been no more than one or two men before him. He didn't think she could fake the satisfaction he had given her. But why else would she hold him off if it weren't for the fact that she had plans to continue a relationship with Gabriel Montoro?

Unless, of course, she was worried about what might happen when she and Alex returned to Alma. Back home, their relationship had been circumspect and businesslike. Maybe Maria didn't want to juggle the inevitable gossip that would ensue if they returned to Alma as an official couple. He could appreciate her reservations even if he thought they were unfounded.

Despite his unsettled thoughts, exhaustion claimed him at last. But his dreams were fractured and troubled and kept him on the run all night.

Maria was sleeping like the dead when Alex's cell phone woke them at seven the next morning. He rolled over and groaned, picking it up to look at the number. Clearing his throat, he punched the button. "Ramon here…" He listened intently. "Yes, of course. Thanks for calling."

Maria sat up, clutching the top sheet to her breasts. She raked her hair from her forehead. "Who was it?"

He rotated his head as if trying to shake off the remnants of too little sleep and too many bad dreams. "It was Rafael Montoro—father, not son. Isabella Salazar has been admitted to the hospital. He wanted me to know, because it may affect our plans to formally offer the proposal to the family this week."

She touched his arm. "Oh, Alex. I'm so sorry."

He avoided her attempt to comfort him and climbed out of bed. "I think I should go to the hospital. As a show of support."

"I'll go with you." Her gaze searched his face.

"Suit yourself," he said. His tone was curt.

The laughing, playful, sexy lover of last night had disappeared. Was it because he was stressed about this turn of events? Or had she angered him by refusing to talk about their relationship beyond this room?

She didn't have the nerve to join him in the bathroom. So she gathered her things and waited until he was finished to take her turn. "I'll be very quick," she said.

He nodded without looking at her. "I'll wait."

As she quickly ran through her morning routine, she wondered if she had hurt his pride. It was too soon for his heart to be involved. But perhaps he was offended that she hadn't jumped at his offer to continue their sexual adventures, even back in Alma.

She would have liked to return to her own room for fresh clothing, but she was pretty sure Alex wouldn't linger. Not in the mood he was in. So she put on the same skirt and sleeveless silk top and examined it in the mirror. Not too bad.

Alex had used the time she was in the bathroom to order toast and coffee and request a car. They ate in fifteen minutes and headed downstairs to the lobby. Although she tried twice to engage him in conversation, Alex was stone-faced.

The hospital in Coral Gables was brand-new and extremely high-tech from top to bottom. Isabella's condition required intensive care, so the family was gathered in the adjacent waiting room. While Rafael III conversed with Alex, Maria sat with Isabella's grandson and the nieces and nephews.

Juan Carlos was the one Maria knew the least. His face was pale, his posture tense. "I'm sorry about your grandmother," she said.

The young man inclined his head. "Thank you, Ms. Ferro."

His manner was formal but polite. Suddenly, his facade cracked as he glared at Rafe. "It's your fault, damn it. She's upset because you won't live up to your responsibilities."

Gabriel bristled. "It's not our country, and it's not Rafe's burden to bear. Back off."

Bella, with a worried look at the stricken Rafe, stepped in to make peace. "We're all upset. Sniping at each other doesn't make it better." She sat down beside Rafe and leaned her head on his shoulder. "Isabella is old and sick and frail. We've all known this day would come."

Rafe jumped to his feet, his eyes stormy with something that looked a lot like fear. "She's not dead yet. And Juan Carlos is right. I was dragging my feet about this decision. I should have said yes or no and ended this."

Gabriel cursed, a vicious nasty word that encompassed the whole of the Gordian knot that bound them all together. "I need some air," he said.

Maria sensed he was close to the breaking point. He

was either going to punch out his cousin or start tearing up the hospital brick by brick. Part of her job was to maintain control of the situation. The last thing they needed at this point was a media circus.

"Mind a little company?" she asked. She wasn't intentionally trying to make Alex jealous by slipping away with Gabriel. She was simply doing what needed to be done. But despite the purity of her motives, Alex shot her a narrow glance that telegraphed his disapproval.

Gabriel shrugged. "Not at all."

Bella gave her a grateful smile. "I'll text you if there's a change."

Outside, in the hospital courtyard, Maria sat on a concrete bench while Gabriel paced. The air was thick and humid, but it was still early enough that the temperature was bearable.

She searched her social repertoire for the right words to defuse his tension but came up with nothing. So she sat in silence. Finally, after fifteen or twenty minutes, he plopped down beside her. "It's a hell of a situation."

"I know. I'm sorry."

Gabriel leaned forward, his head in his hands. "If it were anyone else, I'd say my aunt was faking to manipulate my brother. But she's one of the most honorable women I've ever met."

"And passionate about her homeland."

"Yeah."

"The delegation is set to do a final read through of the official proposal tomorrow. After that, they'll want to meet with your family, or at least Rafe."

"Poor bastard."

"I'm guessing from what he said just now that he hasn't made up his mind?"

Gabriel shook his head. "Damned if I know. Rafe can

mimic the Sphinx when he wants to...but this situation with Isabella makes things harder for him."

"Unless he had already decided to accept."

"I wish I had your positive attitude."

The irony was almost amusing. She didn't feel positive about anything at the moment.

"We probably should go back inside," she said. The sharp edge of Gabriel's anger had been dulled by acceptance and grief. Grief for both his aunt and his brother.

Maria stood up. Gabriel followed suit, shoving his hands in his pockets. "I don't suppose you'd help me run away to Tahiti in a sailboat and tell everyone I'm never coming back?"

She chuckled, liking him more and more each time they met. "You'd regret it if I said yes. Besides, the women of Miami would never forgive me for allowing South Beach's most eligible bachelor to disappear."

"Rafe's the one who's going to be a king. Doesn't that put him at the top of the eligible list?"

"Good point."

They were playing a silly game, trying to take their minds off the very serious events at stake. But nothing could disguise the truth.

She sighed. "You may not be the king," she said, "but you know you can't run away, sailboat or no sailboat. Your family depends on you. Now more than ever. Bella is awfully young. Juan Carlos doesn't have a dog in this fight. And Rafe...well, he's under so much pressure. You can be the glue, Gabriel. They need you desperately, no matter what happens with Isabella."

He cocked his head. "You really care, don't you? About a group of strangers?"

"I've been studying dossiers on each one of you for months. I felt like I knew you before I arrived. But dry facts can only tell so much. Now that I've become acquainted with all of the Montoros, I can see the big picture. And I understand why you're important to Alma." She paused. "To be honest, I think Alma will be important to all of you, as well. But that's something you have to decide on your own."

He hugged her briefly. She felt a faint tremor in his body. There was nothing the least bit amorous about their quick embrace. Gabriel was simply a man at the end of his rope trying to hang on.

When he released her, his expression was sheepish. "You won't tell anyone I freaked out, will you?"

"Of course not. I think you're entitled."

He nodded once, his chin outthrust. "Enough of this. You're right. Let's go back in and see where things are."

Alex saw them move, so he stepped quickly around the corner of the building, unwilling to be discovered. The tableau he witnessed had filled his throat with bile. Despite the fact that Maria had spent the better part of the weekend in Alex's bed, there was no denying the truth. She and Gabriel were in the midst of something.

Body language didn't lie. They were comfortable with each other. Intimate. A connection like that could only happen when two people were very close.

Alex had known Maria for years and yet had never ended up in her bed until now. Gabriel had known her for a couple of weeks, and already the two of them were confidants. Maybe they hadn't had sex yet. Alex didn't honestly think Maria would sleep with two men in the same interval.

But she was not a hundred percent sure about her feelings for Alex. She was worried about how their relationship would play out back in Alma. In some ways, Gabriel must have seemed to her like the easier choice. Or maybe Gabriel represented a walk on the wild side without consequences that would follow her home.

Alex felt the sting of betrayal even as he recognized his response as irrational. He and Maria had made no pledges. They were not exclusive. She had every right, moral or otherwise, to develop a relationship with Gabriel Montoro.

Alex scraped his hands across his face and reminded himself that this changed nothing. Isabella was still desperately ill. The proposal still had to pass muster with the delegation…then the Montoros. And Alex was still the orchestrator of everything.

Bleakly, he stared at a brilliant hibiscus that bloomed riotously in the Florida sun. He'd made a misstep. A bad one. But the situation could be rectified. It *would* be rectified. For a brief moment, he had broken his own personal code. He'd forgotten his responsibilities. He'd let personal desires outweigh the import of his position as head of the delegation.

But it wouldn't happen again.

He braced himself to return to the ICU waiting room, barely able to tolerate the idea of Maria and Gabriel being chummy. But when he walked in, Gabriel and both Rafes were deep in conversation on one side of the room. Juan Carlos had apparently gone downstairs for something to eat. Bella and Maria had their heads together, their expressions grave.

Alex took a chair that wasn't close to anybody and pulled out his phone to check messages. He managed to concentrate for five minutes before stealing a glance at Maria. She was wearing the same skirt and top she'd had on when she came to his room. The same ones from their beach walk.

But all he could see was her naked body stretched out beneath his…her beautiful eyes laughing up at him.

When a nurse entered the waiting area, the anxiety level in the room went up half a dozen degrees. The woman spoke quietly to Rafael III. Then the head of the Montoro family looked at Maria and crooked a finger.

Maria stood, a puzzled expression on her face. "What's wrong?"

Rafael had aged a decade during this crisis, his face gray with fatigue and worry. "My aunt would like to speak with you."

"I don't understand. Why me?"

"I don't know. But she's in a fragile state, and if she wants to talk to you, you will go to her."

The firm tone brooked no opposition.

Maria's panicked expression was genuine. "I'd like someone to go with me."

"I'll go," Alex said.

Maria's look of relief should have been gratifying, but he could scarcely bear to walk by her side.

The room was only steps away. The nurse halted them before going in. "She's somewhat agitated. But she said it was important."

Alex and Maria nodded.

When they opened the door, Alex lowered his voice and whispered in Maria's ear. "I'll be here with you, but I'll stay out of her line of sight. I don't want to upset her if she wants to be alone with you."

Maria's lips trembled. "This makes no sense."

He touched her elbow. "Just go."

Maria approached the bed slowly. "Mrs. Salazar. I'm here. It's Maria."

The old woman was too weak to lift her head, but she smiled. "Thank you for coming, my dear."

"Is there something I can do for you?"

Isabella's skin was sallow and her eyes were sunken. But her smile was a semblance of its original beauty. "I need you to tell me the truth. Is my great-nephew going to accept the crown?"

Maria shot Alex a glance, and he saw her swallow. "Well, ma'am, I believe he's still thinking about it."

"You had dinner with the children. All of them except Juan Carlos. Is that correct?"

"Yes."

Alex wanted to smile at the thought of the Montoros being referred to as children, but he listened to hear what Isabella would say next.

The matriarch was physically weak, but her formidable spirit survived intact. "Why are they so reluctant to accept their birthright?"

Maria bit her lip, her hand reaching out to clasp one of Isabella's. "You should know that they love you very much. And they respect your opinions and wishes. But what you're asking them to do is huge. They were born in this country. They're citizens of the United States. They have business interests and friends and a whole life here."

"That's why I wanted to talk to you," she said with the faintest of twinkles in her eyes. "I knew you wouldn't sugarcoat the truth."

"I'm not saying they won't decide to reclaim the monarchy. I honestly don't know. But for this whole situation to work…both personally and politically, it's my belief that Rafael will have to embrace the throne wholeheartedly or not at all."

The room fell silent. Alex frowned, wishing Maria had been more conciliatory with a patient at death's door.

Isabella squeezed Maria's hand. "I understand what you're telling me. I let my enthusiasm run amok, I think."

"Your feelings are understandable. You were born in Alma. You actually lived there. And your life was torn apart and rebuilt. Everyone values your experience. If it's any consolation, all of them are taking this very, very seriously. The decision may or may not fall the way you're hoping, but I can promise you this…Rafe will do the right thing. He's decent and thoughtful and well aware of the choice being offered."

"But the right thing may not be the throne." Isabella's lips twisted in a wry half smile.

"No, ma'am."

Alex stared at the monitors, waiting for them to go berserk as the elderly woman's blood pressure shot up or down or she flatlined. Maria had just crushed Isabella's dreams.

But the miraculous happened. Nothing changed. At least, not for the worse. Isabella reached out with a trembling hand and found the button that operated the hydraulics of the bed. Adjusting the mattress until she was partially sitting up, she lifted Maria's hand, kissed it and released her.

"You may go now. Please ask all of my family to come in and see me."

In the hall, Maria slumped against the wall, her face pale. She stared at Alex. "Don't make me do that again."

"No one forced you to go in there."

"It's not like I had a choice, and you know it."

He followed her around the corner and found the Montoros waiting anxiously. Maria grimaced. "She wants to see all of you."

When the room emptied, only Alex and Maria remained. He stared at the floor, his hands in his pockets. After a moment's reflection, he retrieved his room key and handed it to her. "Why don't you go on back? I can deal with things here."

"You're angry."

He shrugged. "Not angry. Maybe a little surprised. I saw you with Gabriel in the garden, Maria. And I understand why you hesitated when I mentioned continuing our fling."

She winced at the last word, her eyes wide with distress. "I swear to you, Alex, there's nothing going on between Gabriel and me."

"It's possible you honestly believe that. But I saw the way you two acted with each other, the body language. My personal feelings don't enter into this. If Gabriel has feelings for you, then I, as the head of the delegation, owe it to my country to step out of the way."

Color flushed her cheeks. "So now you're pimping me out for national security? That's insulting and horrible."

"Don't overreact. We can both be mature about this. You and I had a fun weekend. But we're in the midst of a crisis. It's very clear to me that you have a connection with Gabriel—and with the whole family, for that matter. They trust you. So we'll use that to our advantage."

Maria looked at him with naked hurt. "How can you be so cold?"

He stared at her, the ice in his soul freezing every opportunity to back away from this precipice. "It's my job, Maria. And the job comes first. It always has."

Thirteen

Maria shut down, her world in ashes. In the cab on the way back to the hotel, she sat without moving, her hands clasped in her lap. Up the elevator, down the hall to Alex's suite. She had to force herself to insert the key card and go inside.

The rooms carried the faint scent of sex and Alex's aftershave mingled with Maria's light perfume. She couldn't even look at the bed. Stoically, she cleared the bathroom of all her paraphernalia. After that, she rounded up her other personal belongings and stuffed them in the tote she had packed with such excitement on Friday evening.

She made it back to her room before breaking down completely. Sobbing so hard she almost made herself ill, she curled up in a ball on the bed and wondered how she could have thrown herself headlong into such a colossal mistake.

Sleeping with the boss? What a cliché. What a wretched, stupid thing to do. Now, not only was her personal life in ruins, there was a good chance she might have to quit her job. She couldn't face seeing Alex every day at the Department of Commerce. Not knowing what he thought of her.

At the very least, he believed her to be a liar. Far worse than that was the fact he had turned his back on a relationship she thought was incredibly close and special. He'd brushed it aside as if it meant nothing...no more than a blip on the radar.

She'd heard people say that men could have sex without involving their emotions. But she'd never understood exactly what that meant. Now the truth was painfully clear. Alex, either intentionally or as a result of his wide experience with women, had convinced her that what happened in his suite this weekend was the stuff of romantic fantasy.

Fireworks and rainbows and happily-ever-afters. Realizing she had been so painfully naive was both humiliating and heartbreaking. Alex was willing to pass her off to Gabriel like an unwanted pet. No harm, no foul. Whatever was best for business.

She wanted to hate him for his callousness, and she did. But in the end, Alex was simply being Alex.

Suddenly, she couldn't bear the thought of him knocking on her door to ask something about the proposal or anything else. She called down to the front desk and requested a change of rooms, making up an excuse as to why she wanted to be in the completely opposite wing of the large hotel that encompassed two adjoining buildings connected by a skywalk.

A polite bellman showed up and helped her move her things. It wasn't much of a chore. She had packed light to come to the US. The only extras were a variety of small packages...souvenirs she had purchased for her mother and a few friends.

In the new room, she felt safer, but no less distraught.

Changing into the yoga pants and loose cotton top that she had taken with her to Alex's suite, she grimaced. She had envisioned relaxing with him in those simple clothes, maybe watching TV together. Instead, he had kept her naked almost the entire weekend.

Doggedly, she brushed her hair and fixed it in the usual ponytail before donning a baseball cap she wore for jogging to keep the hair out of her eyes. Hopefully, in the casual clothes and the hat no one would recognize her, even if she ran into anyone she knew...which was unlikely.

The members of the delegation were all staying in the other building. The Montoros would either be at the hospital or back in Coral Gables.

She wanted to leave her cell phone behind when she went out. But the tenets of responsibility were too deeply ingrained. This wasn't a vacation. She was here to work. Thus, she had to be available if needed.

For hours, she walked the streets of Miami. South Beach was eclectic and colorful and sophisticated, with its art galleries and restaurants and unique gift shops. Towering high-rises accommodated a wide range of businesses as well as pricey condos. It would be a nice place to live.

At five o'clock, she realized she hadn't eaten lunch. The fabulous smells emanating from a funky Cuban restaurant drew her inside. Fried plantains and shredded beef over rice filled her stomach, but nothing could fix the aching void in her chest.

She felt more solitary than the time long ago when she had been eight or nine and had to come home from school to an empty house. Those were bleak days. Her mother had worked almost constantly. Maria had learned to do homework on her own, to fix light meals on her own and sometimes even to put herself to bed.

The feeling now was much the same. Fear, dread, desperate loneliness. The only thing different was instead of missing her mother, who was the single touchstone for a child living a chaotic existence, Maria was now a grown woman with a broken heart.

She had told Alex if the weekend was all they had, it would be enough. But she'd been fooling herself. She wanted more. So much more...because despite her best intentions, she had fallen in love with him. It hadn't begun in Miami. She'd been headed in that direction for months, maybe years.

Beneath the hot Florida sun, the truth of her feelings for him had blossomed. For one bright, shining moment, she'd thought he felt it, too. But she had confused sex with caring. Alex was a business associate, the head of the delegation, the boss.

And Maria was nothing but a woman who should have known better.

She was sitting on a bench people-watching when her phone vibrated, signaling a text message.

Where the hell are you?

She could practically feel his anger and frustration.

Your key is at the front desk. Is there anything I need to do for the presentation tomorrow morning? she asked. She wouldn't jump to his bidding without a very good reason.

The document is perfect. I asked where you are.

She waited a long time. Maybe an entire minute. Then grimacing, she composed her answer: I'll see you at nine in the morning.

Alex stared at his phone in shock, his jaw slack with astonishment. Never in all the years he'd known her had

Maria ever behaved like this. She'd been at his beck and call, always willing to work late or to go the extra mile. Time and again he had seen her clean up a shoddy project left behind by someone else. She was driven and intelligent and utterly dependable.

But tonight he didn't even know where she was.

He had gone to her room after dinner, hoping to make things easier between them. But a strange man opened the door when Alex knocked. Alex had backed away with an apology and then examined the number on the door a second time thinking he had made a mistake.

The mistake, however, was far more complex than forgetting a room number. He'd let himself get involved with a coworker. It didn't matter that he wasn't her direct supervisor anymore. He and Maria were in Alma on a critically important mission. Personal relationships were inappropriate at best, for the very reason that they made things complicated.

After his anger had cooled somewhat in the wake of their confrontation at the hospital, he felt he owed Maria an apology. It wasn't fair to hold her accountable for her feelings if she really was falling for Gabriel Montoro. The man was charismatic, fun-loving and part of a family who had the potential to change Alma for the better over the coming decades.

Grinding his teeth, Alex tossed the phone on the bed and raked both hands through his hair. If he could have come up with even the flimsiest of pretexts to contact Maria again, he would have. But everything was in order for tomorrow's meeting.

Where was she, damn it? He paced the room, trying to ignore the fact that her image appeared everywhere he looked. Like a hologram taunting him with faux reality, she lingered in his bed, on his sofa, in his shower.

Had she gone to Gabriel? Was she with him even now?

Alex forced himself to consider the possibility, confronting it head-on. The pain almost brought him to his knees. How could he let her go? How could he stand by for the good of his country and watch Gabriel Montoro woo her and wed her?

Maria was *his*. He had touched her, made love to her, shuddered in her arms as she pleasured him.

He dropped down on the bed, his head in his hands. How had he made such a mess of his life?

In the hotel conference room the following morning, Alex greeted the members of the committee as they arrived. Maria was conspicuously absent. Once everyone was seated, he passed out the copies of the finished proposal. Excited chatter rose and fell around the table as heads bent to scan the pages he'd had copied at the nearest office-supply store.

Just as Alex stepped behind the portable podium to begin going over the points of the document— section by section—the door opened once again, and Maria slipped into the room with a muttered apology. Her silky blond hair had been tamed into a sleek chignon. She wore a fashionable but relatively conservative navy suit with a pale pink camisole beneath.

Alex's heart stopped entirely and then lurched into motion, his hands damp as they gripped the edge of the wood. "We saved you a seat," he said, trying for friendly humor and failing miserably.

Maria shot him an inscrutable glance and moved toward the opposite end of the table. Normally, she sat near him in case he needed to confer about details or procedure. Today they were as far apart as possible.

Her skin was pale, her eyes underscored with shadows. Had she slept any more than he had?

The men and women around the table barely noticed her arrival. Interest and excitement ran high knowing that today's meeting put them one step closer to officially courting the Montoros.

Alex forced himself to concentrate. This was not the moment to fumble, not with so much at stake. He spoke calmly and clearly, knowing his audience included some of the finest minds Alma had to offer. The Department of State was represented, as were Treasury and Internal Affairs. Combining the business interests of the Montoros with the economy of Alma would require finesse and vision.

It was clear by the end of the first hour that his team was impressed and pleased with the carefully crafted proposal. With the addition of a few footnotes and corrections here and there, the group voted unanimously to approve the document and move on to the next phase…making an official offer to Rafe Montoro IV to return to Alma and accept the throne.

During a short break when Alex had hoped to speak with Maria, his cell phone rang. After a brief conversation, he gathered his papers and reconvened his group. "That was Rafael Montoro on the phone, our potential head of state. He and the entire family had planned to be present tomorrow, as you know, in this very room, to hear what we have to say. But with his aunt in the hospital, they are understandably reluctant to leave her side."

He paused, knowing there was no protocol for this change. "Rafael has asked to come here and receive an unofficial draft, the one you're holding, so that the family might go over it together and discuss it in private. When

Isabella recovers, we can then meet officially and make the presentation."

Maria spoke up, her gaze impassive. "Do we have the authority to do that?"

A heated debate ensued, culminating in a conference call to the prime minister back in Alma. Fortunately, after a quick transatlantic conversation, Alex's boss gave the nod. Moments later, Alex made a return call to Rafael.

When that was done, he surveyed the members of the delegation. They had all been cooped up in this room, as pleasant as it was, for hours, and everyone was hungry and tired.

"We'll take a break to eat," he said. "Given Rafael's timetable, we should probably meet back here at three o'clock. Are we all in agreement?"

With nods and muttered assents, the group scattered. Maria, surrounded by three other women, was on her way out before he could stop her. "Wait," he said. The four females turned back to look curiously at him.

He felt his neck get hot. "I need to speak to Maria."

The woman to whom he had made wild, passionate love for hours gave him a cool, regal glance, as if princess to peon. "Right now?"

He stared her down, daring her to ignore him, asserting his authority and knowing that he wasn't playing fair. "Yes."

Maria murmured her apologies to her companions and stepped back into the conference room once they walked away. After closing the door, she set her purse and laptop on the table, crossed her arms and stared at him with barely veiled hostility. "What?"

"Where were you last night?"

Her eyes narrowed. "That is not an appropriate question between business associates."

He had a reputation for being cool under pressure, but, damn, she pushed his buttons. "Were you with Gabriel?"

Her expression was impossible to read. "Are you hoping I'll say yes? So you'll know you have a spy in the enemy camp?"

"Don't be ridiculous."

"Is that why you wanted to talk to me? So you could heap a few more insults on my head?"

If he'd expected any kind of negative response from her, he would have guessed anger. But the mood he picked up on was more akin to sadness. "I wanted to apologize," he said stiffly.

"For what?"

He rounded the table. He'd bet his last euro that she wanted to back away from him, but she maintained her position.

"I shouldn't have connected your relationship with Gabriel to the work of the delegation. Whatever goes on between the two of you is personal and private."

"That's very gracious of you."

The words were innocuous. But they were wrapped in a heavy dose of sarcasm that made him wince.

"I'm trying to make amends," he said.

"And failing miserably. I thought when a man had a one-night stand with a woman, he at least owed her a breakup dinner. Or a Dear Jane note."

"It was two nights." Two insanely erotic, tantalizing nights. Even now, the memory made him hard.

"I won't quibble over the details, Alex. All I ask is that next time you want to scratch a sexual itch, you find someone who doesn't mind being shoved aside when your job takes precedence."

"That's not what happened."

"What would *you* call it?" she asked.

"You and I have worked together a long time. There was bound to be an undercurrent of sexual interest. But I was wrong to pursue it, given the circumstances."

"You act as if it was all your idea. I was in the bed, too. So let's call it a dual mistake."

As they exchanged barbs, he moved closer. Now, he snagged one of her hands in his and put his thumb over the pulse point on her wrist. "I'm asking you to forgive me," he said huskily. It was only now dawning on him that physical proximity to the woman who turned him inside out might not be the best idea.

She didn't struggle or try to free herself, though his hold was loose. Because they stood so closely together, she was forced to tip back her head to look up at him. "Forgive you for what?"

Blue-green eyes that were usually guileless and clear were veiled today, the emotions carefully blanked out.

"Stubborn, frustrating woman." His lips hovered over hers, his body straining to get closer. He maintained a safe distance between them, but it cost him.

One kiss. That's all he needed. An apology kiss. That made sense, didn't it? For one quivering, tense second, he knew it was going to happen. He felt it inside his gut. Every cell in his body cried out for him to ignore reason and reality and to take what he wanted.

Maria was frozen in place, her arms still crossed at her waist. The brittle edge of her anger had softened. He was sure of it. "I really am sorry," he muttered. "For everything."

His lips brushed hers with a spark of contact electricity. *Holy hell.*

The jolt rocked him. "Say something, Maria."

Two slender feminine hands struck his shoulders and

shoved hard, catching him off guard, causing him to lose his balance and fall into the nearest chair.

Before he could recover, she was gone.

Fourteen

Maria caught up with her lunch companions at the restaurant downstairs. She was coldly furious, but she wallowed in the icy, cleansing emotion. For the moment, it cauterized the jagged edges of her broken heart. Alex Ramon was an imbecile.

He thought he could manipulate her and use her and get away with his double-talk, avoiding a single consequence to his oh-so-perfect image. Maybe other women had been willing to accept his Dr. Jekyll and Mr. Hyde routine, but not this one.

And he still didn't believe her about Gabriel.

It took all the acting skills she could muster, but she engaged in the conversation among her colleagues without giving a hint at the turmoil that rocked her. She prayed that the Montoros would make their decision quickly, one way or another. All Maria wanted to do was go home.

After lunch she made a quick trip to her room to drop

off her laptop, brush her teeth and freshen her lipstick. An official visit between Rafe Montoro and the delegation as a whole required a certain degree of formality. She wanted to look her best.

Lingering deliberately until the last possible moment, she made her way back to the conference room and took her original seat. The furniture had been rearranged to accommodate a head table. Someone from the hotel had brought in a small vase of fresh flowers.

The tension in the room was palpable.

Her arrogant lover spotted her the moment she walked in, but though he gave her a steady look, he did nothing to summon her attention. Once everyone from Alma was seated, the group fell silent.

Alex stepped into the hallway and returned with Rafael. But the king-to-be was not alone. Gabriel was with him. That came as no surprise to Maria. The brothers were close.

The two Montoros were dressed formally in dark suits and ties. Even Gabriel, rascal that he was, maintained his composure. Alex took a visible breath. "Ladies and gentlemen. May I present Rafael Montoro, IV, and his brother, Gabriel." Facing the siblings, he executed a half bow. "On behalf of the nation of Alma, we welcome both of you this afternoon and look forward to hearing what you have to say."

Alex stepped aside and offered Rafe the podium.

The eldest of this younger Montoro generation spoke pleasantly and confidently. As CEO of Montoro Enterprises, he was accustomed to a leadership role, so he showed no signs of being nervous or intimidated by the fact that an entire roomful of people wanted to make him a king.

Rafael was tall, a couple of inches over six feet. His dark brown hair, cut very short, suited his air of command.

When he was done with his brief, prepared remarks, he fielded questions. Through it all, Gabriel remained quiet but watchful, as if he were trying to assess the character of each member of the delegation.

Other than a couple of polite inquiries, no one introduced any kind of controversial topics. There would be time enough for that later.

Toward the end of the hour, when a note of awkward anticipation entered the mix, Gabriel and Maria exchanged rueful glances. This was a touchy situation, however you looked at it.

Rafael nodded briefly to his audience, for a split second betraying the first hint of agitation Maria had seen from him. "I hope you'll understand that we need to get back to the hospital," he said. "My family and I will read through this proposal and give it our utmost consideration."

He paused. "I am well aware that each of you has gone above and beyond the expectations of your job descriptions. From what Mr. Ramon has told me, you have given your time and talents to this endeavor with varying degrees of personal sacrifice. I am honored by this proposal, and I will weigh the ramifications as honestly as I know how. Thank you."

Quiet applause greeted his last words. The group rose as one, everybody eager to say a word of greeting to the man who might one day reign as their monarch. During the hubbub, Gabriel scooted around the room in Maria's direction. His smile was strained. "This bunch is making me claustrophobic," he said. "Will you come with me for a minute?"

"Of course." He seemed oblivious to Alex's displeasure. They found an empty meeting space across the hall, much smaller than the one they'd escaped, and slipped inside to hide out in the back corner.

Gabriel leaned against the wall and rubbed his face. "I wish I still smoked," he groaned.

"You smoked?" Maria asked with a frown.

His charming grin radiated only half its usual voltage. "For about eight months the year I turned sixteen. When my father found out, he hit the ceiling. He and Rafe took me out on a sailboat and made me smoke two entire packs during one afternoon...in rough seas, I might add. I spent the next hour hanging over the rail barfing my guts out. That was the last day I ever wanted a cigarette. Until now."

She touched his arm. "You've got a lot going on in your family. I know it's hard. How's Isabella?"

"Holding her own. We were all afraid this was it, but she's a tough old bird." He rolled his shoulders. "The timing sucks, though. We need to get the proposal mess settled one way or another."

"How is Rafe leaning? You can trust me. I won't say a word to anyone."

"I wish I knew. I thought Isabella's health crisis would tip the scales, but she made it clear to us yesterday afternoon that she only wants the family to say yes to the proposal if we can do it with unanimity and one hundred percent enthusiasm."

"That sounds like an impossible goal."

"Yeah. So I haven't the slightest idea how this is going to turn out."

"I wish there was something I could do to make it easier."

"That's sweet of you. You're a very nice lady." He flicked her updo. "Was it my imagination, or were things tense between you and Alex at the hospital? I got the impression he'd like to punch me. Has my charade worked? Does he think he'll have to battle me to win you back?"

She blushed. "Oh, that was nothing. We had a difference of opinion about something. It's not important."

Gabriel bent his head and locked eyes with her, his trademark grin wider than it had been so far today. "I have good instincts when it comes to romance. I think the two of you are an item."

"Did we trip and fall into a fifties movie? Don't make me laugh. Alex Ramon is a stuffed shirt. A workaholic. A soulless bureaucrat."

The fact that her voice broke on the last syllable was a dead giveaway. She turned her back on Gabriel, mortified that she was making a scene.

He curled an arm around her shoulders. "You want me to beat him up for you?"

She wiped her face with the back of her hand. "Would you?"

They both laughed, and she felt better, despite the fact that the man she loved was still a jerk.

A cold, rigid voice broke them apart. "Excuse me. I didn't know I was interrupting."

Gabriel whirled around, striding forward to clap Alex on the shoulder. "Not at all. Maria was just commiserating with me about my family's multiple soap-opera-ish woes."

When Alex continued to resemble a silent, stony-faced executioner, Gabriel shook his head. "You've got the wrong end of the stick, Ramon. I don't poach on another man's preserves."

Maria frowned. "What does that mean?"

Gabriel shot her a look over his shoulder. "It means that you and I are buddies, amigos, compadres. But what we are *not* is an item."

His humor fell flat all the way around.

Alex nodded stiffly. "I didn't mean any disrespect."

Gabriel rolled his eyes. "I'm not a prince yet. I don't need bowing and scraping from you." He held out his hand. "Are we good, man?"

Alex nodded, the harsh lines in his face relaxing. "We're good. Thanks for coming today. I think your brother is waiting for you."

"No problem. You've done a good job leading this delegation, Alex. Our family is grateful for your sensitivity and your diplomacy. And, by the by, I want you to call me Gabriel."

"I suppose in the interim it would be okay."

"It will *always* be okay," Gabriel said firmly. "Even if Rafe accepts this king-of-Alma gig, I guarantee he'll only tolerate so much pomp and circumstance. You and Maria have made our family feel as if our wishes and opinions are valid. That goes a long way in the negotiating process. We appreciate it."

Alex nodded. "I'm glad you feel that way."

Gabriel, now by the door, sketched a wave at Maria. "I've got to run, sweet thing. See you soon."

Suddenly the party of three became two.

Maria shifted from one foot to the other. Alex stood between her and an escape route. "Is everyone else gone?" she asked.

He nodded. "Yes."

"Are you pleased with how today turned out?"

Alex weighed his answer. "Not entirely."

"What's wrong? Did Rafe say something? Are they trying to tell you this is going nowhere?"

Alex held up his hands. "Whoa. Slow down the train. I wasn't talking about anything that happened in an official capacity. You asked me if I was pleased with how today turned out, and I said no…because things are at an impasse between you and me."

"Not my fault." Her glare melted his certainty that he could persuade her to see reason.

"I've already apologized," he said. "Can't we move on?"

Memories of her in his bed tangled with the reality of Maria standing in front of him. She was neat and feminine and so damned beautiful in her trendy suit. But her clothing reminded him that they were colleagues first and lovers second…not an order he wanted, but a necessity given the situation with the Montoros.

Her lips trembled. "You don't even get it, do you? I'm not upset because you kicked me out of your bed. I'm furious and astounded that you didn't believe *me* when I told you nothing was going on with Gabriel. Yet when *he* told you the exact same thing, suddenly you take it as fact."

Alex realized he'd screwed up royally. The pun didn't even register as funny. "Perhaps we should take a couple of steps backward and start over." He was aiming for calm and conciliatory. Maria didn't seem impressed.

She walked across the room and went toe-to-toe with him. "There's nothing to start over *with*. We're not anything to each other, Alex. Just a man and a woman who happen to work together."

Deliberately, she elbowed him aside and made for the door.

His temper snapped and flared. "Not so fast."

Dragging her against his chest, he took her chin in his hand and tilted it upward so he could reach her gorgeous, argumentative lips. Instead of angry mastery, he clamped down on his aggravation and gave her gentleness, trying every way he knew how to convey his regret that he had made such a mess of things.

But it was a lost cause. Her body was stiff in his embrace…her lips cold and unresponsive. Reluctantly, he released her. A block of ice settled in the spot where his stomach had been.

She stared at him, her gaze neither stormy nor sweet. Instead, she was indifferent. "Next time you do that, Mr. Ramon, I'll report you for sexual harassment. Good day."

When she walked out on him, Alex was stunned.

He stood in the small empty room for a full five minutes, trying to analyze where he'd gone wrong. All his life he'd been an overachiever. Top of his class in every school he'd ever attended. His father's favorite. A goal-oriented, don't-give-up, type A, hardworking guy who went after whatever he wanted and got it.

Money had never been an issue. His parents had spoiled him, but he had repaid their generosity by consistently making them proud of him. He'd never yearned and ached for something he couldn't have, had never faced real, honest-to-God disappointment and failure.

This was a hell of a moment to learn an unpleasant life lesson. Apparently he wasn't infallible after all. There was at least a fifty-fifty chance that the Montoros were going to decline the request to reclaim the monarchy. Which meant that Alex and the delegation would have wasted weeks and months of planning and positioning.

Going home to Alma empty-handed, with the proposal unsigned, would not only be a personal defeat, it would constitute an embarrassing misstep in Alex's career. People had depended on him. His *country* had entrusted him with a mission of incalculable importance.

Forcing himself to take a painful look at his behavior this past weekend was mildly reassuring. Even though he had let his personal life intrude during a time he should have been concentrating on the Montoros, he honestly didn't think making love to Maria had been any kind of dereliction of duty.

His worst sin lay in allowing her to believe that he didn't respect or value her as a person and woman.

That had never been his intention, but looking at the situation from her point of view, he could now see how badly he had bungled things. She was hurt that he thought she was a liar. Nothing could be further from the truth. But when she told him nothing was going on with her and Gabriel, he'd assumed she simply didn't recognize the other man's interest.

The truth was, Alex couldn't imagine any red-blooded male being immune to Maria's charms.

When he had handed her his room key and asked her to remove her things, he'd been operating from hurt and jealousy and anger. Though he'd told himself it was the right thing to do because of his position as head of the delegation, the truth was, he'd been reeling from seeing her in the garden with Gabriel.

Alex had never cared enough about any woman to be affected one way or another if the female in question found someone else. His work had always been at the forefront of his priority list. Satisfying his physical needs had come second. He liked sex as much as the next guy and enjoyed women and their soft bodies and interesting minds.

But not once in his life had he ever experienced this gnawing feeling of emptiness and loss.

Hubris brought down many a man. Recognizing his failings had certainly chastened and humbled Alex. Now he faced a double-barrel shotgun ready to destroy much of his life. If this had happened six months ago, he would have been obsessing over how he could save face and salvage his career.

At this moment, however, he didn't give a damn about

losing his reputation or his job or anything else that might be part of the Montoro fallout.

His only regret was that he had screwed up the one exquisitely wonderful, warm and perfect relationship he'd ever experienced. He had lost Maria's good regard, her friendship and any prospect of having her in his bed.

And there was a dollop of bitter gall on top of this mountainous fiasco. He knew one truth beyond any shadow of doubt. He was in love with Maria Ferro.

Maria didn't know what to do. She was not an indecisive person, but she felt as if the walls had caved in on her.

Her first impulse was to call the airline to see about changing her ticket. But when she tried, the cost was ridiculous, and even then, she couldn't get a seat until the following week because of a baggage handler strike.

The impulse to run was overpowering. She didn't want to face Alex and would try to avoid him for as long as possible. When they were eventually together again, would he be able to read heartbreak in her face? Would he guess that she was in love with him?

When flying home early didn't work, she decided it was for the best. To leave without saying goodbye to the Montoros would be terribly rude, particularly with Isabella in the hospital.

Two days later, Maria sat in a coffee shop a few blocks from the hotel and scrolled through emails halfheartedly. The past forty-eight hours had dragged by. The only news of note was that Isabella had improved dramatically and would be returning home. Her diagnosis, of course, was still terminal, but doctors gave her an open-ended amount of time to live, so everyone involved was thankful.

While all that was happening, Maria had read books,

walked on the beach and even taken a bus tour of the city. Anything to pass the time.

Waiting was excruciating. She could only imagine how Alex must feel. Today was even worse, and it wasn't yet noon. She and her mom chatted online for a bit. Hearing about events back in Alma seemed strange…as if the world should have stopped while Maria was in Miami.

Finally, just as she was ordering a sandwich for her lunch, a text came through. From Gabriel.

Don't say a word to anyone, but we're close!

Her heart stopped. Immediately, she wanted to call Alex, but of course, she couldn't. She answered quickly.

Will there be a monarchy?

It looks that way. God help us…

She had a feeling Gabriel meant those last three words literally. The task set forth before Rafael was enormous, but the entire family would be affected in so many ways.

Does Isabella know? she texted.

Not yet. Rafe and Dad want to make sure all the t's are crossed and i's dotted.

Makes sense.

If this all comes to pass, big party planned. Other news for the Montoros to announce.

Tell me. Tell me.

My lips are sealed.

She could almost see his smirk.

Thanks for the heads-up.

You bet. See you soon.

Maria paid for her sandwich and sat down to eat it, but she had lost her appetite. If she and Alex hadn't argued, Alex would probably have included her in all of this last-minute hush-hush negotiation. As it was, she'd been left out in the cold. She was surprised at how much that hurt.

Her phone lay on the table. Surely Alex would tell her when it happened. Or maybe things had fallen apart. She shoved her half-eaten lunch aside and bit her fingernail, a bad habit she'd given up in high school.

It was thirty-seven minutes from Gabriel's text until the next time her phone dinged quietly. This time the message on the screen was from Alex. It was simple and to the point.

We have a king!

Tears sprang to her eyes. She knew exactly how Alex would look right now. Jubilant. Relieved. Incredibly handsome.

He had not texted her privately. One by one, the replies came in until it became clear he had included the entire delegation in a group message. Maria was one of the crowd.

Knowing she had to say something or risk seeming oddly silent to her colleagues, she bit her lip and slowly composed her answer.

A great day for Alma. I am proud to have worked alongside all of you.

Then she shut off her phone. There was only the minut-
est of chances that Alex would call her, but she couldn't
take a chance. Hearing his voice would tear her apart.

Grabbing up her things and her tote bag, she tossed the
remains of her lunch in the trash and set out to walk the
streets of Miami. Maybe she could outrun her demons.
And maybe the moon was made of green cheese.

Her life had changed. It would change even more back
in Alma. She had some big decisions to make.

Fifteen

Alex couldn't remember the last time he'd been this tired or this satisfied. Or this frustrated. He barely knew what to think from one moment to the next.

When Rafe Montoro rang to say he was signing the document but with a few caveats, a firestorm of phone calls had ensued. The prime minister had to be roused from his bed back in Alma. The time difference would make the next few days challenging as the two parties resolved minor differences.

As a show of good faith, Rafael IV planned to make a quick trip to Alma very soon to sign a new agreement between Montoro Enterprises and a major refinery in Alma to ship oil to the US.

After the long days and weeks of waiting and wondering, suddenly it was all happening very quickly.

Alex tried Maria's phone three separate times, but the calls went straight to voice mail. Where the hell was she?

With Gabriel? Even if nothing romantic was going on between the two of them, it was clear to Alex that Gabriel
and Maria were becoming very good friends.

Alex had thought, once upon a time, that *he* and Maria
were close. But now she had deliberately put distance between them. Knowing that the situation was his own fault
didn't help.

For the remainder of the day until late in the night he
fielded communications between Alma and the soon-to-be
royal family. Decisions had to be made about the timing of
public announcements. In the interests of good business,
it was important to protect the Montoros' image here in
the States as well as abroad.

The stock market didn't like change or uncertainty, and
Montoro Enterprises was a publicly traded company. All
the kinks needed to be ironed out before revealing this
extraordinary news.

For the next seventy-two hours, Alex worked pretty
much nonstop, existing on four to five hours of sleep a
night. Though he and Maria communicated via text and
email, when they labored side by side at the table, there
was always someone else in the room.

Alex could have forced the issue, demanding that they
meet in private. But he had done enough damage already.
So he chose to bide his time.

The truth was, he didn't have the luxury of worrying
about his personal life at a time like this. All of his attention had to be focused on Alma and the Montoros and the
changes to come.

But when he finally fell into bed during the wee hours
of the morning, he lay in the darkness remembering the
feel of Maria's body pressed up against his and imagining he could still detect the scent of her perfume on his
pillow.

* * *

Maria smoothed the skirt of her fire-engine-red gown and wondered if she had made a mistake. Looking in the bathroom mirror, she tugged at the bodice, hoping to cover at least half an inch more cleavage. Her breasts were modest in size, but with the cut of the fabric and the sewn-in boning, everything she had was up and out on display.

When the news leaked that the Montoros were accepting Alma's proposal, all heck had broken loose. Maria had spent long hours with her laptop preparing press releases in a variety of formats. Some for Alma, others for the local Miami market, and still more for the entire United States and the rest of the world.

A political event of this magnitude had repercussions that would echo for years to come. It was exciting and challenging to be part of the process. All her education and training and hard work had led to this pivotal moment. She should be proud. And she was.

But all the job satisfaction in the world did little to mend a broken heart, especially in light of the knowledge that she would most likely have to look for other work when she went home.

Already, she realized that she couldn't be in the same building as Alex and pretend that she didn't care. She wasn't the first woman to be mistaken about a man, and she wouldn't be the last.

But the hurt ran deep.

What she needed to do in the meantime was to compartmentalize. Personal feelings—locked away. Fun-and-games Maria—out to play. Tonight's party at the Montoro compound in Coral Gables was likely to be the glitziest, most glamorous affair she'd ever attended. To hell with Alex Ramon and his arrogant judgmental attitude. Maria was going to enjoy herself.

In between frantic work sessions, she had slipped away yesterday afternoon and found a boutique at one of the nearby hotels that showcased the work of a local designer. Although of runway quality, the woman's designs were still relatively unknown and the prices were not astronomical.

In addition to the pale aqua dress she wore at the opening reception, Maria had brought with her from Alma two easy-to-pack outfits for formal occasions that might arise, but neither was particularly exciting. So when she had spotted this sexy red number, she'd had to try it on. Even the saleslady had been visibly impressed. The color was perfect for Maria's skin and hair.

The splendid creation made her feel like a princess. Which was not a bad thing on an evening when a monarchy was about to be reborn.

She eyed the tiny straps and fitted waist. Though she couldn't see the entire silhouette, she ran her hands down her hips, feeling the way the silk hugged her curves. Below the knees it fanned out in a mermaidlike froth of tulle and satin.

Maybe she would meet a handsome local who would sweep her off her feet. Maybe they would dance until dawn.

It was a nice image, but even as she turned away from her reflection, she had to blink back tears. She would not cry for Alex Ramon. Not tonight. Tonight was a time for celebration.

Maria was in the lobby, bags packed, at five o'clock. Bella had insisted on coming to pick her up in a limo. The entire delegation, as a courtesy, had been offered accommodations in the various guest villas at the Montoros' Coral Gables estate for the weekend.

Several cars were being dispatched to the hotel to ferry

Alma's guests of honor to the soiree. Fortunately, Maria didn't have to worry about an uncomfortable encounter with Alex.

Bella's eyebrows went up when she walked in and saw Maria. "You look fantastic."

"Thank you," Maria said. "You're good for my ego." As the driver stowed Maria's bags, Bella and Maria settled on opposite sides of the wide seat and fastened their seat belts.

Bella frowned. "Don't take this as a criticism, but you look like you've been crying."

Her matter-of-fact assessment sent Maria scrambling for the small, mirrored compact in her evening purse. "Do I?"

As she scanned her face hurriedly, Bella chuckled. "That was just a test. If you'd told me you hadn't been crying, I'd have known you were okay. But I can see it in your eyes. You and Alex haven't made up, have you? Gabriel told me what's going on."

Maria gave her a sour look. "Not funny. And there's nothing to make up. Alex and I are fine."

"Never kid a kidder." Bella reached into the small refrigerator and poured a glass of champagne, handing it to her with a sympathetic smile. "Chin up. He may take one look at you in that dress and keel over at your feet…"

Unfortunately, Bella's blithe pronouncement was way off the mark. When Maria first spotted Alex, he was deep in conversation with a local news anchorwoman who looked far more interested in her interviewee than in the Montoro story.

Although Alex spared a brief glance in Maria's direction, his gaze didn't linger. So much for the red dress.

Instead of bemoaning something she couldn't change, she chose to soak up the splendor of the evening. The backdrop for tonight's festivities exhibited all the glamour and drama of a movie set. Lush lawns lay like green velvet, punctuated with every manner of tropical bush and flower amid towering palm trees.

White tents, strung with lights that would eventually twinkle against the night sky, provided shelter in case of inclement weather, but so far, the clouds only served to accentuate what would be a dramatic sunset.

Caterers were hard at work setting out china and crystal and, most impressive of all, heavy silver utensils bearing the Montoro crest. The precious metal dated back to the eighteenth century and had been hidden away in a root cellar by a faithful servant when the Montoro ancestors fled for their lives.

Most recently it had been on display in a museum in Alma but, under Alex's directions, had been flown across the ocean for tonight's party. Maria gave a moment's pause to wonder how safe it was to actually use such priceless artifacts, but security was heavy and visible.

Everyone had been required to enter through a special gate where professional teams of men and women used hand wands and other means to ensure that only invited guests were allowed in.

Bella glanced at her watch. "I hate to abandon you, but I promised my father I'd take care of a few things."

Maria smiled, shooing her away. "I'm fine. Go. I may hide out in my room for a bit if you'll tell me where I'm staying." The limo driver had absconded with her luggage.

Maria's smile was rueful. "I wasn't in charge of the lodging assignments. The housekeeper put you and Alex in the same villa you had before."

Maria gaped. "Please tell me you're joking."

"Sorry." She seemed genuinely apologetic. "Every bed is taken."

"Never mind then," Maria said grumpily, her panic barely under control. "I'll make myself useful somewhere."

Bella walked away, leaving Maria to wander the grounds in limbo until the main event started. Did Alex already know they were sharing a villa? Was he angry about it? Was that why he had barely looked at her when she arrived?

If she had imagined being bored during the wait, nothing could have been further from the truth. Perching on a fabric-covered chair in an out-of-the-way corner, she had a perfect view of the guests as they arrived. It was almost like the red carpet at the Oscars.

Since she wasn't from Miami, or even an American, many of the faces were not recognizable to her. But it was easy to spot the ones who graced the covers of the tabloids. Rock legends and rappers. Television personalities. Stars of stage and screen. The Montoros were infinitely more well-connected than she had realized.

At the far end of the lawn, with the ocean as an azure background, a small stage had been erected along with a high-tech sound system. At seven o'clock, the evening was to kick off with formalities. After that, on to dinner and dancing.

She had waved at Gabriel from a distance, but he had two gorgeous women with him, one on each arm, so she didn't intrude.

By the time the dignitaries took the stage, Maria was a nervous wreck. She wanted to give Alex a word of encouragement, but with the discord between the two of them, it was probably best to keep her distance. Personal feelings had to make way for the important business at hand.

She wished desperately that she were one of the carefree partygoers with nothing but pleasure on her mind. The festive crowd mingled and moved like a vibrant, colorful flock of birds, the men's black-tie apparel providing a backdrop for the female plumage.

A hush fell as Rafael Montoro III, his three children

and Alex ascended the shallow steps and took their seats. Only the eldest member of the group remained standing. He approached the podium and looked out over the sea of faces, his expression full of emotion.

He cleared his throat. "It is my great pleasure to welcome each of you into the heart of the Montoro family this evening. We are proud citizens of the United States of America, and Florida has been our home and our sanctuary. Nothing will ever take away that bond. But life is full of surprises, and as you all understand, the only constant is change."

He paused as laughter greeted his remarks.

"For any of you who do not know me," he said, "I am Rafael Montoro III. On the podium with me tonight are my three children—Rafael IV, Gabriel and Bella. We look forward to chatting with as many of you as possible during this wonderful evening. There is much to celebrate. I am proud to say that as of this week, Montoro Enterprises has officially been listed in the Fortune 500 for the very first time."

This time the response was wild and loud, punctuated with cheering and high fives.

He waited, smiling, for the hubbub to die down. "Now I would like to introduce Mr. Alex Ramon, deputy prime minister of commerce for Alma, and also the leader of the delegation from that country."

Alex and Rafael exchanged a half handshake, half embrace before the older man sat down. When Alex adjusted the microphone to accommodate his greater height, Maria's palms were as damp as if she were standing there beside him.

But when he spoke, his words resonated with such passion and conviction and sheer charisma, she forgot for a moment that he had shared life's most intimate act with her. Instead, she listened intently, filled with pride and admiration for the man who had accomplished so much.

After a brief explanatory statement, Alex smiled and asked Rafe to join him. "It is my great honor and privilege to present to you the next king of the nation of Alma, Rafael Montoro IV."

Rafe, perhaps unnerved by the import of the moment, nodded, his features tense. But his shoulders relaxed somewhat when Alex indicated that he should say something.

"It's early days yet," Rafe finally said, "and I am deeply cognizant of the honor bestowed upon me by the people of Alma. But I want you to know that I take this commitment very seriously, and I will do everything in my power to ensure this new relationship brings progress and benefit to the people who are entrusting me with their leadership."

This time, the applause had a different tone. Everyone in earshot had an inkling of what Rafael faced. It was not an easy thing to rule, and they offered him their respect along with their congratulations.

To Maria's surprise, Rafael sat down, and Alex once again took the podium. "I would be remiss tonight if I did not recognize each member of the official delegation from Alma. You'll find their names printed in your programs. I hope you will take the time to greet them this evening and express your appreciation for their hard work and dedication to the idea of restoring Alma's monarchy."

He stopped talking abruptly, and, for a split second, Maria felt as if he were staring straight at her. "The thing is," he said, the words contemplative, "politics and business negotiations encompass far more than dry statistics and formal agreements. In the end, it's all about relationships. About people. About trust and integrity. One member of our group seems to understand that truth at a most basic level, and I am not sure we would be standing here tonight were it not for the wise counsel and collaborative efforts of the lovely lady in the red dress, Ms. Maria Ferro. Thank you, Maria, for all you have done to build bridges and bring consensus to the table."

She never heard the applause this time. Her heart was beating too loudly in her ears to take in anything else. People around her shook her hand and kissed her cheek and offered words of congratulations. It was all a blur.

Suddenly, Alex was at her side, looking darkly handsome and so very dear. His firm jaw and classic features made him stand out, even in an assembly of very good-looking men.

He didn't touch her. But the searing look he gave her made her shiver. "I nearly swallowed my tongue when you walked into my line of sight earlier," he muttered, the words husky. "You and that dress should be an illegal combination."

"Did you mean what you said?" she asked. "Or did the delegation tell you to spout all that?"

"God, sweetheart. I really screwed up, didn't I? Of *course* I meant it. Every word."

It was gratifying to know that he valued her work, but his compliments didn't erase the fact that he didn't trust her.

Suddenly, she became aware that several people were standing close enough to take interested note of what they were saying.

Alex took her arm, his fingers warm and strong on her bare skin. "Let's get out of here."

She eluded his hold. "No. I don't have anything to say to you. You've never believed me when it comes to Gabriel, and that hurts."

"I do believe you," he said urgently. "But I thought you

were fooling yourself about *his* feelings. Turns out I was dead wrong. About everything."

"Gabriel and I are friends."

"I know that now. I've been a total ass. And I'm sorry. I was jealous and stupid. I don't deserve it, but I'm asking you to forgive me."

She gaped in surprise at his unequivocal about-face. Alex took advantage of her shock to hurry her along.

They made it as far as the last tent before she dug in her heels. *"Alex,"* she said urgently. "I forgive you. I really do. But this is your night. This is Alma's night. Everything you've dreamed of and worked for the last eighteen months. You can't walk out on the party."

He kissed her softly, lingering long enough to make her breath catch and her knees go weak. "Watch me, my love."

Grabbing an empty golf cart, he pulled her onto the seat beside him and started the motor. She wasn't sure she'd have been able to find her way through the maze of paths, but Alex took them straight to the small, charming villa where they had stayed on their first visit to Coral Gables.

When he removed his foot from the pedal, the cart rolled to a stop, and Maria felt her belly quiver. She tried to speak, but her throat was so dry the words stuck there unvoiced.

Perhaps Alex sensed her agitation, or perhaps he was simply in a hurry. Either way, he took her by surprise when he scooped her up and carried her around to the front door. The villa wasn't locked. They found the key inside on a table with a note of greeting from their hosts, a basket of fruit and an arrangement of fresh flowers.

Alex secured the door with one hand, not even breathing hard.

Finally, she found the words she wanted to say. "Thank you."

He frowned. "For what?"

She touched his chin. A tiny nick on the left side of his jaw told her his late-day shave had been hurried. "For saying all those nice things. And for groveling so sweetly."

Finally, a note of humor lightened his face. "If you think *that* was nice, you ain't seen nothin' yet."

He bypassed the luxurious living room and went straight down the hall, only hesitating between the two bedrooms. "Your place or mine?"

Maria decided it was about time to rein in all that assured masculinity. "Aren't you assuming a lot, Mr. Ramon?"

He kicked open the door to the room that had been Maria's on their last visit. Dropping her on the mattress, he took her small purse from her nerveless fingers and tossed it aside. Coming down beside her, he leaned on one elbow, his expression sober. "I was an ass and an idiot, but I adore you, Maria. My life means nothing if you aren't in it. Say you love me. Say you forgive me. Marry me and give me babies."

The arrogance was still there. Nothing but demands. Her heart swelled anyway. "You may be a diplomat, but you're terrible at groveling."

He slid off the bed and knelt on the rug, his dark eyes sober. Reaching out, he took her hand in his. "We got off to a rocky start. I wish I could have wooed you in private, at our leisure, not in the midst of a ticking political time bomb. You deserve so much better."

"I *like* working with you," she said softly, curling her fingers with his.

She saw his throat work when he swallowed. "My only excuse is that it took me by surprise."

"*What* did?"

"The fact that I'm in love with you."

She stopped breathing for at least five seconds. "You really love me?"

"Isn't that what I've been saying?" His masculine indignation made her smile.

"Somehow, when you distill it to those three words, it seems more real. I love you, too, Alex." She sat up and leaned forward, curling a hand behind his head to kiss him. "I think I probably have for a long time."

"If you like real," he muttered, "you're going to like what I've got planned next."

He ripped off his tux jacket and jerked at his shirt, sending studs flying. Her pulse sped up and stuttered. "Shall I help?"

"No. Come here."

Poor man. He couldn't help himself. He was accustomed to being in charge. But they could work on that.

She shimmied off the bed and stood in front of him. Though he was taller, her heels put them eye-to-eye. Tracing a finger from one side of his collarbone to the other, she sighed. His hard, broad, warm chest was a thing of beauty. "I'm kind of sorry we didn't stay," she murmured, kissing the spot where a pulse beat in his neck.

His hands fisted at his sides. "Why is that?" The words were little more than a croak. Between them, his erection tented the front of his trousers.

Curling her arms around his neck, she rested her cheek on his shoulder. "I had dreams of dancing with you."

"Hold that thought," he said.

He released her and searched his jacket until he came up with his phone. Clicking icons as he concentrated, he found what he wanted. Moments later a classic love song began playing softly.

"Oh, Alex…"

He took her in his arms and teased gently. "Oh, Maria."

"I'm still not sure how this is going to work back at home," she fretted. "People will talk."

"The only thing people will say is how smart I am to have snagged you before some other guy found you first."

His hand on the bare skin of her back was firm and hot. "Have I told you how much I love this dress?"

"That's a lot of the *L* word floating around from a man who has a reputation for being buttoned up."

He stepped back and held out his arms, a sexy grin tilting the corners of his mouth. "Does *this* look like I'm buttoned up?"

"Good point." She wrapped her arms around his waist this time, swaying to the romantic melody.

Alex dipped her without warning. "Are you attached to this dress?" he asked, lifting her upright again.

Dark color slashed his cheekbones. His eyes glittered with emotions she recognized. Hunger. Need. Desperation. It might as well have been years since they had made love, so urgent was the wave of yearning that pulsed between them.

She licked her lips. "It cost a lot of money. I was going to wear it all evening."

"I'll be careful with it then," he muttered, lowering her zipper before she could do more than squeak. "And the night's still young. We might make it back to the party…"

"Fair enough." He was lying, and she didn't even care.

Slipping the narrow straps of her red fit-for-a-princess gown down her arms, he groaned when he realized she wasn't wearing a bra. Her nipples tightened as he stared at her breasts.

"I want you."

It seemed as if he had been reduced to caveman syllables, but she understood entirely.

Holding his hand as she stepped out of her bikini undies, she faced him wearing nothing but stilettos and a tentative smile. "I want you, too. All these years we've known each other I admired you, but it took me a while to realize that my feelings went way beyond that. You're a difficult man to resist."

"Then don't even try, sweetheart."

He dragged her up against him until nothing separated them but the fabric of his tux pants. The feeling was exquisite. But she had a feeling it could be even better.

Her fingers stroked his lower back. "I need you naked. Hurry."

"Whatever the lady wants."

Alex pulled away and managed the task with clumsy speed and harsh breathing.

When he was done, he tumbled them both onto the mattress, making her laugh. "I like this wild and crazy Alex," she said.

He reached for his pants that he'd tossed on the corner of the mattress. Extracting a small box, he handed it to her. "Marry me, Maria. Please."

The raw, almost awkward proposal caught her off guard and sent her heart spinning. The ring was gorgeous, a single solitaire, large enough to signal ships at sea. "It's beautiful."

He slipped it on her finger. "That's not an answer."

"Yes," she muttered, emotion making it difficult to speak. "Yes, Alex."

He stroked her from throat to belly, his warm, slightly rough touch igniting sparks everywhere he went. "Don't ever leave me again," he muttered, his expression darkly serious.

His intensity humbled her. She brushed her thumb across his lower lip. "I won't. But you know we'll still fight once in a while. We're both bullheaded."

He moved over her and into her with firm, gentle possession that made her lift against him, sighing, her legs wrapped around his waist.

Alex rested his forehead on hers. "Fighting is okay. As long as we call a truce every night."

She bit her lip when his thrust hit a certain spot. The physical sensation was second only to emotional bliss. The fact that he was here with her in this bed spoke volumes. Barely a quarter mile away, the high point of his professional career played out among the rich and famous. But Alex had made his choice.

His love humbled and elated her.

When the moment of no return neared, rational thought gave way to sensation. Heat. Tenderness. Skin to skin. Heart to heart. Damp skin to damp skin.

Her body jerked as the climax hit, sending her tumbling amid the sparks. Alex held her tightly.

His end came moments later, a raw groan of stunned pleasure.

Lying together in a tangle of arms and legs, they breathed raggedly.

As she ran her toe up the back of his calf, she grumbled. "We can do this all night, I swear. But they need you at the party, Alex. Honestly, they do."

A mighty sigh rolled through his chest. "I know."

"The sooner we get dressed, the sooner we can come back here."

"A bribe, Maria?"

"Did it work?"

He bit the side of her neck. "Yes, damn it."

She smiled, even though he couldn't see it. "I love you, Mr. Ramon."

Alex rolled out of bed and picked up her red dress, his

scowl dark as he eyed her naked body. "Put this back on before I change my mind."

"Patience is a virtue."

"Patience sucks."

Laughing, she dressed and smoothed her hair, watching covertly as Alex did the same. His nudity made him appear even more powerful than usual, every inch of him an alpha male.

At last, they were both presentable.

She held out her hands. "One last kiss before we go."

Alex backed away, his expression harried. "I can barely look at you, much less kiss you. Don't be surprised if I drag you behind a palm tree later and take you standing up."

It was hard to tell if he was kidding or not.

Re-dressed in his tux, he was masculine beauty personified. "My prince," she whispered, love squeezing her heart painfully.

His searing gaze swept her from head to toe. "I adore you, Maria. I can't wait to spend the rest of my days with you. You've taken my drab life and added sparkle."

The vulnerability in that statement, coming from a man so big and strong and definitely "unsparkly" made her want to weep. She went to him and wrapped her arms around his waist, laying her head on his shoulder. "I love you."

She felt the muscles in his throat work. He kissed the top of her head. "Let's get this over with, princess. I have plans for you. Big plans…"

Her heart was filled to bursting. Maybe fairy tales did sometimes come true. "Ditto, boss. Anything you say…"

* * * * *

CARRYING A
KING'S CHILD

KATHERINE GARBERA

This book is for my Facebook posse who are always willing to chat about hot guys, good reads and the general craziness of life.

One

Emily Fielding was shaking as she stepped off the elevator into the foyer of Rafael Montoro IV's penthouse in South Beach. The Montoros had settled in Miami, Florida, decades ago, when as the royal family of Alma, they had to flee their European island homeland because of a coup. Now the dictator who'd replaced them was dead and the parliament of Alma wanted the Montoros back.

With Rafe as king.

Great. Happy ending for everyone. Well, everyone except for Emily, the bartender who was pregnant with the soon-to-be-king's baby. Or at least that was what her gut told her. Her gut and three home pregnancy tests. She wasn't easy to convince.

She had debated not telling Rafe about the baby, but having grown up without knowing who her father was, she just couldn't do that to her own child. Sure, she'd had to lie to get up here to his very posh penthouse apartment, and she knew her timing sucked because Rafe had a lot of royal duties to attend to before his coronation, but she was still here.

Getting past security hadn't been that easy, but she'd made a few calls to friends and found that one of them had a connection to Rafe via a maid service. So she'd used Maria's pass to get into the gated community and her key to get into his building.

Sneaking around wasn't her style. Normally. But nothing about this situation was normal.

She was shaking as she stood on the Italian marble floor and let the air-conditioning dry the sweat at the small of her back. Luxurious and well appointed, the apartment was exactly the sort of place where she expected to find Rafe. His family might have fled Alma in the middle of the night, but they'd brought their dignity and their determination with them to the United States and this generation of Montoros had truly flourished.

Rafe was the CEO of Montoro Enterprises. He had been featured in *Forbes* long before the recent developments in Alma. He'd earned the wealth she saw around him, and the fact that he played as hard as he worked was something she could respect. She played hard, too.

She forced herself not to touch her stomach. Not to draw attention to the one thing that changed everything. Since she'd looked at that stick in the bathroom and realized she was going to have a baby, everything had changed.

Pretending that there was more to her visit than ensuring that her child would know who its father was would be stupid. A wealthy businessman she could have had a shot with, she thought. But not a king.

Still…

She'd seen photos of Alma. With its white sand beaches and castle that looked like something out of a dream, it was a beautiful place. The kind of place that she might have dreamed about as a little girl. A fairy-tale kingdom with a returning prince. Sounded perfect, right?

Except that Rafael Montoro IV was a playboy and they'd had a fling. She wrinkled her nose as she tried to come up with something else to call it, but a two-night stand didn't cover it, either. One weekend spent in each other's arms. She could lose herself in the memories if she wasn't careful.

Hell, she hadn't been careful. Which was precisely why she was here. Pregnant and determined. She walked down the hallway toward the sounds of Jay-Z playing in the distance. She paused in the doorway of his bedroom.

She'd had to charm her way upstairs, but no way could this wait another moment. Rafe needed to know before he left. She needed to tell him.

She felt queasy and swallowed hard.

There were right and wrong ways to deliver this news, and as appealing to her sense of outrage as it would be to throw up on his carpet, she was hoping for a little sophistication. Just a tiny bit.

After all, she'd seen pictures of his sister and jet-setting mother, though his mother wasn't really in the picture since her divorce from Rafe III. Still she was an elegant woman.

She cleared her throat.

She listened to Jay-Z and Kanye West singing about how there's no church in the wild. She almost laughed out loud as she watched Rafe stop packing his suitcase and start to rap along. She leaned against the doorjamb and admitted her anger was really fear. She wasn't mad at him. She just wanted him to be a different kind of guy so that she could have the fairy tale she wanted.

Not a castle and a title, but a man who loved her. A man who wanted to share his life with her and raise children by her side.

And no matter how fun Rafe was, his path lay somewhere else. He was duty-bound to become the constitutional monarch of Alma. She was determined to return to Key West and live out her life. She wasn't interested in being involved with a royal; besides, she'd read in the papers that the heirs would have to marry people with spotless reputations.

He was really getting into dancing around the room and rapping.

She applauded when he finished and he turned to look at her.

"What are you doing here?" he asked, shock apparent on his face.

His body was tense. She suspected he was a tiny bit embarrassed to be caught rapping. Nerves made her mouthy. She knew that. So she should just say she was sorry for using her friend's key to get into his penthouse.

But that wasn't her way.

"Hello to you, too, Your Majesty. Should I curtsy or something? I'm not sure of the rules."

"Neither am I," he admitted. "Juan Carlos doesn't

like it when I am seen doing something…well, so American but also undignified."

"Your secret is safe with me," she said. "Who is Juan Carlos?"

"Juan Carlos Salazar II, my cousin, head of the Montoro Family Trust and advocate of decorum at all times."

"He sounds like a stuffed shirt," she said. "I doubt I'd meet with his approval."

"Emily, what are you doing here? And how did you get up here? Security is usually very hard to get past."

"I have my ways."

"And they are?" he asked.

"My charm," she said.

He shook his head. "I'm going to have to warn them about feisty redheads."

"I actually used a key that I procured from your maid service."

"You've been reduced to criminal behavior. Curiouser and curiouser. Why are you here? Did you decide that you wanted to give me a proper send-off?" he asked. He strode over to her, his big body moving with an economy of motion that captivated her. The same way it had when she'd first glimpsed him in the crowded Key West bar where she worked as a bartender.

He was tall—well over six feet—and muscly, but he moved with grace and she could honestly watch him all day long.

"Why are you here, Red? You said goodbye was forever."

Goodbye.

She'd meant it when he'd left. He was a rich guy from Miami and experience had shown her they were only in Key West for one thing. Having given it to him she'd wanted to ensure she didn't give into temptation a second time.

"I did mean it."

"Help me, Red. I don't want to jump to conclusions," he said.

She chewed her lower lip. Up close she could see the flecks of green in his hazel eyes.

He was easily one of the most attractive men she'd ever seen. He'd make a killing in Hollywood with those thick eyelashes and those cheekbones. It wouldn't matter if he could act, just putting him on screen would draw the masses in.

She wished she were immune.

"I'm pregnant."

He stumbled backward and looked at her as if she'd just started speaking in tongues.

Pregnant!

He stepped back and walked over to the Bose speaker on the dresser to turn off the music. A baby. From what he knew of the tough-as-nails-bartender, he could guess she wouldn't be standing in his penthouse apartment if he wasn't the father. His first reaction was joy.

A child.

It wasn't something he'd ever thought he wanted. He hardly knew Emily so had no idea if she was here for money or something else. But knowing his child was growing inside of her stirred something primal. Something very powerful. The baby was his.

Maybe that was just because it gave him something to think about other than the recent decision that had been made for him.

He'd been dreading his trip to Alma. He was flat-tered that the country that had once driven his family out had come back to them and asked him to be the next king, but he had grown up here in Florida. He didn't want to be a stuffy royal.

He didn't want European paparazzi following him around and trying to catch him doing anything that would bring shame to his family. God, knew he worked and played hard.

"Rafe?"

"Yeah?"

"Did you hear what I said?" Emily asked.

He had. A baby. Lord knew his father hadn't been the best and as a result, Rafe had thought he'd never have kids. It wasn't as if either of his parents had set a great example. And he was still young, but damn if he wasn't feeling much older every day.

"Yeah, I did. Are you sure?" he asked at last.

She gave him a fiery look from those aqua-blue eyes of hers. He'd seen the passionate side of her nature, and he guessed he was about to witness her temper. "Would I be here if I wasn't?"

He held his hand up.

"Slow down, Red. I didn't mean are you sure it's mine. I meant…are you sure you're pregnant?"

"Damned straight."

"I get it. I had to take three at-home pregnancy tests and visit the doctor before I believed it myself. But trust me, Rafe. I'm positive I'm pregnant and that the baby is yours."

"This is a little surreal," he said.

"I know," she said, with just a hint of softening on in her tone. "Listen, I know you can't turn your back on your family and marry me and frankly, we only had one weekend together so I'd have to say no. But…I don't want this kid to grow up without any knowledge of you."

"Me either."

She glanced up, surprised.

To be honest, he sort of surprised himself. But he knew all the things not to do as a dad thanks to his own father. It didn't seem right for a kid of his to grow up without him. He wanted that. If he had a child, he wanted a chance to share the Montoro legacy…not the one newly sprung on him that came with a throne, but the one he'd carved out for himself in business. "Don't look shocked."

"You've kind of got a lot going on right now. And having a kid with me isn't going to go over well."

"Tough," he said. He still wasn't sure he wanted to be king of Alma. He and his siblings hadn't grown up with the attitude that they were royalty. They were regular American kids who'd never expected to go back to Alma. "I still make my own decisions."

"I know that," she said. She tucked a strand of hair behind her ear. "I've just been so crazy since I realized I was pregnant and alone. I didn't know what to do. You know my mom raised me by herself…"

He closed the gap between them again and pulled her into his arms. He hadn't realized she'd been raised by a single parent. To be honest, a weekend of hot sex didn't really lend itself to sharing each other's past like that. "You're not by yourself."

She looked up at him. That little pointed nose of hers was the tiniest bit red and her lip quivered as if she were struggling to keep from crying. That's when he realized how out of character it was for Emily to be unsure. The baby—his baby—had thrown her for a loop as well.

"Thanks. I just need…I have no idea. I mean, a kid. I never expected this. But we used protection."

"I didn't the third time, remember? I was out and we…"

She blushed and rested her forehead against the middle of his chest, wrapped her arms around his waist and held him. He'd thought he hated being trapped, but in Emily's arms this didn't feel constricting.

"Ugh. My mom was right."

"About what?" he asked. He looked over her head at the man in the mirror and remembered how many times he'd wanted to see some substance reflected back. Was this it? Of course it was. The baby would change things. He had no idea how or why, but he knew this moment was going to be the one that helped forge his future and the man he'd become.

"She said all it takes is a sweet-talking man and one time to get pregnant."

"I'm a sweet-talking man?" He tipped her head up with his finger under her chin.

"You can be."

"What are we going to do?" he asked at last. It was clear she'd run out of steam as soon as she entered the room. Marriage was the noble thing to do. He knew that's what Juan Carlos would suggest, but he and Emily were strangers, and tying their lives together didn't seem smart until they knew each other better.

She pushed away from him and walked over to the window. He knew the view she was afforded. This place had been hard-earned. He'd worked just as his siblings had to make Montoro Enterprises into the success it was today.

"I just wanted you to know. Beyond that I don't need anything. Someday the kid is going to ask about you—"

"Someday? I'm going to be a part of this," Rafe said.

"I don't see how. You're going to be jetting off to Alma to take the throne. My life is here. The baby's life will be here."

He rubbed the back of his neck. The timing on this sucked. But he didn't blame Emily. He'd been running when he went to Key West, afraid to admit that he was in over his head. He'd just gotten word that his family was definitely interested in returning to Alma and as the oldest son he was expected to take the throne.

He was the oldest son. He was Rafael the Fourth. He should have been in command all the time. But the truth was, he was lost.

He wanted his own life. Not one that was dictated by rules and the demands of running a country. If he'd made the decision to return to Alma on his own he might feel differently but right now he felt strong-armed into it.

But somehow in Emily's arms he'd found something.

Emily didn't really feel any better about her next steps, but now that she'd told Rafe her news she could at least start making plans. She didn't know what she expected… Well, the fairy-tale answer was that he'd profess his undying love—hey, their weekend together was pretty spectacular—then sweep her off her feet to his jet, and they'd go to Paris to celebrate their engagement.

But back in the real world, she was staring at him

and wondering if this was the last time she'd be alone with him. It didn't matter what the fantasy was or that she knew how he looked naked. They were still strangers.

Intimate strangers.

"You are looking at me in an odd way," he said.

She struggled with her blunt nature. Saying that she knew what he looked like naked but not how he'd react to their child would reveal too much insecurity. So she searched for something light. Keeping things light was the key to this.

"Well, I never heard you rap along with Jay-Z and Kanye before. Sort of changed my opinion of you."

"I'm a man of many talents," he said.

"I'd already guessed that."

"Did you?"

"Yes."

He walked over to her, all sex on a stick with that slow confident stride of his. His hazel eyes were intense, but then everything about him was. Last time they were together, she'd sensed his need to just forget who he was, but this time was different. This time he seemed to want to show her more of the man he was.

The real man.

"What else have you guessed?" he asked in a silky tone that sent shivers down her spine.

He had a great voice. She knew he had flaws, but as far as the physical, she couldn't find any. Even that tiny scar on the back of his hand didn't detract from his appeal. "That you are used to getting your own way."

"Aw, that's so easy it's almost like cheating."

"Have you figured out that I'm used to getting my own way, too?" she asked. Suddenly she didn't feel as if things were just happening to her. She was in control. Of Rafe, the baby and this entire afternoon. The pregnancy had thrown her. Brought up junk from her childhood she'd thought she'd moved on from, but now she was getting her groove back.

"Oh, I knew that from the moment I entered Shady Harry's and saw you standing behind the bar."

"Did you?" she asked. "I thought it was my Shady Harry's T-shirt that caught your attention."

The spicy scent of his aftershave brought an onslaught of memories of him moving over her. She'd buried her face in his neck. Damn, he'd smelled good. Then and now.

"Well, that and your legs. Red, you've got killer legs."

She looked down at them. Seemed kind of average to her. But she wasn't about to argue with a compliment like that.

"I like your ass," she admitted.

He winked at her, and then turned so that she could see it. He wore a slim-fitting suit that looked tailormade. Given who he was, it probably was.

He was going to be king.

She had no business flirting with him. Or even staying here a moment longer.

"Sorry."

"What?" he asked. "Why? What happened?"

She shrugged. No way was she admitting she was intimidated by his title. But that was the truth. She wasn't in control of that. No matter how much she wanted to be.

"This suit doesn't do anything for me, does it? I asked Gabe if these pants made me look fat but he said no."

She had seen pictures of his entire family in the newspaper and knew that the Gabe he referred to was Gabriel Montoro, his younger brother.

She laughed, as she knew he wanted her to. But inside something had changed. She no longer owned this afternoon. "I should go."

"Why? What happened just now?"

"I remembered that you aren't just a rich guy from Miami who came to Key West for the weekend. That your life isn't your own and I really don't have a place in it."

His expression tightened and he turned away from her. She studied him as he paced over to his bed and looked down at the expensive leather suitcase lying there. She'd interrupted his packing. He probably didn't really have time for her this afternoon.

"You said you never knew your father." With an almost aristocratic expression, he glanced over his shoulder at her. She had the feeling she was seeing the man who would be king. And she had to admit he made her a little bit nervous. Maybe it was simply the fact that she knew he was going to be a king now. But it seemed as if he was different. More regal in his bearing than he had been during their weekend together.

"Yes. I don't see what that has to do with anything."

"I did know my father and my grandfather and great-grandfather. From my birth I was named to follow in their footsteps. I've never deviated from that expectation, and to be honest, I took a certain pride in carrying on our family name and trying to set an example for my brother and sister."

"I'm getting a poor little rich boy feeling here. You have been given a lot of opportunities in your lifetime and now you have the chance to lead a nation," she said, but inside she sort of understood what he was getting at. His entire life had been scripted since birth. She understood from what she'd read in the newspapers that the Montoros may have left Alma in the middle of the night, but they hadn't left their pride behind.

"All my life I've done what is expected of me. I haven't shirked a single duty. I'm the CEO of Montoro Enterprises and now I will be king of Alma, but for this one afternoon, Red, can I be Rafe? Not a man with his future planned but your lover? Father of your baby?" he asked.

He came back over and dropped to his knees in front of her, wrapping his arms around her hips. Then he drew her closer to him and kissed her belly. "I want you to be able to speak to our baby about me with joy instead of regret."

She looked down at him as he rested his head against her body. Tunneling her fingers into his thick black hair, she understood that from this point on, when she left this penthouse they couldn't be this couple again.

She sighed, and the woman she'd always been, the one who lived by the motto Never Say Never, took over. Rafe and she might not have more than this time together. And she wanted this one last time with him.

She hadn't expected to be a mom this soon. She had made all these plans for her life and then when she'd taken those pregnancy tests it had all gone out the window.

But for this moment she could forget about tomorrow. She hoped this would be enough, but feared one more afternoon in his arms would never be enough to satisfy her.

Two

Rafe pushed aside all of his thoughts and just focused on Emily. It was amazing that she'd come to find him. She was strong enough, independent enough to keep the baby from him if she'd wanted. It embarrassed him a little, humbled him, too, that he would never have known about the baby if she hadn't shown up.

He'd been focusing on the royal legacy and managing everyone's expectations. Especially people he didn't even know and hadn't cared existed until last month. Funny how he'd gone from worrying about financial targets and managing a multinational company to worrying about a little thing like protocol.

But as long as Emily was here he could forget all that. Concentrate on being the man and not the king.

He held her tightly as he stood up, lifting her off her feet and letting her slide back down his body. She was curvy and light, his woman, and he wanted to be just her man. He carried her to the big brass bed and stood next to it, just waiting for a signal from her.

She owed him nothing.

She sighed and then lowered her head and brushed her lips over his, and something tight and frozen inside him started to melt. She kissed him not like the bold bartender she was when they'd met, but like a woman who wanted to relish her time with her lover.

They both knew without saying it that this was the last time they'd be together like this. Maybe if they'd met two years from now after he'd been on the throne and had time to figure out what being king meant, their path would have been different. But they hadn't.

They had this afternoon and nothing more.

He wanted these memories of the two of them to keep for himself as he moved into a life that was no longer his own.

He pushed his hands into her thick red hair, cradling her head as he took control of the kiss. He thrust his tongue deep into her mouth, tasted peppermint and woman. Her arms slipped lower and she stroked her hand down his back as he deepened the kiss.

Though he knew this long, wet kiss was just the beginning, he wanted to savor it. Dueling desires warred inside him as he wanted to make every touch last as long as possible. The intensity of his lust for her was almost unbearable; he needed to be hilt-deep inside her right now.

He lifted his head, rubbed his thumb along the column of her neck. Her pulse was racing and her eyes were half closed. Her creamy skin was dotted with freckles and the faint flush of desire.

He dropped nibbling kisses down her neck. She smelled of orange blossoms and sea breeze. She was like the wildest parts of Florida, and he felt as if he could hold her for only a fleeing moment and then she'd be gone. Tearing through his life like a hurricane.

He slid his hands down her back, tightening them around her waist, and lifted her off her feet again. She wrapped her legs around his waist and put her hands on his shoulders. Then she looked down into his eyes with that bright southern-Atlantic-blue gaze of hers. He felt lost. As if he were drowning in her eyes.

She nipped at his lower lip and then sucked it into her mouth and he hardened. He was going to explode if he didn't get his damned tailored pants off and bury himself in her body.

He reached for his fly but she shifted on him, rubbing her center over his erection. He shook, and the strength left his legs as he stumbled and fell back on the bed. She laughed and then thrust her tongue into his mouth again. And he gave up thinking.

She was like the wildest hurricane and all he could do was ride this storm out. She moved over him and made him remember what it felt like to be alive. The same way she had four weeks ago in Key West. She made the rest of the world pale, and everything narrowed to the two of them.

The heat flared between them and his clothes felt too constricting. He needed to be naked. Wanted her naked. Then she could climb back on his lap. He tore his mouth from hers, his breath heavy as he drew her T-shirt up and over her head and tossed it aside.

She wore the same beige lace bra she'd had on the last time they'd had sex. He traced his finger over the seam where the fabric met skin, saw the goose bumps spread from her breast over her chest and down her arms. Her nipple tightened and he leaned forward to rub his lips over it as he reached behind her back and undid the bra.

The cups loosened, but he didn't lift his head from her nipple. He continued teasing her with light brushes of his tongue over it until she reached between them and undid his tie, leaving it dangling around his neck as she went to work on his shirt buttons.

He shifted back, taking the edge of her bra between his teeth and pulling it away. She laughed, a deep, husky sound he remembered so well. And he got even harder. He had thought there was no way he could want her more, but he'd been wrong.

She pushed the fabric of his shirt open and peeled it down his arms, but she hadn't undone his cuffs so his own shirt bound him. His hands were trapped.

"Undo my hands."

"Not yet, Rafe. Right now, I'm in charge," she said. She scraped her fingernail down the side of his jaw to his neck and then over his pectorals. He sat there craving more of her touch, but damned if he was going to ask her for it. Control and power were two things he always maintained. But with Emily it was as if they'd flown out the window.

She took what she wanted, and though he'd never admit it out loud, he didn't want to stop her. It felt good to just let go.

Flexing her fingers, she dug her nails into his chest and then shifted forward so that the long strands of her hair brushed against him. He shuddered with need, turning his head to try to catch her mouth with his, but she just laughed again and shifted back on his thighs, looking down at him with those eyes that were full of mysteries he knew he'd never really understand.

She drew one finger down the center of his chest, following the path of the light dusting of hair. She swirled her finger around his belly button in tiny circles that made everything inside him contract.

She stroked his erection through the fabric of his pants, and he canted his hips.

She rocked against him and smiled when he moaned her name. Wrapping her arms around his shoulders, she caught the lobe of his ear between her teeth and bit it lightly before whispering all the things she was going to do him. He felt his control slipping with each thrust of her tongue as she flicked it into his ear and then shifted backward on his thighs to reach between them, stroking his length through his pants again.

Cursing, he tried to reach for her but his bound arms wouldn't let him. She rotated her shoulders and rubbed her nipples against his chest. She closed her eyes as she undulated against him, and this time he pulled his arms forward with all of his strength and heard the tear of fabric. She opened her eyes and then started laughing.

He grabbed her waist and rolled to his side, pulling her with him. He rolled over top of her, carefully keeping his weight on his elbows and knees so she wasn't crushed under him. He took both of her hands in his and stretched them high over her head and then rubbed his chest over hers and heard her moan.

Damn, she felt good. Better than he'd remembered her feeling, and that said a lot because he still had erotic dreams of their weekend together.

He lowered his head and sucked her nipple into his

mouth, holding both of her wrists above her head with one of his hands. He reached lower between their bodies and undid her jeans, pushing them down so that he could cup her in his hand. He rubbed her mound, and then traced the seam of her panties. Her legs scissored underneath his and he shifted until he lay between them. He let go of her wrists as he slowly kissed his way down her body.

She was covered in freckles; up close he could see that they were all different sizes. He flicked his tongue over each of them as he moved lower and lower until he found her belly button ring. The small loop had a starfish dangling from it. He tongued it and traced the circumference of her belly button.

He moved lower, catching the top of her bikini panties with the tip of his finger and drawing them slowly down. She shifted her hips and he pushed her jeans and panties down to her knees. She kicked them the rest of the way off.

He traced the pattern of freckles from her thigh to her knee, circling her kneecap and the small scar there before caressing his way back up the inside of her thighs. He felt the humid warmth of her body and traced her feminine core with his fingertip. She shifted on the bed, her hands reaching for him, but it was his turn to tease her. Plus if she touched him, he feared his control would splinter into a million pieces and this would be over too quickly.

He parted her folds and then leaned down to taste her. He closed his eyes as he sucked her intimate flesh, causing her to draw her legs closer around him and her hands to fall to the back of his head. She gripped his hair as her hips lifted upward toward his mouth and his tongue.

She was addicting. He couldn't get enough of her. He pushed one finger into her body and heard her call his name. She was wet and ready for him. He fumbled, trying to free himself from his trousers. He lifted his head, looked up at her and saw that she was watching him. Her eyes were filled with passion and desire.

He stood up, shoved his pants and underwear off in a move that definitely couldn't be called graceful, and then he lowered himself on top of her. He slowly used his chest and body to caress hers as he moved over her. She shifted her legs so that her thighs were on either side of his and he moved his hips forward, felt the tip of his erection at the opening of her body. He hesitated. This time was different from their weekend in Key West, but the passion in her eyes was the same.

Slowly he entered her, trying to make it last because she felt so damned good. She gripped his rock-hard flesh as he entered her and drove himself all the way home and then forced himself to stay still once he was fully seated in her body.

Her hands were on his shoulders, running up and down his back and then reaching lower to cup his butt and try to get him to move. But he needed a moment before he did that. A moment to make sure that she was with him. He lowered his head to her neck, and then bit her lightly before moving lower, kissing the full globes of her breasts.

She tightened as she arched underneath him. She looked up at him and whispered dark, sexual words that made his control disappear along with his will-power, and he found himself thrusting deeper into her body. Driving toward his climax and carrying her along with him.

He pushed her legs higher, putting her feet on his shoulders so he could go deeper, and pounded into her faster and faster until he heard her calling out his name and he spilled himself inside her. He thrust into her three more times before he let go of her legs and fell forward, bracing himself on his arms. He kissed the pert pink nipple on her left breast as he rested his head on her shoulder and tried to catch his breath.

He got up and left her for a few moments to wash up and then came back and lay down next to her on the bed. He was aware of the time and knew he should already be at the private airport and getting on his family's jet so he could travel with them to Alma, but he couldn't make himself leave.

He knew that this wasn't love. He wasn't going to lie to her or himself. But she was pregnant with his child and this fired him with an enthusiasm he just couldn't muster when he thought of being king. He didn't want the throne, but his father, who couldn't inherit it because he'd never had his marriage annulled after divorcing Rafe's mother, had been very clear that he thought Rafe needed to do his duty.

He stroked his hand down Emily's arm. She had turned on her side and had her head on his shoulder.

"What are you thinking?"

"That I'm glad you came here today. Did you ever think of not telling me?" he asked.

He suspected he knew the answer, but wanted to hear it from her.

"No. It wasn't easy to track you down—you're pretty secretive about this penthouse bachelor pad, aren't you?

But Harry has lots of friends who have connections. It only took him six hours to find you."

"Harry scares me," Rafe admitted. The owner of Shady Harry's bar had been fun and gregarious when Rafe had been partying and buying rounds for the entire place. But the next morning when he'd spotted the older man as he'd left Emily's cottage, Harry had given him a look that said to watch his back. "What's he to you?"

"He and my mom dated for a while," Emily said. "He's sort of like my stepdad. Why?"

"I have a feeling if I show up in Key West he's going to be waiting with a shotgun."

"You're not going to Key West, you're going to Alma. I've seen pictures. It's really beautiful," she said.

Not as beautiful as she was, Rafe thought. He leaned up on his elbow, put his hand flat on her stomach and realized he couldn't control this any more than he could say no to the people in Alma who'd asked his family to come back and rule the country.

"It is. They've had a rough time since the revolution and I guess…I have to go," he said.

"I know. I told you I wasn't here to ask you to stay. I just needed you to know."

"Why?"

"I didn't know my dad. My mom has never mentioned his name to me. I asked her one time about him and she started crying. I want more than that for our baby. It's not that I had a deprived childhood, but I always wonder. I have this emptiness inside me that nothing can fill. It's that empty spot where everyone else has a dad."

He was humbled by her explanation. He knew he wanted to be more than a name and a face to their kid, though. "We need to figure this out."

There was a knock on the bedroom door.

"Rafael? Are you in here? Your father is in a car waiting downstairs and if you're not down in ten minutes he's coming up here and getting you." It was his personal assistant, Jose.

Jose was his right-hand man at Montoro Enterprises and at home. He took care of all the details.

"I have company," Rafe said. But Emily was more than just company. She was his lover. The mother of his unborn child.

"I am aware of that," Jose said.

"Tell Father I'll be down when I'm down," Rafe said.

But the mood was broken and Emily was getting up and putting her clothes on. She had her jeans on and buttoned, but he stopped her before she put her T-shirt on. He pulled her into his arms. It seemed the sort of gesture that would reassure her, but since he was already thinking of everything he had to do, it felt hollow. He knew she noticed it, too, when she pulled back and shook her head.

The mantle of being a Montoro was tightening around him. "I—"

"Don't. No excuses and definitely no lies," she said. She reached into her back pocket and pulled out a business card for Shady Harry's; he turned it over and saw she'd written her name and number on the back. "If you want to know about our child, contact me."

"I do. I will," he said.

She smiled up at him. "I know that the next few weeks are going to be crazy for you, so no pressure."

She pulled her shirt on and then tucked her underwear into her purse and started for the door. He watched her walk out. Part of him wanted to run after her and make her stay so he could talk her into trying a relationship or maybe even marriage. Another part wanted to scoop her up and run away with her to some Pacific island where no one would know their names, far enough away from his family and everyone they knew.

But Emily was a brave sort of woman, and running had never been his style, either, so he had no choice but to get dressed and head down to the car.

His father didn't speak to him the entire way to the airport. Rafael III had wanted the throne enough to try to convince his ex-wife to come back, but Rafe's mother wasn't interested in doing anything to help out her former husband. To say the two of them had a strained relationship was putting it mildly.

They were a prime example of how getting married to the wrong person didn't make for a happy family. Rafe had the childhood to prove it.

During the ride, his cousin Juan Carlos spoke too much. Telling him what was expected of the next king of Alma.

Juan Carlos had been orphaned and seemed to be fixated on the monarchy as a way of proving to himself and the rest of the family that he could carry on his parents' legacy. Perhaps if Rafe's parents hadn't divorced and been horrible to each other, he'd have felt the same way about the family honor.

Rafe freely admitted to himself that if Emily's pregnancy became public knowledge it would create a scandal that would make protecting that legacy even more difficult. But Rafe tuned Juan Carlos out and tried to figure out what he expected of himself as a man.

Three

Key West was a tourist town and there was no getting around that. The atmosphere was laid back and everyone had a sort of hungover look. There was something about being on the edge of the ocean that inspired indulgence in sun, sand and drinks.

Emily sat on the front porch of her flamingo-pink and white cottage with her feet propped on the railing, desperately needing to absorb that laid-back attitude. She'd left Miami and Rafe behind. She'd done what she'd set out to do, namely tell him he was going to be a father. That had gone well—differently than she'd expected, but the end result was the same. She was back here.

Alone.

"Em. Your mom asked me stop by," Harry said as he walked around the side of the house.

He was tall, at least six five, and wore middle age well. His reddish-blond hair had thinned a little but was still thick enough, and he wore it cut short in a military style. His beard was equal parts red, blond and gray, and he had an easy smile. He was the closest thing she had to a dad. So she was glad to see him.

"Why?" Emily asked. Though she knew why her mom had sent Harry. If anyone could make her forget her troubles it was the jovial bar owner.

"She thought you might need some company. She's on her way back to port but won't be here until tonight."

Emily sighed. "I don't really want any company."

"Figured you might say that, so I brought you a cup of decaf and a blueberry bagel. We can both sit here and eat and pretend we're alone."

Decaf.

Seemed like a little thing, but she always drank full-on caffeine. Now she knew that her mom had spilled the beans about her being preggers. Harry handed her a bakery bag from Key Koffee with the bagel and the coffee.

"You know?"

"I know. It was that slick guy from South Beach, right?"

She tipped her head back and closed her eyes. "He's not that slick."

Harry laughed. "They never are. Talk to me, kiddo. Do I need to take my .45 and head to Miami?"

She opened her eyes and lifted her head. "You would have made a really good dad," she said, smiling at him.

"I think I have been to you," he reminded her.

"You have. But no to the .45. Besides, you'd have to fly to Europe to find him."

Harry took a bite out of his everything bagel and settled down on the top step, turning sideways with his back against the railing to face her.

"Europe? He seemed American to me," Harry said.

"He's Rafael Montoro IV. Part of…I'm not sure what to call him. But his family was royalty in a tiny Mediterranean country called Alma. They were kicked out decades ago but now they want them back. He's the oldest son and heir apparent to the newly restored monarchy."

"Complicates things, doesn't it?" Harry said.

"You have no idea," she said. "But I didn't expect him to do anything when I gave him the news. You know?"

Harry took a sip of his coffee and then gave her one of those wise looks of his that she hated. He knew when she was lying, especially to herself.

"Okay, fine, I wanted him to be, like, we'll do this together. Instead, I got…he was sweet but clearly torn. He can't let his family down. And he and I only had one weekend together, Harry."

"Sometimes that's all it takes," he said.

"It wasn't enough for the guy who fathered me," she said. "Please don't tell Mom I said that. But really, that complicates everything. I've always thought I was okay with the fact that I don't know who he was, but this baby…" She put her hands on her stomach. "It's making me realize I'm not."

Harry didn't say anything. And after a few minutes Emily looked away from him and back to the foot traffic on the street near her house. What could he say? He was her substitute dad who'd stepped up when he didn't have to. Harry must have thought that she was making a mess where there didn't need to be one.

"I get it, kiddo. It's hard to not want the best for your baby. We all do that," he said. "Try to fix the problems in our past so that our kids don't have to experience them."

"Did you do that for Rita and Danny?" she asked. Harry had two kids who were both more than fifteen years older than her and lived in Chicago. They came down for two weeks each spring to visit Harry.

"I tried. But I ended up making my own mistakes and they have done the same. It's all a part of being human," he said.

"I'm getting Zen Harry this morning," she said. But his positive attitude helped take her mind off Rafe and the sadness she'd been feeling.

It wasn't that she'd expected anything else from him, but that she'd wanted something more. She shook her head as she realized that what she'd wanted was to be wanted.

For him to want to stay with her.

It was unrealistic, but a girl could dream.

"Well, I do have all this wonderful advice and no one to share it with," Harry said with a wink. "You'll be okay, kiddo. You'll make decisions and choices and some of them are going to be fabulous and others you're going to regret. But I do know one thing."

"What's that?" she asked.

"You're going to love that baby of yours, and in the end that's all that really matters."

"You think so?"

"I do. Your own mom did that for you. Look how you turned out," he said.

"Not bad," she admitted. She liked her life. She could have followed her mom into a similar career—

she was a marine biologist—but Emily liked being on the land and not out at sea. She had a degree in hotel and restaurant management and one day hoped to open her own place. She knew she had a good life, but a part of her still missed Rafe.

Another part of her knew she just missed the idea of Rafe. So far every time they'd been together they'd ended up in bed. It wasn't as if he was even a friend.

She wanted that picture-perfect family that she kept in her head. She wanted that for this baby she was carrying. She didn't want her child to have the piecemeal family that she did. No matter that she loved her mom and Harry fiercely. For her child she wanted more.

And being the bastard of a European king probably wasn't what her child would want. She was going to have to be very protective. Raise the baby to know its own strength and place in the world.

She noticed Harry watching her, realized she wasn't alone and that made the loneliness she felt when she thought of Rafe a little less painful.

Alma was breathtakingly beautiful. The island was surrounded by sparkling blue seas and old world charm seemed to imbue every building. They'd landed at a private air field and were driving to the royal palace in the urban capital of Del Sol.

Rafe had heard there was a lively nightclub scene and before Emily's visit had sort of thought of checking it out. But now that he had the dual mantle of monarchy and fatherhood hanging over him, he figured he should rethink that.

Del Sol was even more striking than the black and white photos he'd seen in the albums his *tia* Isabella kept. While there were modern buildings dotted throughout the city many of the old buildings remained. Tia Isabella had been a young woman when she'd been forced to flee Alma with the rest of their family. When Rafe and his siblings and cousin had been growing up they'd been entertained by her stories. Tia Isabella had spent a lot of time talking about the old days and what it had been like to grow up on Alma. But Rafe thought he understood why his grandfather hadn't talked that much about it. Rafe would have been sad to leave this homeland, too.

As the royal motorcade made its way into Del Sol, Alma's capital, people on the streets craned their necks to get a glimpse of the Montoros. Rafe was used to a certain level of fame and notoriety in Miami, but not this. There he was one of the jet-set Montoros. The young generation who worked hard and played harder.

Here he was the future monarch. He'd be the face of Alma to the world. And while his ego was sort of jazzed about that, another part of him wasn't.

"Maybe you should put the window down and do that princess wave," his sister Bella said with a sparkle in her blue eyes. Their father and the rest of their party were in a separate vehicle.

"Princess wave? That's more your cup of tea," he said. "Maybe I'll throw up the peace sign."

She giggled. He'd always been close to his little sister, and making her laugh helped him to relax.

Bella looked like a fairy-tale princess with her pretty blond hair. Not anything like Emily. He wondered what Emily would think of Alma. It was an island not that unlike her hometown of Key West, but the laid-back attitude in the Keys was a world away from this charming European nation.

For a country that had been ruled by a dictator for decades, the people in the streets seemed happy and prosperous and the buildings were clean and well-maintained. Rafe didn't see any signs of financial ruin. But economic danger lurked whenever there was a change of regime. And if there was one thing he was good at, it was making money.

But would the government here listen to him?

To be honest he wasn't the kind of person to negotiate for what he wanted. That was one of the reasons Montoro Enterprises had thrived under his leadership. He made bold decisions. Sometimes they didn't pay off, but most of the time they did.

"You okay?" Bella asked.

He started to shrug it off. There was no way he was going to mention Emily or the fact that she was pregnant to his sister. Not until he had a chance to figure it out for himself. But the family stuff was also getting to him, especially how Juan Carlos was going really crazy about protocol and proper image and all that.

"This return to Alma is throwing me," he admitted to her.

"How?" she asked. "You've always handled whatever the family has dished out. This will be no different. Pretend you're the CEO of the country."

As if. Being the king was a "name only" position. No power. Maybe that was why he hesitated to fully embrace it. He was a man of action. Not a figurehead.

"Good suggestion," he said, glancing out the window as they approached the castle. Surrounded by glittering blue water on three sides, it rose from the land like a sand castle at the beach. He groaned.

"What?"

"I was hoping the castle would be in disrepair."

"Why?"

"So I could hate it."

Bella laughed again. "I love it. It's everything I thought it would be," she said.

"What if there's not a hopping club scene? Will you still love it then?" he asked. Bella liked to party. Hell, they all did. They hadn't been raised to assume the throne. They were all more likely to show up in the tabloids in a compromising position than on the society pages at a formal tea. The closer he got to the throne the less sure he was that he wanted to be there.

He felt Bella's hand on his shoulder. "You're going to be fine. I think you'll make a great king."

"Why? I'm not sure at all."

"You've been a great big brother and always ensured our family's place in business and in society."

"Business is easy. I understand that world," Rafe countered.

"I never thought the day would come when you'd admit that you aren't sure of yourself," she said, taking her phone from her handbag.

"What are you doing?"

"Texting Gabe that you have feet of clay."

"He already knows that."

"We all do," Bella said. "Why are you acting like you are just figuring it out?"

"I'm going to be a king, Bella. It's making me nutty," he said.

"You weren't as thrown by it a week ago," she said.

"What happened yesterday to make you delay your flight?"

Nothing.

Everything.

Something that could change the man he was. If he let it.

"Business. Running Montoro Enterprises does take a lot of time," he said.

The car pulled to a stop and an attendant in full livery came to open the door for them. Bella climbed out first but looked back at Rafe.

"Lying to me is one thing. You can keep your secrets if you want to," she said. "But I hope you aren't lying to yourself."

He followed her out of the car, and the warm Mediterranean air swept around him. She had a point. He knew in his gut that this didn't feel right. He should be in Miami with Emily. He missed her.

The porte-cochere led to an inner brick-lined courtyard. There was a fountain underneath a statue of Rafe's great-grandfather Rafael I. He was surprised it hadn't been torn down when the dictator had taken over. Bella stopped walking and spun around on her heel, taking in the beauty of the palace.

For the first time he felt a sense of his royal lineage settling over him. If their family hadn't been forced to flee he would have grown up in this palace. His memories would be of this place that smelled wonderfully of jasmine and lavender. Where was the scent coming from?

His father came up beside him and put his hand on his shoulder not saying a word. Something passed between them. An emotion that Rafe didn't want to define. But Alma became real to him. In a way that it hadn't been before. In Miami it had been easy to say he wasn't sure if he wanted to be king but seeing this palace—he felt the history. And he sort of understood Juan Carlos's perspective for once. Rafe didn't want to let down their family line.

If Alma wanted the Montoros back on the throne than Rafe would have to put aside the feelings he felt stirring for Emily and figure out how to be their king.

That surprised him. He hadn't expected to feel this torn. He was isolated from the rest of his family who seemed to think this return to royalty was just the thing they needed. They were all caught up in being back in the homeland. But as much as he felt swept up in the majesty of their return to Alma he knew he was still trying to figure out where home really was.

Emily worked the closing shift at Harry's and walked home at 2:00 a.m. Key West wasn't like the mean streets of Miami, but she moved quickly and kept her eyes open for danger. It was something she'd teach her kid.

She was starting to find her bearings with this pregnancy more and more as each day passed. Being a mom was going to take some getting used to, but as her own mom had said, she had nine months to make the adjustment.

Her cell phone vibrated in the pocket of her jeans and she reached back to pull it out. Glancing at the screen, she saw it was an international call. She only knew one person who was traveling internationally right now. She did some quick math and figured out that it was early morning in Alma.

"Hello?"

"Hey, Red. Figured you'd be getting off work. Please tell me I didn't wake you." Sure enough, it was Rafe.

"You'd think you'd be more careful about disturbing a pregnant woman's rest," she teased. She didn't want to admit it but she'd missed him. Three days. That was all it had been since she'd seen him, but it had felt like a lifetime. His voice was deep and resonated in her ear, making her feel warm all over.

"Well, maybe I did call the bar earlier to determine if you were working tonight," he admitted.

That sounded like Rafe. He was a man who left little to chance. "What can I do for you?"

"How are you feeling?" he asked. "How's Florida?"

"I'm feeling fine," she said. "I have had a little bit of morning sickness, and it's not just limited to mornings. I've been getting sick midafternoon."

She saw her house at the end of the lane and got her keys out. She'd left the porch lights on and it looked so welcoming. The only thing that would be better was if Rafe was waiting for her. And to be honest, as he talked to her on the phone, it was almost as if he was there with her.

"Makes sense since that's when you wake up," he said. "Is there anything you can do to help that?"

"No," she said. "It's not too bad. How's Alma?"

"Nice. You'd like it. It's all sand and sea for as far as the eye can see and quaint little villages. Not as laid back as Key West but still nice."

"Any places to go paddleboarding?"

"Not yet. Why, do you think you'd move here and start a business?" he asked.

It was the closest he'd come to suggesting that she

be near him in the future, and she felt numb even contemplating it. She had her own plans to open a restaurant around the corner from Harry's. Not to be Rafe's hidden mistress in some far-off European country.

"Not at all. I've got a place picked out for my future restaurant," she said.

"Is that what you want to do?"

Once again she realized how little they actually knew of each other's lives.

"Well, I can't be a bartender forever."

"I guess not. Tell me about your dreams," he said.

She thought she heard the sound of footsteps on a tiled floor on his end. "Where are you?"

"Not ready to share that much with me?" he asked, countering her evasion.

In a way she wished they were playing a game. It would make everything easier. She could concentrate on winning and not really have to think about the emotions. But the truth was she was tired and still a little unsure of what she was doing. Sure, just hearing Rafe's voice made her feel not so alone. But she didn't want to allow herself to become dependent on him.

Not to turn her life into one big sob story, but usually when she started to feel comfortable with someone they left. It wasn't that they abandoned her, just moved on and left her to her independent self. Even her mom and Harry. And she didn't want that with Rafe.

"Nope. I want to hear about Alma. I read a little online yesterday. Seems like the change of regime is going to have a big impact on the economy. I know you are good at making money. Is that why they chose you and your family to come back and lead the country?" she asked.

"Our family ruled the country before the coup that installed the late dictator, Tantaberra. That's why we were chosen. But my parents are divorced so Dad, who would be next in line, can't assume the throne. They want someone with the right pedigree and the right reputation."

"Um…I'm guessing if they found out about me that could put a wrench in things."

"Possibly. I'm not going to deny you exist, Emily."

"Really?"

"Yes. Would I be on the phone with you if I didn't care?" he asked.

"I don't know," she said honestly. "We're strangers."

"Who are about to be parents to a baby," he said. "Let's get to know each other. And while we have half the world between us maybe I can talk to you without being distracted by your body and that sexy way you tilt your head to the side. You always make me forget everything except wanting to get you naked."

Her breath caught as she sank down into the big armchair where Rafe had sat the one time he'd been to her place. They'd made love in the chair and she felt closer to him now. She tucked her leg up underneath her and let those memories wash over her.

"Red? You still there?"

"Yes. Dammit, now you've got me thinking about you naked."

"Good. My evil plan worked," he said. "Tell me something about yourself."

"What?"

"Anything. I want to know the woman who's going to be the mother of my child."

She thought about her life. It was ordinary: nothing

too tragic, nothing too exciting. But it was hers. "When I was six I thought if I spent enough time in the ocean I'd turn into a mermaid. My mom's a marine biologist and we were living on her research vessel, *The Sea Spirit*. She made me a bikini top out of shells and sent me off every day to swim."

"I'm glad you didn't turn into a mermaid," he said with a quiet laugh.

They talked on the phone until Emily started drifting to sleep. She knew she should hang up, but she didn't want to break the connection. Didn't want to wake up without Rafe.

"Red?"

"Yes?"

"I wish I was there to tuck you into bed," he said.

"Me, too," she admitted. Then she opened her eyes as she realized that she was starting to need him.

"Good night, Rafe," she said, hanging up the phone before she could do anything stupid like ask him what he'd wanted to be as a boy. Or to come back to Key West.

Four

Rafe secluded himself from the rest of the family in the office area of the suite of rooms he'd been given. The deal he'd struck for Montoro Enterprises to ship Alma's oil was taking a lot of his time.

Alma was a major oil producing country to the north of Spain. Montoro Enterprises would be shipping the oil to its customers in North and South America where the bulk of their business interests were. It made good business sense but he also wanted it because he'd get a chance to explore the country of his ancestors. When he'd first done the deal he'd anticipated his father becoming King not himself.

Plus truth be told, he'd been so focused on work because he was avoiding his family and the coterie of diplomats who seemed to be lurking whenever he stepped out of his suite. He didn't want to talk about his coronation or about the business of running the government. Yet.

But sitting around and hiding out went against the grain, so he'd been working nonstop. He hadn't shaved in the three days, and Mozart had replaced Jay-Z and Kanye on the stereo because no one would ever be tempted to stop working and rap to Mozart. He hadn't even contacted Emily, though he'd thought of her night and day.

She was an obsession. He knew that. He had the feeling that if he were in Miami maybe it wouldn't be as fierce, but he was far away from her and thinking of her was nice and comforting in the midst of this storm that was brewing around him.

He banged his head on the desk.

"I can see I'm interrupting," Gabe said as he entered without knocking.

"I'm working."

"Yeah, I noticed," Gabe said, nodding toward the empty cans of Red Bull that littered the desk and the floor. He walked to the window and pulled back the drapes.

Rafe blinked against the glare of the sunlight. "What time is it?"

"Four in the afternoon. You're expected for dinner tonight and if you don't show up Juan Carlos is going to have a stroke. I know he's been a pain lately with all this royal protocol, but we don't want our cousin to have a stroke, do we?"

Rafe shook his head. "No." He scrubbed his hands over his face. His eyes felt gritty and the stubble on his jaw felt rough. He was a mess. Truly. "This sucks."

Gabe laughed that wicked, low laugh that Rafe had

heard women found irresistible. He just found it annoying.

"Yeah, it does. Not so cool being the older brother now, is it?"

Not at all. "I should walk away…that would leave you holding the bag."

A fleeting glimpse of panic ran across his brother's face. "Dad would disown you. I'm pretty sure the board would fire you from Montoro Enterprises. Then what would you do?"

Run away to Key West.

Seemed simple enough, but to be fair he wasn't sure what type of reception he'd receive if he just showed up on Emily's doorstep.

"I think I'm too American to want to be a royal, you know? Maybe Dad still wants it, but it feels weird to me. I don't want to be called 'Your Majesty' or 'Your Highness.'"

Rafe watched his younger brother. If there were the slightest sign that Gabe was interested in being king, Rafe would just walk away and let his brother have it. But Gabe rubbed the back of his neck as he paced over to the window. "Me neither."

"Then I guess I'd better stop acting like a jerk and get out there," Rafe said. "What's the plan?"

"Dinner with some supporters. And a family who'd love for you to meet their daughter," Gabe said with a wry smile.

Rafe shook his head. He'd do his duty to his family, but he was already involved with a redhead who wouldn't take kindly to him catting around. He was getting to know her, starting a relationship with the woman who was going to be the mother of his child.

What if she didn't feel possessive toward him the way he did toward her? And he did feel possessive. Emily was his. "I'm not interested."

"Are you interested in someone else?"

"It's complicated, Gabe."

"I never thought I'd see the day when you said that. Is she special?"

"She could be," Rafe said. Or at least that was what his gut was saying. The rest of him wasn't too sure.

Once his brother left and Rafe had wrapped up what he was working on for the day, he started getting ready for the state dinner. When he got out of the shower, he saw that he had a text message from Emily.

It's official. Just got word back from the doctor's office. I'm due in January.

Would he be able to get back to the States in January?

Being with Emily would mean giving up the monarchy… and possibly his job, depending on how much it pissed off his family. Montoro Enterprises and Alma were now all linked together. Could he walk away from one without walking away from them all?

But what kind of man walked away from his own child?

Not one that Rafe wanted to be. He knew that but as he'd said to Gabe earlier, it was complicated.

He braced his hands on the bathroom counter and looked into his own hazel eyes searching for answers or a solution. But there was nothing there.

And that really pissed him off. He needed to take control of his personal life the way he did the boardroom. No more doing what everyone else wanted unless it fit with his own inner moral compass.

Except that he'd been a playboy for so long he wasn't too sure he had one. Everyone had one, right? Then shouldn't the answer be clearer than this?

When he was finished shaving, he took the towel off his hips and tossed it at his image in the mirror before he walked into the bedroom to dress.

He hit the remote for his sound system and switched from Mozart to "The Man" by Aloe Blacc . He stopped in his tracks. Right now it seemed as if everyone had a piece of him and the man Rafe had always wanted to be had been lost.

He knew what he had to do. No use pretending he was going to do anything else. It wasn't that he thought the path would be easy, but then when had he ever taken the easy path? It was simply that spending time with his siblings made him realize that family was important to him.

His mind made up, he grabbed his phone and began typing, hitting Send before he could have second thoughts.

I'll be there. When is your next appointment? I'd like to go with you if I can.

He owed it to himself and to his child to at least see if he could be a real partner to Emily. And be a real part of the baby's life.

Really? Okay. If you do this then I don't want you making promises you can't keep.

That right there showed him how little she knew of him. Hell, what did he know about her? He knew how she looked in his arms. He knew that she had wanted to be a mermaid when she was little. He smiled at that one. He knew she was having his baby.

I'm a man of my word, Red. I'll be there.

Two days later Emily woke up to a beautiful sunny morning. Since it was her day off, she decided to take her paddleboard and head to a quiet cove on Geiger Key where there weren't many tourists. She'd been too much in her head since she'd found out she was pregnant and needed to forget for a few hours.

After she'd had her daily bout of morning sickness, she took the prenatal vitamins the doctor had prescribed and then got dressed in her usual bikini. She stood in front of the full-length mirror mounted on the back of her walk-in closet door and looked at her body. No signs of her pregnancy were visible. In fact, she looked a little bit thinner than she had before. Her boobs were getting a little larger, though.

She'd always sort of been…well, smallish, but now she was actually filling out the top. Not bad, she thought. She patted her stomach and shook her head. She definitely needed today for herself.

Someone knocked on her front door. She grabbed her board shorts, putting them as she went to answer it.

There was a man in a suit waiting there.

"Hello, Ms. Fielding. I have a package for you from Rafael Montoro. He asked me to deliver it to you personally."

She took the package from him. "You look a little fancy for a deliveryman."

"I'm Jose, his assistant at Montoro Enterprises," Jose said.

"That explains the suit," she said.

She wanted to ask more questions, debated it for a moment, and then decided to heck with looking cool. "So when will he be back in the US?"

"I'm not at liberty to say."

"Really? He sent you here but you can't tell me that?" she asked. "I know it's your job to protect his privacy, it's just that he said…never mind. Thank you for getting up early to deliver this. Are you driving back to Miami?"

"Nah. I took the company chopper."

Of course he did. Men like Rafe—and his assistant, for that matter—didn't drive almost four hours to Key West like other mere mortals.

"Safe travels," she said, turning around to go back inside.

What had he sent her?

"Ms. Fielding?"

She glanced over her shoulder at Jose. "He's hoping to be back next week but that all depends on the people in Alma."

She smiled at him. "Thank you."

"Don't rat me out," he said with a wink, and then left.

His assistant was nice. She wondered if that was a reflection of Rafe as a boss, but she knew no matter who worked for him he might still be a jerk at work. "Jose!"

"Yes."

"What kind of man is Rafe to work for?"

"Demanding. He won't settle for a job half done. But he's also very generous when a project is over. He's a good man," he said.

"Thanks," she said.

He walked away and she thought about it. A good man. Was she a good woman? Hell, yes, she was. She sat down on what she was now calling the Rafe chair and opened the package. When she pulled back the sides of the cardboard box there was a pretty paper inside with the words *Handcrafted in Alma* printed on it in scrolling letters.

She carefully pulled the sides of the paper back to reveal something in Bubble Wrap. Lifting it from the box, she carefully removed the Bubble Wrap and caught her breath as she saw that it contained a stained glass mermaid that looked a lot like her.

She traced her finger over the details and tried to downplay the importance of the gift. But she couldn't avoid the fact that he'd taken her childhood dream and given it to her.

She took a picture and then attached it to the text message.

She's even prettier than I imagined a mermaid could be. Thank you for this wonderful gift.

The response was almost instantaneous.

I'm glad you like it. I'm just coming out of a meeting. Do you have time to chat with me?

She thought about the paddleboarding she'd planned

for the day, but as her mom always said, the ocean wasn't going anywhere. Plus a part of her realized she'd been running away from her house and her situation so she didn't have to deal with it on her own. Talking to Rafe was a solution. She didn't want it to be, because she'd always prided herself on being independent and handling anything life threw at her. But she knew she wanted him by her side.

Yes. I can talk.

Good. I'll call in a few minutes.

She paced around her living room and ended up back in the kitchen. She took the stained glass mermaid and held her up to the back window, where she got the light from the morning sun, and realized she'd fit perfectly there.

She jotted down the supplies she'd need and then made herself a mango and passion fruit smoothie. By the time she was finished with it, he still hadn't called.

He was a man who would be king, she thought. Obviously his time wasn't his own. She waited another thirty minutes before she turned the ringer off on her phone, got into her car and drove to Geiger Key.

She tried to shake it off. She'd known that the only one she could count on was herself, but it stung just the tiniest bit that he hadn't messaged her back to say he'd been delayed.

Rafe was in a bad mood by the time he escaped the royal palace in Del Sol and drove down the winding coastal road to his family's beach compound in Playa del Onda. He'd spent the entire day either in meetings or being cornered by Dita Gomez.

Dita was the oldest daughter of one of the best families in Alma. Her parents were part of the newly forming royal court and they were hoping for a royal match. Dita was a lovely lady, no doubt, but as his man Kanye might say, she was a gold digger. Rafe wasn't entirely sure how she had access to his schedule but everywhere he went, she was there.

He'd been so busy dealing with getting rid of Dita that he hadn't been able to call Emily. And he knew her well enough to know that giving the excuse that he'd been dodging the advances of a beautiful blonde wasn't going to go over well.

Wanting to punch something, he shoved his hands in his hair. This was too restricting. He hadn't felt a connection to Alma or to the people the way that Bella seemed to. While he was busy plotting ways to get back to Miami early, she was happy to stay for a little while longer.

He wondered if something had happened to make Bella so happy with the land that time forgot. He made a mental note to talk to her, but he had no idea when he'd get a chance. His schedule was grueling.

He glanced at his watch; it had been seven hours since he said he'd call Emily. That meant it was probably midafternoon in Key West. He dialed her number and waited. It rang twice before he got a text message that had obviously been tailored for him saying she didn't want to talk to His Majesty.

First he was angry. Screw her. He was doing his best to keep all the balls in the air. Family, business, kingdom. He'd expect her to understand.

Then he remembered what she'd said to him a few days ago. *Don't make promises he couldn't keep.*

So he dialed her number again and this time she answered. But she didn't say anything—all he heard was the rush of wind and the faint sound of music in the background.

"Don't hang up. I'm sorry. My days over here are insane and I ended up being cornered by someone from the royal court. This is the first time I've been alone since I texted you."

After an excruciating pause, she finally spoke. "It's okay. I know you're busy. But even busy men can take a moment to text."

"Point taken. Honestly, Em, I feel like I'm running from one thing to the next and I can't catch up. I'm not used to this. And I feel like I have to play nice and by their rules. This means a lot to my family."

That was the problem. He wanted to tell them what he'd do and then say take it or leave it. But that wasn't an option. Tia Isabella was so excited to be returning home. He couldn't and wouldn't disappoint his great-aunt or any of his other relatives by ruining this for them. They'd looked to him for leadership and he was stepping up.

But he was losing himself.

"I'm trying to figure this out."

"Who says you have to do it all?" she asked. "Being the monarch and the head of a huge company is a big task for anyone. I think in most countries that isn't allowed."

"I know. But I like running the company. There I'm only answerable to the board and I have a certain degree of anonymity to deal with problems on my own.

Here…I sat in a meeting today about what color napkins we should have at the coronation."

She laughed. "What color did you decide?"

"I have no idea. I tuned out," he said. "I'd never do that at a board meeting."

"Well," she said at last. "I'm no expert on that sort of thing but I think you're going to have to find what makes being king exciting to you. I bet at Montoro Enterprises there are tasks that would normally bore you but you do them because you want to be successful."

She was right. "Good advice."

"Thanks. And thank you again for the mermaid. I hung her up after I got back from paddleboarding and am looking forward to seeing my kitchen lit up when the sun sets tonight."

"I wish I was there with you," he said.

"Don't."

"Don't what?"

Don't say things like that. Let's keep this light," she said. "That way I don't start thinking something else and you don't have to worry about calling me."

Hell. "I do want to call you, Em. I like talking to you and you make me…you're the only thing that feels real right now."

"That's because I have nothing to do with Alma or the throne. And you know with me it's just about the baby and getting to know each other. But that's running away from your obligations in Alma. And I think that for a little while that might suit you, but eventually it won't."

"I'm not sure what you mean by that," he said. Afraid very much that he did know what she meant.

"That once you decide to commit to Alma and the

people there, you will realize that you can't have me. I'll have been the distraction you needed to make the decision, and then I'll be left by the wayside."

Damn. He knew she was right. He didn't want to admit it to her, but then with Emily he didn't have to. "That's not my intention."

"Whether that's true or not, you can't change who you are and with you, Rafael Montoro IV, it's all about your family legacy. And we both know you aren't going to turn your back on it."

She was right. She'd taken the debate he'd been having with himself and boiled it down to its essence. He was a man who was all about family; it was the compass he used in every decision he'd ever made. Now he just had to decide if he could shift away from the Montoro legacy to pursue his own future with Emily and their child. And the decision would be a tough one.

After he hung up with her he went to his office to work. He put on a little Jimmy Buffett because he needed to hear some sounds of home.

There was a knock on the door and he rubbed the back of his neck. "Come in."

"Sir, I have a few more questions for the coronation," Hector said as he entered. Hector was the head of the Coronation Committee. Since Alma hadn't had a monarch in several decades, they were anxious to make sure the coronation had all the bells and whistles.

"Please have a seat," Rafe said. This was what he'd be giving up, he thought as Hector talked about where foreign dignitaries would be seated. Alma was going to be a world player. Lots of countries were interested in doing business with them since their previous ruler had kept the country isolated. Rafe's skills in business made him uniquely suited to help Alma get the most from their entry into the global marketplace.

"Do you like that?"

Rafe had to start paying attention. As Emily said, he needed to find the things about it that excited him. "You know better than me, Hector. No offense, but I'm not at all interested in color schemes or seating arrangements."

"None taken. You're a man of action and need to be doing something," Hector said.

"True. I'm going to let you make all the choices. If something doesn't look right then I will tell you."

"Thank you, sir."

"Clearly you know what you're doing," Rafe said.

Hector stood up to leave, but turned back when he got to the door. "I mean, thank you for coming back here. It means a lot to our people."

Hector left.

Rafe felt humbled. He knew that he wasn't going to find it easy to choose between Alma and Emily. He needed her and the people needed him.

Five

"I toured the countryside today. I have to say that it is beautiful. There's a little cove that I know you would like," Rafe said.

It was 10:00 a.m. Emily sat at one of the corner tables in the coffeehouse on Duval Street talking to Rafe. It had become their date. He hadn't missed calling her one time since the day he'd sent the stained glass mermaid a week ago. She hated to admit it, but she looked forward to his calls every day.

She took a sip of her herbal tea and looked out the window, but she didn't see Key West. Instead she saw the countryside of Alma as he described the rolling hills and hedgerows. The sheep on the hillside munching on grass.

"How's the weather there?" she asked. "I've never been farther north than Georgia."

"It's nice. The island isn't that big and so the sea breezes keep it cool. I think you'd like it."

He said that almost every time they talked, but she'd read the papers and online articles and knew there was no way she could ever visit him there. There was even speculation online that he'd chosen a bride from one of Alma's aristocratic families. She knew that came with the territory of being a monarch.

"Met any nice locals?" she asked before she could stop herself.

"A few. The head of the Coronation Committee is a great guy. He's helped me find things I like to do," he said.

She noticed he didn't mention any women, even though she'd seen his picture with more than one. It still made her sad.

Not sad enough that she stopped taking his calls or looking forward to talking to him.

She suddenly understood how a woman could willingly become a man's mistress. Because she had the feeling that if he asked her to, she'd be tempted to say yes. She was falling for him and he wasn't even here with her. But the silly thing was it was more intense by not actually having him physically here. They didn't argue over the little things like what to get for dinner because they only had a few hours together each week, and then it was only by phone.

"You still there?"

"Yes," she said. "Just imagining Alma."

"What's your view like today?"

"Sunburned tourists in swimsuits and flip-flops. There was a guy last night at the bar who had a few too many and kept coming on to this group of coeds.

They ignored him and so he started stripping. Can you imagine? I was laughing because he was harmless. A sunburned middle-aged man. I wanted to see how far he'd go. But Harry put an end to it."

"Sounds interesting. Did you think he'd look good naked?" Rafe asked.

"Nah. He didn't look anything like you. It was the expression on his face that had me hooked. He wasn't going to stop until those women acknowledged him."

"So he didn't look like me… Does that mean you like the way I look naked?" Rafe asked. "Because I haven't slept a single night without remembering how you felt in my arms that last time in Miami."

She took a sip of her tea and put her feet up on the chair across from her. She'd thought of little else but the way Rafe looked with his shirt off or how he'd moved when he'd been rapping to Jay-Z in his bedroom at the penthouse. She hadn't realized that she could be so lusty with this pregnancy, but she was.

"Tell me about it," she said.

"I will tonight. Why don't you call me when you get off work? I'll be waiting up for you."

She liked the sound of that. She glanced around the coffeehouse and noticed a man watching her. He looked away as she spotted him. Weird.

"Okay. I'm working an early shift because Harry is worried that late nights aren't good for me."

"They probably aren't. As a matter of fact, why don't you quit your job there?"

"Why would I do that?" she asked. She'd be bored stiff if she had nothing to do, and her savings would only last her three months. Then she'd have to look for another job. Though she knew Harry would take her back.

"I don't like the idea of you working late nights," he said. "I can support you so you don't have to work."

She put both feet on the floor and leaned forward as a wave of annoyance swept over her. "I don't need your money, Rafael. I'm not about to become your kept woman."

"Slow down, Red. I just meant that if you are tired, I'd help you out. It's nothing any man wouldn't do for the woman carrying his baby."

"That's not true," she said. Her own father had done a lot less. He'd just walked away and left her mom and her alone. "I guess you hit one of my triggers. I don't do needy."

"Hell, I know that. I don't do overprotective usually, but with you I want to. I know that's not what you want from me, so I'm keeping my distance," he said.

"Yeah, right, you're 'keeping your distance' because of your obligation to your family. You're just as afraid of committing yourself to me as you are of committing yourself to the throne."

There was silence on the line and she wondered if she'd gone too far. A part of her almost wished she had because then he'd just break it off with her and she'd know she was on her own.

These calls, this bond that was developing between them couldn't last. She knew it and if Rafe was being honest he'd admit to it too. The way things stood, they couldn't co-parent their child. Didn't royal babies have nannies or something?

She was going to be a hands-on mom and every time

she talked to Rafe she fell a little more for him, started to picture him as a hands-on dad.

"You're right," he said. "But I'm also not rushing back to your side because if I do I'm not sure what sort of reception I'll get."

"What sort do you want?" she asked. She had no idea how she'd act if he showed up on her doorstep, but frankly she imagined she'd be tempted to throw herself into his arms. And she had no idea how he'd react to that.

"You."

She caught her breath. "You don't have to keep this much distance between us, you know."

"I know. But you are unpredictable and I'm not on solid ground right now. Just know I wouldn't be calling you this often if you weren't important to me."

He didn't have to keep quite as much distance as he was for her sake. But getting to know him this way was safer. That was one of the issues she kept pushing to the back of her mind. "Okay, sorry for overreacting. It's just…a lot of things are changing in my body. You know how scary that is for a control freak like me?"

"I do. Red, that's how I feel about this entire constitutional monarchy thing in Alma."

She laughed. He was the only man she knew who'd compare being king to being pregnant. Mainly because he was the only man she knew who wasn't afraid to admit that he had doubts. That he liked to control things. That he was human. He didn't front with her and she knew that was one of the reasons she liked him.

"Okay, so about this late-night call. What do you say we use that video chat function? I miss seeing you," she admitted.

"Finally. I thought you'd never admit to missing me."

"I guess you're not as smart as everyone gives you credit for being," she said.

"Probably not," he said. "But I'm not concerned with what anyone thinks about me but you."

Those words made her heart beat a little faster and made her feel all warm and fuzzy inside. It wasn't love. Not yet. But she knew if he kept calling her every day she was going to start really falling for him, and she was starting to struggle to remember why that was a bad idea.

After hanging up with Emily, Rafe left the royal palace in Del Sol and walked around the well-manicured gardens. As he walked, he had his iPod set to his Key West playlist, which was really his Emily playlist. But he knew better than to actually name it that—he didn't want to leave any evidence of his affair for others to observe.

He listened to Jack Johnson sing about waking up and making banana pancakes together. Pretending the world outside didn't exist. And Rafe wanted that. But then as the days went by and he met more people in Alma he started to see how much the country needed him, or at least his family, here, too. Rafe guessed they were all so relieved to have the monarchy back.

After years under a dictator he understood that. It was sort of how he'd felt when he'd turned eighteen and left his father's house. He had acted like a wild man in college for about three months before he realized that he wanted his life to be about more than tabloid headlines. So he'd gotten serious and proven to himself that he could stand outside of his father's shadow and still be a part of the family.

"Hey, big brother," Bella said, coming up behind him and linking her arm through his. He pulled his earbuds out and smiled down at his baby sister. She'd really thrived in Alma and had an affinity with the people here that bordered on mutual admiration. For the Montoros, and Juan Carlos in particular, it was as if they'd come home. They were a part of Alma and Juan Carlos was busy bringing them back into the fold. There was sincere joy in all of them at being here. Even Rafe. Though he was torn, with his love of Miami and his lover in Key West.

"Hello, Bella. What's up?"

She led him to one of the wrought iron benches nestled next to a flowering jasmine bush and sat down. He sat down next to her and looked at his sister for the first time in days. She smiled easily.

"You seem distracted lately and I'm going to do the meddling kid sister thing and ask why."

"I'm trying to figure out how to be royal after years of being so ordinary," he said. It was his pat answer, and he'd been saying it to himself for so long that when he finally heard it out loud he realized how hollow the words were.

Maybe Bella wouldn't notice.

"Yeah, right," she said. "I'd think you'd have a better excuse than that."

He wasn't in the mood to discuss this with her and started to get up. But she stopped him with her hand on his sleeve.

"I think you have someone back home," she said.

"A woman who isn't from here and can't fit into this world."

"I have a lot of women back home," he said.

"Lying to me is one thing," she said with that honesty that made him feel exposed. "But lying to yourself is something else. If you have a woman, then marry her. Then take the throne."

If it were as simple as that he'd do it. But he knew from the meetings he'd been in that a smooth transition was needed. He was expected to marry someone who'd strengthen the Montoros' claim to the throne. Someone who'd make the people of Alma and its enemies believe that the restored monarchy would be around for a long time. That they were the only ones who could return Alma to its former glory.

And a bartender from Key West who didn't know who her father was wasn't going to be approved by the committee.

"Thanks, Bella, but it's not that simple," he said.

"It is if you know what you want."

He realized anew that he was lost. Hearing his little sister boil down his problems and come up with a solution was humbling. But he couldn't do what she suggested. He hadn't even seen Emily since he'd learned he was going to be a father. Their daily calls were great, but he needed to hold her in his arms again. Look into her eyes and see what, if anything, she felt for him.

Aside from lust. Sex between them had been raw and electric since the moment they'd met, and now he had to figure out if what he felt for her was more than that. Was he just using her as an escape to get away from the mantle of kingship that he didn't want? And he *really* didn't want it.

Because if he did it would be easier to make a decision about Em. Force her to take some money from him and set her and the baby up and then keep his distance. But he wanted more than that.

"I…thank you," he said.

"For what? I didn't say anything that you don't already know for yourself. Tell me what's going on."

He shook his head. "You've done enough."

"I have?"

"Yes. I just needed to hear someone else say it. I've been afraid of screwing up and embarrassing the family so I've stopped being myself. I've been trying to be regal and we both know I'm not."

She laughed and punched his shoulder. "You're not succeeding at being regal. I saw you roll your eyes when the Gomezes mentioned what beautiful babies you and Dita would have."

"I thought I showed a lot of restraint by not mentioning that the babies would probably be born with a tail and cloven hooves."

Bella laughed. "You're not that evil."

"Imp, you think it's funny having someone come after you because of your position? Wait until the princess royal or whatever title they decide on for you has to make a good marriage."

"Don't even joke about that, Rafe. I'm too young and pretty to be tied down to a man." She batted her eyelashes.

He hugged her close. "Damned straight. Besides, only one of us should be shackled by this monarchy thing. I'll do what's needed to protect you, Gabe and the rest of our family."

"Don't sacrifice yourself for us. We're stronger than you think we are."

"I know that. But I want you both to be happy."

Emily's shift was long. Her feet hurt and she felt as if she was going to be sick until she stepped outside into the balmy June air. It was only eleven—so not that late—as she walked through the crowds toward her cottage.

She had been looking forward to chatting with Rafe all evening. But once again she'd seen him on the local news on one of the televisions at the bar. He was with a blonde woman and she hoped like hell that it was just for publicity purposes. But a part of her realized that she had no hold on the king of Alma.

But that Rafe was different from the man who she spoke on the phone with and she hadn't asked about the woman because she really didn't want to hear that his obligation to his family might force him to marry someone else.

The US press, especially the local Miami reporters, loved anything to do with royalty and since the Montoros were raised in America, the media were obsessed with them. It seemed she didn't have to try too hard to find out about Rafael, Gabriel and Bella. She learned about the private schools they'd gone to and had seen Rafe's college roommate on CNN talking about how the Montoros were all about family.

She got it. As far as the media were concerned Rafe was going to make a great king. It had been a long time since an American had claimed a foreign throne, and despite the fact that most patriots were all about democracy they did like a fairy-tale story like this now and then.

She rubbed the back of her neck as she let herself into her house. She kicked off her Vans and left the lights off as she walked to her bedroom. She'd wanted him all day. Looked forward to the time when she could be alone and talk to him, and now she wasn't sure.

She wasn't sure how much more of Rafe she could take before he became so embedded in her soul that she wouldn't be able to survive without him.

She was sure part of it was the hormones from being pregnant with his baby. The other part was that she'd never had this kind of interaction with a guy. They talked every day. Most of her boyfriends had been busy with their own lives and had called only when they were horny or lonely.

Which had suited her.

She'd never wanted anything solid and lasting until now.

Until Rafe. And he wasn't available for her to claim.

Her phone rang. She glanced down at the Skype icon and knew that it was Rafe doing what she'd asked: calling her for a video chat this time.

She missed him. She didn't want to.

But she swiped her finger across the screen, unlocking the phone to answer the call. The image on the other end was dark with just a pool of light in the background.

Her own image popped up as a dark square in the bottom corner of the screen. She hadn't turned on the light.

"I guess you changed your mind about seeing me," he said.

"I just got home," she said. She fell backward on her bed and reached over to flick on the lamp on her nightstand. "I can't see you, either."

He turned the phone and she saw him sprawled on his back on a big bed with some sort of padded brocade headboard behind him. His shirt was unbuttoned and he had one arm stretched up over his head. He was holding the phone up above him with his other hand.

"Better?"

She sighed. She shouldn't do this late at night when her defenses were down. And they were down. She was feeling mopey and alone. Her mom was due back tomorrow and maybe that would help. But for tonight she had Rafe.

"I miss you."

"You do?"

"I do. You look like you had a formal event tonight," she said. She'd seen him on the news entering a gala with the blonde on his arm earlier this evening.

"I did. Listen, if you saw any pictures on the news of me with a woman, it was just state business. She's nothing to me."

"Does she know that?" Emily asked. Because that woman had seemed as though she had her claws sunk into him.

"Would I be here with you if she didn't?" he asked.

She looked at him in the shadows. "Would you?"

"No. I thought you knew me better than that," he said.

She had made him angry but she needed to know if he was the kind of man who'd cheat on her. "We don't have anything official between us. I...are you a one-woman man?"

He leaned in toward the camera, so close she could see the green and dark brown flecks in his hazel eyes. "I am."

"Then stop having your picture taken with foreign blondes," she said.

He sighed. "It's not that easy. She keeps showing up everywhere I am."

Emily was tempted to go to Alma and—

Do what?

She was Rafe's baby mama, not his fiancée.

This was something she had no idea how to handle. But she wanted him to be hers. For the world to know that he belonged to her. But she didn't want to say that to him. Admit that all these late calls had made her start to fall for him.

"How was your day?" She toed off her socks and grabbed a second pillow to prop her head up.

"Interesting. My baby sister is worried about me."

"Why?"

"She said I don't seem happy," Rafe said.

"Are you?"

"Happy isn't exactly something I aspire to. I think that is a path to crazy," he said. "I'd like to be content."

"Happiness equals crazy?" she asked. "I've never thought that."

"I mean trying to be happy all the time. Life isn't about always being happy. There are quiet moments and the normal grind. That's what makes the happy times memorable."

"So is this a quiet moment?"

"It's so much more than that, Red. You're my reward for being the good son and doing what's expected of me here in Alma."

It wasn't what she wanted to hear, but it warmed her up and made the feelings that had been dogging her all night dissolve. She realized that she'd been edgy and mopey because she didn't like seeing Rafe with that blonde woman.

"I was jealous."

"Of?"

"That blonde." She made a face and put her thumb over the part of her phone that showed her end of the video chat. She didn't want to see her own face.

"Don't be."

"I want this to be light and easy, Rafe. But it's not. It hasn't been for a while."

"You want the truth, Red?" he asked, rolling to his side and propping his phone up on something so that he wasn't holding it any more.

"You know I do."

"This hasn't been light or easy since the moment I first kissed you. I'm not a one-night-stand guy and we both know you don't take guys home all the time. We've both been trying to pretend that it was nothing more than a moment, but I think it's time we stopped pretending."

She swallowed hard. Had she been pretending? Was that why she'd been jealous and lonely?

"What do you suggest?"

"That we figure out what we both want. I know I want you. Not just for sex."

"Me, too."

Six

It was somehow easier to talk to her when he saw her face. She looked good, with that smattering of freckles across the bridge of her nose and the weary hope in her blue eyes. She seemed to want him to be the man he wasn't sure he could be.

He wanted to be a man of his word, but that was complicated. Making promises to her was out of the question because he had to figure out a solution that would take care of his family's future. Or did he? He was tired of walking on the tightrope between what he wanted and what he should do.

He thought of his mom, who'd divorced their father when Bella turned eighteen. It was as if his mother had served her time raising them and was ready to do something for herself. He didn't want to wait like that... Besides, assuming the throne was for life.

"What are you thinking? You got all intense all of a sudden," Emily said.

"I was thinking about my mom," he admitted quietly. "How she raised us until Bella was eighteen and then moved on with her life. What kind of mom will you be?"

"Not that kind. But I'm independent," she said. "I imagine my child will be too."

"It's our child."

"You're going to be ruling Alma, Rafe. I'm the one who will raise our child."

He didn't like her point. But he knew better than to argue it. He wasn't in a position to win. And he was tired of losing.

"You look nice. No sign of the pregnancy yet," he said.

"Thanks. A Shady Harry's T-shirt and jeans aren't exactly haute couture but they suit me."

They did suit her. He wanted to suit her as well. Be a part of that life. Yet he was torn. How could he be?

"I've got to get changed. I smell like the bar."

"Can I watch?" he asked. Seeing her brought all of his senses into sharp focus and made the life he'd been living these last few days look as if it were in black and white. He had been on autopilot doing what was expected of him and doing it well, but now he truly felt the first spark of excitement...of life.

"Is that what you want?" she asked. There was a teasing note in her voice and he caught a glimpse of the woman who'd bound him with his own shirt in South Beach.

If she only knew the power she wielded over him.

"It is."

"Well okay then," she said. "It's not going to be very exciting. I mean I've never worked in a high-end strip club or anything."

He shook his head. "I didn't think you had."

"Have you been to one?" she asked.

"Are you going to go on a feminist rant if I say yes?" he asked.

"No, I'm not. The women who work in places like that usually earn a good living. And it's their choice to make," she said. "So you have been to one."

He shrugged. Some nights that was where the crowd he ran with back in Miami had ended up. "It's not my favorite place to hang out."

"That's good to know. You should know I've only gotten undressed in front of a few guys."

"You should know I have no interest in any of the other men in your life," he said. "I want to be the only one."

He knew he had no right to say that. That he might not even be able to claim Emily but, hell, this was the twenty-first century and he wasn't going to marry another "suitable" woman when he felt this strongly about her.

She touched her finger to the screen and he imagined he felt her light touch on his face. "As of right now you are."

She got to her feet and his screen was filled with the image of her ceiling until she got to the bathroom. She flipped on the light switch and she propped the phone up on the counter. "I need a shower, too."

"How about a bath? If I were there, I'd fill that big claw-foot tub of yours with warm water and bubbles and have it waiting for you when you got home."

He wanted to take care of her. She was the first person outside of the circle of his family he'd ever felt this way about.

"Okay. Give me a few minutes."

"Don't take your clothes off until I can see you."

"Do you have a bathtub in your big palace?" she asked. "I saw some pictures of your entire family walking around the gardens on CNN last night. Looked nice."

"I do have a very nice bathroom here. The tub is controlled by a computer," he said.

"Join me in the bath?" she asked. There was a hint of vulnerability in her words. He found it both enchanting and a little bit unnerving. Emily was a very strong woman who didn't really need anyone. But tonight he caught a glimpse behind that attitude and saw that she did need him.

That made him feel like Atlas, strong enough to carry the weight of the earth on his shoulders. And like the mythological being he couldn't simultaneously protect Emily and shoulder his burden. He had no idea where any of this was going. He was used to being the strong one. The one who knew exactly what needed to be done—

And he did this time. He needed to let her go, but for once wanted to be selfish and keep her. For tonight he was going to do just that.

"Okay," he said, getting up and going to his own opulently appointed bathroom. He selected the temperature from a computerized keypad on the wall and soon the water started flowing into the tub. He flicked on the overhead light that just illuminated the tub and then glanced back at his phone screen to see where Emily was.

She was sitting on the edge of her tub biting her lower lip as she fiddled with the taps.

Then she stood up and undid her jeans.

"Hey. Not so fast, Red. I want to see every inch of you," he said.

"Fair enough. Take your shirt off. Not that you don't look sexy with it unbuttoned and your chest showing."

He'd undone his shirt earlier because he felt uncomfortable and hadn't really known what to wear for a video call with her. He lifted his arms. "You see these buttons?"

"Yeah?"

"You're supposed to undo them first. That way I don't have to rip the shirt," he said.

"I like it when you rip your shirt," she said with a wink. "In fact the next time I see you I've got a new shirt for you to try on. One that is made of tougher material."

Arching one eyebrow at her, he tossed his shirt toward the corner and then stood there, feeling a bit ridiculous.

"Damn, you look good," she said.

The open admiration in her eyes as she looked at him made him feel ten feet tall. He rubbed his hand over his chest. And then flexed his muscles for her. He heard her intake of breath. And suddenly all those reps he did at the gym were worth it. He worked out because he lived in South Beach and owned a very successful business. He wasn't about to have a photo of himself looking like a sloth turn up anywhere. But knowing she liked his body gave him another reason to do it.

"Your turn. I want to see your…muscles."

She laughed. "I did help unload a beer delivery this afternoon, so I think my arms are looking a little buffer than usual."

He frowned. "Why are you unloading anything? Harry should know better."

"He does. He was pissed when he got there. But the delivery guys weren't our usual ones and they were piling the beer in the sun…no one else was there. Harry ripped them a new one and they apologized to me."

Good. Still, Rafe didn't like that she'd had to deal with those guys. She should be pampered while she carried his child.

She pulled the Shady Harry's T-shirt up over her head and he immediately noticed her breasts swelling around the sides of the cups of her bra. She reached behind her back and unhooked the bra and let it slid down her arms and onto the floor. Her nipples looked bigger and a darker shade of pink than he remembered. Signs of the changes his baby was having on her body. She skimmed her hand down to her stomach and he noticed just the smallest bump there.

She unhooked her jeans and pushed them down her legs with her panties. And just like that, she was standing there naked.

He touched the image on his phone and realized that seeing her like this was a double-edged sword. He wanted to be there with her.

And that's when he came to his decision. He was going home first thing in the morning. He didn't care what the parliament thought; he needed to be back in Florida with Emily. Even if it was just for a few days.

"Dammit, Red. You get more beautiful each time I see you naked."

She blushed, and he observed that the color started at the top of her breasts and swept up her neck to her cheeks. She shook her head. "I had to unbutton my jeans at work tonight. It's not like they are too tight… well, okay, they are, but it was uncomfortable for the first time."

"I can see the little bump," he said. He traced his finger over her body on the screen. The changes were small, but this was their child making itself known in their lives. Well, mostly hers as of right now. He was missing out.

"I see a little bump in your pants as well," she said with a wink.

He guessed she didn't want to talk about the pregnancy, and he let her change the subject. "Little? Woman, look again."

He undid his pants and carefully shoved them down his legs until he stood there naked. He heard her sharp intake of breath and then her wolf whistle. She was good for his ego. And she kept things light. Was he ever seeing the real woman?

"Not so little."

"Not around you," he said.

"I didn't mean for this to be phone sex," she said.

"I never mean for it to turn into sex with you, but damn, Red, you turn me on like no one else ever has."

She smiled at me. "I feel the same. But I smell like the bar."

"Not to me. To me you smell like Florida sunshine and a day at the beach."

She walked over to the tub with the phone, her heart-shaped face filling the screen. Her eyes were sparkling, and unless he missed his guess, she was happy. While he might not think happiness was a good goal for every second of his life, he was glad to see her smiling.

She propped her phone up on the ledge of the tub and then climbed in. She closed her eyes and let her head fall back against the pillow she had there. The edges of her long hair fell into the water. She looked like his mermaid.

His.

He climbed into his tub, balled a towel up behind his head. The water felt hot and luxurious against his sensitive skin.

"This is nice. But I'm always by myself," she said.

"Me, too."

"Even in that crowd that's always with you?" she asked.

"Yeah."

"If I was there, I'd climb in behind you and rub your shoulders," she said. "You seem stressed."

"I'd like that. But only because I'd feel your naked breasts against my back."

"Maybe I'd lean over you and kiss your neck. Nibble on your earlobe. I know you like that, too."

He stretched his legs to make room for his growing erection and rubbed his hand over his own chest. He wished she were here so he could touch her. But his imagination was doing a good job of filling in the gaps.

"I'd probably pull you around in my arms and kiss you. I can't resist your mouth," he said.

"That's good. I like the way you taste, Rafe. No other guy I've kissed has tasted so right."

Damned straight. He wanted to be the only guy who

felt right to her. In all things. A wave of pure possessiveness overwhelmed him and he knew he wanted to claim her as his. But this damned situation with his family was keeping him from doing it.

"I'd put my hands on your waist and lift you up a bit until I could reach your breasts. Are they more sensitive now?"

She nodded.

"Show me."

"How?" she asked. She shifted up on her knees and leaned toward the phone. "I like your mouth on me."

Damn. He did, too. Her nipples felt so right in his mouth, and nothing made him harder than when he swirled his tongue around them and she gripped the back of his head.

"Touch yourself. Run your finger around your nipple and pinch it. Pretend I'm biting you," he said as she shifted back. "Just talking has made your nipples hard."

She nodded and gave him a slow smile. "I've been thinking about you touching me. Remembering how your mouth felt against my nipple."

"Show me," he said again.

She brought her hand up from the water, the droplets sparkling in the light as they fell from her arm. Then she cupped her breast and trailed her finger around her nipple. It puckered as she touched it, and he got even harder watching her as her head fell back and she let out a moan.

"Feel good?" he asked, his voice husky and low. His skin was so sensitive that each lap of the water brought him closer to the edge. He was going to come. But he didn't want to until she did. He wanted to keep watching her for as long as he could. And draw out the pleasure so he could feel as if they were together. He needed this. Needed her.

He'd been trying to deny it, but there it was. The truth that he'd been afraid to admit to himself.

She was cupping both of her breasts and he groaned as he reached for the screen of his phone and touched it. He remembered the way she felt underneath him. How her limbs felt wrapped around his.

"Not as good as when you do touch me," she said. "If I were there I'd caress your chest and then slowly tease you by working my fingers lower."

"When you do that it makes it difficult for me to think," he admitted.

"Really?"

He nodded. Words were sort of beyond him at this moment.

"Are you hard for me?" she asked.

"I am." He stroked himself, remembering how she fit him like a glove when he thrust into her.

"Show me," she said. "Let me see how hard you are."

Her words were like a velvet lash on his skin and he shuddered. This was excruciating. He wanted to come inside her and each time she said something so sexual he couldn't contain his groans.

"Red…"

"Show me, Rafe. I want to see you. See how much you want me."

He groaned, but did as she asked, shifting until he was out of the water and she could see him. He stroked his hand up and down his shaft.

"Swipe your finger over the top," she said. "Pretend it's my tongue on you."

He did as she instructed and then shuddered as he realized how close to the edge he was.

"Are you ready for me? Show me," he said.

She parted her legs and showed him. Pushed her finger up inside and moaned as she did so. "It's not the same as when you do it."

"Does it feel good?" he asked.

"It does."

"Come for me, Red."

This was too intimate and yet not intimate enough.

"I want to touch you, Rafe. If I were there I'd take you inside me. I need you," she said.

"Me, too, Red."

She moaned. "I'm so ready for it. For you."

He was, too. He remembered the way it had felt the last time they were together. How she'd gripped him as soon as he entered her body. How deep he'd gone and the way her eyes had opened and he'd met her gaze. Felt her wrapped around him all the way to his soul.

"Rafe."

Hearing her name on his lips made him come. He closed his eyes and put his head back as his orgasm washed over him. He opened them to see her doing the same. She gave him a slow, sexy smile.

"That's my kind of bath," she said, smiling.

"Mine, too," he said. "When I get home I want to do this again."

"But together in the same tub."

He hit the button to drain the tub and got to his feet. She stayed where she was, watching him, and he realized that in her eyes he was enough. He didn't have to prove anything to her. Or at least he hoped he didn't have to. Because he was coming to realize he didn't know who he was anymore. He hadn't known in a long, long time.

"Come to bed with me, Red. Let's talk until we both fall·asleep."

She nodded. She got out of the tub and dried herself off and he just watched, absently toweling himself dry. He caught his breath when she padded naked back to her bed and climbed between the sheets. She'd washed the sheets but not the pillow case he'd slept on.

"This pillow smells like you," she said.

"It does?"

"Yes. I've been pretending you are here with me every night… Tomorrow I'm going to deny that. But tonight I need you here with me."

He understood. When the sun was out there were oceans between them and problems that wouldn't be easily solved. And while he wanted to do what Bella said and put himself first—maybe marry Emily so that the rest of the world would have to accept her—he knew she wouldn't go for that. She didn't want a man who could be hers only halfway.

And that was all he could offer right now. But he knew he wanted to call her his and he needed to figure out a way.

He climbed into his own bed and curled on his side. "I don't have a pillow that smells like you."

"Sorry, babe."

She smiled sleepily at him and he watched her as she started to drift off to sleep. "Thank you for being here tonight."

"You're welcome, Red."

He watched over her until he knew she was sound asleep and snoring slightly. Maybe he kept the line open for longer than he should have before disconnecting the call.

He knew he couldn't do this any longer. He was tired of making do with phone calls to Emily. He'd thought that the video call would make it easier but it hadn't. Instead it made him long to touch her. Really touch her.

He got out of his bed, pacing to the window and looking out at the sea. The ocean was endless and as he glanced up at the moon that was almost setting he realized that in Emily's part of the world the moon was rising. He wanted to be in the same place she was. See if there was anything really between them.

Honestly he knew this wasn't real. How could it be? He was painting her the way he wanted her to be. And not to be oedipal or anything, but he was making Emily into the woman he wanted while imagining her as the mother he never had.

He got dressed and walked out of his room down the hall to Gabe's. He figured Gabe would be easier to talk to than Juan Carlos. But there was no answer when he knocked.

He rubbed the back of his neck.

Damn.

He walked to Juan Carlos's room and wasn't surprised when his cousin answered the door wearing a dressing gown with the Alma royal seal monogramed on the breast.

"What is it?"

"I...I have to return to the States."

"Why? You know that royal protocol states—"

"Screw royal protocol, J.C. I had a life before Alma came to us and I can't just walk away from it."

"You gave your word. Our family gave our word. You are the oldest."

"I wish I wasn't."

"Stop being so selfish. This country needs a leader. It needs someone who can take it from the isolated kingdom it's been into the twenty-first century. You are the man."

"I didn't choose this," Rafe said. "I'm not sure I want this."

"Too bad, Rafael, you're birthright has brought you to this. Sure, it would have been easier if we'd been brought up on the island but that doesn't make our legacy any less important."

Juan Carlos would be so much better at this than him, Rafe thought. But he wasn't from the right family line and Rafe really couldn't—

"I have to return to the States," he said again. "I'm the one who will be king so my decision is final."

"This is ridiculous."

"Why?"

"Because already I can see that your loyalty isn't to your people. And they will see it too."

"I can't take care of the people of Alma until I figure out this part of my life."

"Is there a woman?"

"Yes. Yes, there is, and I haven't had a chance to resolve anything with her."

"Is she…would the court approve a marriage to her?"

Rafe doubted it. Hell, he wasn't even sure he wanted to marry her. He had to get back to her and figure this all out.

"I have no idea if I want to marry her or not. I need some time to myself to figure this out."

"Hell. I'll go with you."

"I don't want the entire family to know," Rafe said. "Why would you come with me?"

"As you said, you can't be a good ruler until you know where you belong. I want that, Rafe. I know I seem all tied up with royal protocol, but I want what is best for all of us. You're like a brother to me."

"You are to me as well," Rafe said. Juan Carlos had grown up in their home after his parents had died. "I do need to be in Miami to take care of the details of the new shipping deal I just signed. I will let the court and the coronation committee know that's why I'm returning."

"I will back you up," Juan Carlos said. "Just be sure you make the right decision."

Rafe nodded. His impromptu decision to leave had to be delayed until he could talk to the court advisors and his family. Since it was early morning it would take time for the entire Montoro clan who were in Alma to be ready to go.

But sure enough, later that day, they were all on the plane and headed toward Miami.

Seven

Emily went to Key Koffee for a cup of decaf and sat at the corner table again. Last night with Rafe had been different. It had been fun, but also, in the safety of the darkness and with the distance between them, she felt he'd shared more of himself than he had before.

Caution, she warned herself.

Her mom was always warning her about racing headlong into action before thinking about it first. But she felt as if it was too late to change. And last night had made her fall a little more for Rafe.

Which was probably why she was up early even though she had to work later. But her mom was also due to dock at the marina at nine, and Emily wanted to be there to greet her.

"Give me a double espresso and a lemon poppy-seed muffin to go as well as my usual order," Emily said to Cara behind the bar.

"Sure thing. Feeling hungry this morning?"

"A little, but the extra stuff is for my mom. She's back in port today," she told Cara.

"How about your man?" Cara asked.

Emily shook her head. "I don't have a man."

She couldn't claim Rafe as her own until he indicated he was ready for that. And she knew despite their closeness when they were alone that he wasn't. That knowledge sort of tinged her day. She frowned a little. The smell of the espresso was strong this morning, and she felt bile rising in the back of her throat.

She swallowed hard to keep from getting sick and then realized it wasn't going to work. She ran for the bathroom but made it only as far as the hallway before she began retching. She forced herself to keep moving into the bathroom and threw up. She was heavy and aching and knew this wasn't one of the times when she could say she was enjoying her pregnancy.

Cara followed her into the bathroom with a wet towel. After Emily rinsed her mouth and splashed water on her face, Cara walked her back to her table. Emily felt as if everyone was staring at her. Cara just smiled at them.

"She's pregnant. You don't worry about our food."

Everyone nodded and went back to their papers and electronic devices.

"I sort of wasn't planning on telling anyone yet," Emily said.

"Sorry, Em. But I can't have people thinking it's my food."

"It's okay," Emily said.

"Your man should be here with you," Cara said in

a kind way. "I saw you two together. He's not the kind of man who'd just walk away."

Cara tucked a strand of Emily's hair behind her ear. "Have you told him?"

She wasn't that close to Cara, but they were friends. They'd gone to the same high school and had even taken a road trip to Georgia together one time. But she didn't want to discuss Rafe with her. "Yes. It's complicated."

"Fair enough. Park yourself right there. I'm going to get your order for you."

Emily looked up and noticed a man watching her. The same guy who had been eavesdropping on her telephone conversation with Rafe the other day.

"How you feeling?" he asked, coming over with a packet of Club crackers that they kept on the tables for when Key Koffee serve conch chowder in the afternoon. "These always helped my wife when she was expecting."

She smiled her thanks and took them, weakly opening the pack and taking out a cracker. She munched on one and tipped her head back as her body stopped rioting and started to calm down.

"Are you reading this?" he asked.

She glanced down at the *Miami Herald,* which was flipped open to the society page with a picture of Rafe and his family in Alma.

"No."

"I can't believe how obsessed everyone is with that family," the guy said. "I'm Stan, by the way."

"Emily," she said. "Well, it's a fairy tale, isn't it? American royalty becomes real royalty."

"True enough. I've heard that Rafe comes down to Key West," Stan said.

It seemed to her that he was fishing for information. She didn't know if he was some obsessed royal watcher or just making conversation. "I guess he does. It's not that uncommon."

"No it's not. But surely now that he's going to be king he won't be," Stan added.

"I have no idea," Emily admitted.

"Mind if I take this paper?"

"Be my guest," she said.

"Thanks," he said, walking out.

"Here's your breakfast to go," Cara said, coming over. "What did he want?"

"The newspaper," Emily said. She started to get up but Cara pushed her back down. "Sit for a little while. I called Harry to come and get you."

"Cara."

"What? You're family, Em. We take care of our own here," she reminded her.

She felt tears burn the back of her eyes and blinked so they didn't fall. She'd always felt as if Key West was her home, ever since she was three years old and her mother moved them there. The people she knew were like family to her, but she had always figured it was a one-way street. The feelings of a girl left too many times by a mother whose job was her life, her obsession.

"Thanks, Cara. But I'm a big girl."

"Even big girls deserve to be looked after," Harry said, walking into the coffee shop and approaching their table. "We got time for me to grab a cup of coffee?"

"No need to wait, Harry," Cara said, handing him a cup and a bakery bag.

Unless Emily missed her guess, that bakery bag would have a toasted everything bagel in it. Cara was right. They were all family.

This place was as much a part of her as the baby growing inside her. And though she didn't need the reassurance, it was nice to know that she wasn't alone. That if Rafe made the choice that any sane man would and took the throne of Alma half a world away from her, she'd still have family around her. Her baby would grow up with the family she'd chosen for herself and not the one she'd been born into. The family her mother had chosen for them when she'd moved them to Key West.

"You okay, kiddo?" Harry asked.

"Just morning sickness."

"Another thing that I will bring up to Rafe Montoro the next time he shows his face here."

Rafe stretched his long legs out in front of him as he settled in for the flight. His cousin Juan Carlos—the one in the family who was the best suited for royal life since he seemed to know so much about it—sat across from him reading a book on the history of Alma from the 1970s to today.

His father, brother and sister were all sitting in the back of the plane talking quietly amongst themselves. They were happy enough to follow his lead especially when he mentioned that the oil deal needed his attention in Miami.

Rafe had been surprised by Juan Carlos's understanding but now he realized he shouldn't have been.

He knew his cousin as well as he knew Gabe…though he had to admit that he'd known both men better when they were children. But the bond among all of them was still strong. And Rafe felt less isolated that he had before. Felt a little more as if his family had his back.

Rafe read the book last week, since the government people wanted to make sure that everyone in the Montoro camp was familiar with the past. The common consensus being that maybe then they wouldn't make the same mistakes again. Rafe didn't want to have to flee the country in the middle of the night and start over with nothing.

At least his great-grandfather had his wife by his side, and his family. Something that was becoming more and more important to Rafe.

"Juan, what would you do if you were going to be king?" Rafe asked. "I'm tempted to invest Montoro Enterprises money into the manufacturing sector so that Alma isn't just reliant on oil."

"That's a start. They really need stability so that Alma's citizens will start staying on the island instead of emigrating to countries in the EU. I think we should try to become a member of the EU as well," Juan Carlos said.

"It's one of the prime minister's top priorities. He has me scheduled to go to Brussels next month for meetings on the subject," Rafe said, rubbing the back of his neck.

"I can go with you if you like," Juan Carolos said. "I'm not as impatient as you are at the negotiating table. Of course, you are always very shrewd at getting the best deal for Montoro Enterprises."

"That would be great. I'd love to have you there with

me," Rafe said. One thing about his family that had
been made clear during the last few weeks as they'd
traveled to Alma and gotten a handle on their new lives
was how they all banded together. "When is Tia Isabella going to join us in Alma?"

"Soon, I hope," Juan Carlos said. Juan Carlos's
grandmother suffered from Parkinson's and had her
good days and her bad days. "We are waiting for her
doctors to okay the visit."

"How is she doing?" Rafe asked. "You talk to her
nurse every day, don't you?"

"Yes, I do. I think the thought of returning to Alma
has rallied her spirits, and though medically I'd have to
say there have been no changes, she seems healthier."

Rafe smiled to himself. The very thing that felt like
a burden to him was a dream come true to Tia Isabella.
She had longed to return to her home for decades and
now it was possible.

That almost made his royal sacrifice worthwhile.
But there was also a lot to be said for the old-world
charm of Playa del Onda. And for Juan Carlos's excitement over their all being part of the royal aristocracy again as well.

It just made everything more difficult for Rafe. He
wanted to keep his family happy. He was the eldest
and had the power to do it. But then he remembered
Emily and he was torn.

Had been torn for too long. When he got to Miami
he needed to see her and figure this entire thing out.

"Do you think that the government would accept a
commoner as my wife?" Rafe asked his cousin. They
were still negotiating the constitution that Alma's parliament had brought to them. Rafe had been asking for

little changes because he wanted to see how far they would go to get him and his family back in the country.

"Is your woman a commoner?" Juan Carlos asked.

"Not many royals in the States, Juan Carlos." He didn't want to talk about Emily with anyone else. Not yet. Why then did he keep bringing her up? He clearly needed to talk even if he didn't want to. Not until he had her sorted out. God, she'd kill him if she knew he thought that way about her.

"I don't know. I think they want you to marry a woman who will reinforce the monarchy, and a commoner wouldn't do that," Juan Carlos said at last.

Rafe nodded at his cousin and then leaned back and closed his eyes. He'd figured as much. There was no way to have it both ways. Why was he still trying to?

Because he couldn't walk away from Emily.

There it was: the truth he'd been trying to pretend didn't exist for too long. And letting his family down, well, that wasn't something he was prepared to do, either. He wasn't even sure if he walked away from the throne that they would let him keep his job at Montoro Enterprises. Though truth be told, he was a genius at making money, so he had no doubt he could start his own company and make it a success.

But that would mean walking away from everything and everyone. His family was so deeply rooted in his life, he truly wasn't sure what he'd do without them. When they'd lived in the Miami area, he saw them every day at their Coral Gables compound. He worked hard for all of them so that they wouldn't have to worry.

That was why he hesitated. Then there was Tia Isabella. With her deteriorating health, Rafe didn't really want to do anything to upset her. If he walked away, would he find a way to make peace with the family before her illness got the better of her? Bella would be forced into a difficult position as well. His father would more than likely try to come between her and Rafe, and that would cause her stress. She liked to keep the peace.

Gabriel would be none too pleased with him. Gabe lived a nice and easy lifestyle, enjoying the many beautiful women who flocked to Miami. No-strings relationships were his MO.

Rafe laughed to himself. Gabe always did whatever the hell he wanted. He'd be plenty pissed at Rafe if he walked away from the throne and Gabe had to take it. That would be a nightmare for all concerned. His younger brother was a player. Not the image that Alma wanted for their new king.

So Rafe was back to the exact same position he'd been in since he left Miami. Except this time he was leaning more toward Emily. Hell, last night had changed something between them.

He no longer saw her as the fun-loving bartender who had gotten pregnant, but more as Emily, the woman who was going to be the mother to their child. *Their child.* If he had a son he'd be Rafael V. Or would he? Would Emily want to name him something else? There was still so much for them to discuss.

He closed his eyes, trying to picture what their child would look like. Would the baby have his dark hair and eyes or Emily's bright blue ones? He tried to picture the little tyke, maybe with her red hair and his hazel eyes.

He wanted to be a part of that. Be a part of his child's life. He had to find a way to have it all. Perhaps he needed introduce Emily to his family so they could start to get to know her. Once that happened, they would be on his side. And marrying a commoner wouldn't be such a big issue.

At first Emily might be reluctant about this plan of action, but Rafe was confident he could change her mind and bring her around to his way of thinking.

He'd seen that look in her eyes as she'd drifted off to sleep last night. She cared for him. He was gambling that she wanted him in her life as much as he wanted to be there.

He'd never been much of a gambling man. He preferred to take risks where he could control the outcome. But there was no controlling Em. She was a force unto herself and no matter what happened, she was never going to be coerced into doing anything she wasn't comfortable with.

Emily, her mom and Harry spent a pleasant day together at her house. It was nice to forget about everything and just enjoy having her mom home.

Jessica Fielding had the same blue eyes as Emily but her hair was blond and cut short in a low-maintenance bob. She'd had a look of mild concern on her face ever since she docked earlier today. "So how far along are you?" she asked.

"About eight weeks. I'm not really showing yet but have lots of morning sickness," Emily said as her mom got up and brought her a glass of homemade lemonade and a gingersnap. Emily had been ordered to sit on the padded chaise longue in the shade of a big magnolia tree in the backyard while Harry manned the grill preparing fish for their dinner and her mom bustled around doing things for Emily that she could do herself.

She'd protested at first, but then figured her mom

was only in town for a few days and it was okay to let her spoil her. Well, fetching drinks and fixing dinner was probably going to be the extent of the spoiling. Her mom wasn't one of those in-your-face, hands-on parents.

"Tell me about the father," her mom said. "Is he totally out of the picture?"

Emily took a sip of her lemonade. "Not entirely. Was my dad when you were pregnant?"

"Em," Jessica said.

"Mom, I want to know more about him. I'm not going to suddenly show up on his doorstep—how could I? Is he even alive?" These were the questions she'd kept hidden away for years but the truth was, she needed to know now more than ever. She'd always wanted to know for herself but really felt as if she had to know the answers to share with your child.

"No, you can't show up on his doorstep, Emily. He's dead. He died when you were three," Jessica said at last. She rubbed her hand over her forehead and Emily almost felt bad for asking about him.

But she had a right to know. Someday her child was going to want to know about Rafe, and Emily planned to have the answers ready.

"Why didn't you ever tell me this?"

"You never asked."

"I didn't ask because you seemed sad whenever I said anything about my father," Emily said.

"Sorry, sweetie, I just thought you were too young to understand and then as you got older you never brought it up so I kept quiet."

"Is that why we moved here?" Emily asked.

"That was part of it. Also, I had the grant so I needed

to live someplace where I could do my work and be home every night for you," Jessica said

She got that. Work had always been her mother's driving force. Emily had been swimming before she learned to walk and had understood boat safety by the time she was six. Her life had been on the water and as an assistant to her mother's work. The work always came first, and Em had understood that at a very early age.

Emily was beginning to think of what she would do once her baby was born, and though she hadn't talked to Harry yet, she was pretty sure she wouldn't be tending bar.

"Did he want me?" Emily asked. It was the question that had weighed on her mind for a long time.

"He did, sweetie, but he had another family. He was a married man," Jessica said at last. "He saw you from time to time before he died. But really he knew that he couldn't leave his wife."

That wasn't what she'd expected. A married man. Had her mother known he was married? It didn't fit the picture she had of her mother, of the woman she'd always thought her mother was. Then the thought struck her that she might have another family.

"Do I have siblings?" she asked, mildly alarmed by the thought of strangers who might share her DNA.

"No. His wife was infertile and they never had children. He offered to adopt you and raise you with his wife, but I couldn't let you go."

Harry left his position by the grill and went over to her mother, putting his hand on her shoulder. Emily realized now why her mom had never spoken of her father. But she was glad to finally know something about him.

She went over to her mom and hugged her tightly. Her mom hugged her back, and then kissed the top of her head.

"I love you, Mom."

"I love you too, honey. I'm sorry I never talked about him."

"It's okay," Emily said. "Thank you."

"For what?" she asked, tucking a strand of hair behind Emily's ear.

"Telling me. I hated not knowing. I always felt… Well, that doesn't matter now," Emily said. But she'd always felt an emptiness inside her where a father should be. Now she knew. Their situation had been complicated. More so than her own?

She wasn't too sure.

"Tell me about the father of your child," Jessica said.

"He's Rafael Montoro IV," Emily said. Then she realized that she always used his full name when she told people about him so they'd get why he wasn't with her. She was sort of making excuses for coming second in his life. "We had a weekend together and then I got pregnant. His family got called back to Alma to restore the monarchy before I knew I was going to have his baby."

"Harry filled me in on a few of the details via our calls on the satellite phone."

Jessica sat down on the end of the chaise longue and lifted Emily's legs, drawing them over her lap. "Well, I can see why you said it was complicated. What did he say when you told him about the baby?"

"I caught him on his way out of town, Mom. We

really didn't have any time to talk. I wanted him to know he had a kid coming but I never expected anything from him."

Her mom nodded. "You're strong enough to raise the baby on your own, and you have me."

"And me," Harry said.

Emily smiled over at Harry. "I know. But I think he wants to be a part of the baby's life."

"And yours?"

She bit her lower lip. She'd been telling herself that he did, but what if she was just seeing something that wasn't there? Emotions and bonds that she wanted to see because she'd started to care about him. And not just because he was her baby's father.

"I don't know. He's been calling me every day while he's in Alma. He sent me that beautiful mermaid that's hanging in the kitchen."

Her mom smiled. "Remember when you wanted to be a mermaid?"

She nodded.

"You told him?" her mom asked. "Oh, baby, I'd hoped you wouldn't fall for a man who wasn't available."

She had, too. Of course until this afternoon she'd had no idea how much her own life might parallel her mother's, but it was clear now that the Fielding women always seemed to go for men who were already spoken for.

"I'm not sure I've fallen for him."

"You are starting to," her mom said.

"Mom." Her mom always had to push her when she wasn't ready.

"Dinner's ready, ladies," Harry said, interrupting the fight that he could sense brewing.

They went to the table and Harry served the fish her mom had caught that morning and fresh mango with grilled green onions. It was delicious and Emily forgot her ire at her mother as they finished eating.

This was turning out to be one of the best days she'd had in a while. She'd talked to Rafe this morning and felt closer to him than ever. She'd learned the details of her own parentage and felt closer to her mom than ever before.

Her mom picked up the dishes and went into the kitchen to watch the evening weather forecast, something she did every night so she'd know what to expect on the water the next day.

"You better come in here and see this," her mom said as she leaned out the window.

Emily got to her feet, looking up at the evening summer sky and wondering if it looked similar in Alma.

She stepped inside and noticed that that instead of the local fishing report the television was tuned to E! News. She'd been watching *Keeping up with the Kardashians* earlier. Now the words *Montoro Baby Mama!* were on the screen and Emily felt as if she was going to be sick.

Eight

Rafe turned his phone to flight-safe mode once they were getting ready to land. There was a tingle of excitement in the pit of his stomach as he made plans to bring Emily to his family. She was stubborn, so he knew it wouldn't be easy to convince her to leave Key West, but he was fairly confident that he had his ways of persuading her.

They landed at the private airfield the Montoros always used. As Rafe got off the plane and started walking across the tarmac, he noticed there seemed to be a swarm of reporters waiting. Had something happened in Alma in the last ten hours while he'd been on the plane? He slowed down, as did the rest of the party, all looking at one another as they flicked on their phones and scanned headlines.

Gabe was the first one to spot it and cursed under his breath.

"Your baby mama is headline news," Gabe said.

His baby mama.

Damn.

"It's not like that," he said.

Juan Carlos looked pissed but he was quiet as he simply turned away from Rafe and walked toward the hangar. He couldn't have known that the press would find out about Emily while they were in the air. Rafe shoved his hands into his pockets and rocked back on his heels.

Gabe clapped a sympathetic hand on his shoulders before following the rest of their party into the hangar. Rafe's phone finally connected and he saw he had a dozen missed calls from Emily along with seven text messages that all said the same thing. Call me.

She'd already seen the news.

Of course she had. For a brief moment he wondered if she'd leaked the news, but then he remembered how fierce she was about keeping to herself. It was doubtful that she'd rat herself out.

When Rafe got into the hangar, Gabe immediately introduced him to a tall, dapper man in a white linen suit. Geoff Standings was a British press agent who'd once worked for the British royal family. Apparently he'd been sent by the royal advisers back in Alma to meet Rafe's plane and start doing damage control.

Gabe didn't look as amused as he had a few minutes ago.

"We need to fix this," Gabe said.

"Duh."

"No, I mean if the people of Alma decide that you are too hot to touch, then I'm going to have to take your place as king. We need to fix this. Now."

"Fine. Geoff, what do you recommend? I have been planning to introduce Emily to the family, and was even thinking of having a dinner next week where she could meet the members of my family who came with me on the trip. Do you think we should get engaged? Should I marry her?"

"Well, marriage usually is the right step for an illegitimate baby. But in your case I'm going to have to figure this out. I have already sent my assistant to start researching her lineage. Maybe we can find a relation—however distant—to a royal somewhere."

"If that doesn't work?" Rafe asked.

"I think we can make a case for you as a love match. Prince William married a commoner and perhaps Alma won't mind so much if we can make her into a style icon the way Kate is."

Style icon? Rafe doubted Emily would go for that. He loved her style but it was bohemian and beachy. Not exactly what Geoff was talking about.

Geoff was frantically typing away on his smartphone. "Either way, I'm going to book you some shows so you can get out there. Yes, you need to be engaged to her. I'd like to send a press release out that says she's your fiancée, not just your 'baby mama.' Who do you think leaked this?"

Good question.

"I have to ask her before you say she's my fiancée. She might get stubborn if she sees that online or in a paper before I ask," Rafe said.

"Fair enough. Any ideas on the leak?"

"None," Rafe said. "I think she's told her mom and her boss and that's it. Neither of them would tell a reporter."

"Let me look into it and see if I can find out where the information came from. Where will you be?"

"Key West. You've got my cell number, and here is Jose's as well. He's my assistant based at Montoro Enterprises headquarters in Miami and he's at your service."

Juan Carlos returned. "I'll take the family out the front of the airport. I've had your car brought around. Resolve this, Rafe. This needs to be made right."

"I know," he said. "I'll be back in the office in a couple of days to take care of the details of the Alma shipping deal, but I need to go to Key West."

He didn't like answering to his cousin and normally wouldn't have but if Juan Carlos was upset Rafe knew the court advisors in Alma would be as well.

"I was trying to keep this under control," Rafe said.

"I realize that. That's why I'm going to help you as much as I can. Alma needs the Montoros back on the throne."

Juan Carlos gathered the rest of their family. Bella gave Rafe a hug and Gabe shook his head but clapped him on the shoulder before they headed toward the main airport area and the waiting reporters.

No one said another word as Rafe strode out of the airport to his waiting Audi. His phone rang as soon as he was inside. He synched it to Bluetooth and hit the button to answer it.

"Jose here. Have you seen the news? I'm getting calls from morning news shows asking you to come on and tell your story. What should I do?" Jose asked.

"Coordinate with Geoff. He's the PR expert that the Alma court hired to make the scandal go away. I need some media prepared and he's the expert. They are all going nuts over this. Any idea where the leak came from?"

"No, sir. She wasn't visibly pregnant when I delivered your gift and I didn't see any reporters hanging around her place."

"Thanks, Jose. I'm going to leave the phone off while I drive to Key West.

"Why don't you take the chopper? I already have it ready and waiting at the Coral Gables compound."

"I'm trying to decide if I need more time alone to clear my head," he said.

"It's up to you, sir."

If he took the chopper he'd cut his travel time in half and be at Emily's side that much sooner. But he was still not sure what he was going to say when he got there. The plans he'd been hatching as he flew back from Alma were all moot now. He was in damage control, and so was the rest of the family.

"I'll take the chopper."

"I'm turning around and will be in Coral Gables with your bag in a few minutes."

"Where were you headed?"

"Key West," Jose said. "I also have procured two jewelers to meet you. They are waiting in Coral Gables."

"Thanks, Jose." Rafe disconnected the call.

Jose had thought of everything, which was why Rafe paid him the big bucks. Still, Rafe was uncertain. Having the chopper and his bag and even a ring might make going to Key West easier for him, but he had no idea what kind of reception he was going to get when he saw Emily. How was he going to tell her that they had to be engaged? He knew he needed to have that conversation in person and not over the phone. In fact, the sooner he could get to her the better. He needed to think about what he was going to do.

With Em he tended to react first and then do damage control later. This was one time when he needed to plan with his head and not his groin. He wanted her, but he needed the details to be right. There was no more choosing between the throne and Emily.

What kind of king would the people of Alma think he was if he abandoned his child? In a way it was the perfect solution to the debate he'd been having with himself. There was no more keeping Emily and the baby hidden.

Emily gave up trying to call Rafe and convinced her mom and Harry to go home around 11:00 p.m. She changed into a big T-shirt she'd gotten during the last hurricane to hit the Keys with the slogan It Takes More Than a Little Breeze to Shake Me on it.

Harry had called his buddies at the Key West Police Department and together they'd cleared the reporters from her yard and were keeping them at the end of the street. She'd heard a chopper fly over and hadn't turned on the local news because she was afraid she'd see her home on it.

She felt as if this story about being Rafe's "baby mama" was enough to shake her though. She had an idea that the source might be that creepy guy from the coffee shop who'd watched her and made awkward conversation with her. But how had he known about Rafe?

Not that they'd done much to keep it secret. They had been flirting at the bar that weekend he'd been on Key West. Everyone had seen them together. She guessed it wouldn't take Sherlock Holmes to figure out that she and Rafe had hooked up.

But baby mama? That was insulting. She guessed it was meant to be. If it was that creep from the coffee shop, did that rat bastard have a vendetta against Rafe? She vowed to get to the bottom of it tomorrow. She rolled to her side feeling very alone as she stared out the window.

She'd done everything to pretend that it was normal. That she wasn't bothered by the fact that he hadn't called her back.

Why hadn't he?

Surely he knew she hadn't gone to the papers. Didn't he?

There was nothing in it for her if she did. Or maybe he hadn't heard about it yet. But that seemed far-fetched to her, even if she wanted it to be true.

What if he'd decided he'd had enough and the paparazzi were the last straw? It didn't seem like the man she knew to just retreat. More than likely he was coming up with some plan. Maybe he'd ask her and the baby to leave town. Disappear for a while so he could get on with his coronation plans.

Tired of listening to her own thoughts, she got out of bed and wandered through her empty house to the kitchen. She found the carton of frozen yogurt she'd shoved into the back of the freezer when she got home from the grocery store earlier. She'd been trying to hide it from herself because the last time she'd opened a pint of the key lime pie flavor, she'd eaten it in one sitting.

But if ever she needed the cold comfort of fro-yo, it was tonight.

She didn't want to leave Key West, to start over on

her own. But she wasn't alone, was she? She had this little pod in her belly.

She dipped her spoon into the carton and took a big scoop, putting it in her mouth as she leaned against the counter. Letting the frozen dessert melt on her tongue was bliss.

She didn't care what was happening outside her little cottage. She'd just stay here with her fro-yo until she figured out how to fix this.

She'd never met a problem she couldn't solve. It was just late-night loneliness making her feel blue. That and the fact that she was getting total radio silence from Rafe. Why didn't he return her call?

She had a feeling this was going to be one of those nights when sleep evaded her. Part of it she blamed on the habits formed by spending her entire adult life working nights, but the other part was worry. She never admitted she was scared. But she was very afraid that this thing with the news might have helped Rafe decide he didn't need her or their baby in his life.

She wasn't thinking that because he was a jerk or anything. It was just that she understood that royals, especially those in a volatile newly reestablished monarchy, probably needed to be above reproach.

Her mind went to the video chat they'd had two nights ago. He hadn't exactly been staid on that call. She guessed that was what appealed to her about him.

She rubbed her stomach as she walked into the living room. Without turning on the lights, she went to her couch and turned on the television and the DVR to watch her comfort movie. But there was a knock on her door before the opening credits started to roll. She paused it and put her frozen yogurt container on the coffee table, grabbing her baseball bat from the hall closet before she went to the front door.

She pushed aside the curtain on the small, narrow window next to the door and peeked out, not sure what she'd find.

Rafe.

Illuminated by her front porch light, he stood there in faded jeans that fit in all the right places and a T-shirt that molded to his chest like a second skin. Not very regal tonight, was he. Very American and very real, though, she thought.

She unlatched the door and let it swing open, keeping her bat in one hand.

"Rafe."

Was he really here?

"Red. Planning to hit me with that bat?" he asked, pulling her into his arms and hugging her tightly. "I'm sorry I didn't return your calls."

"Why didn't you? When did you get back to the States?" she asked. She felt shell-shocked after everything that had been going on this evening. She hated to admit it but she was very glad to see him.

"No. The bat is not for you. I thought if I found that rat bastard reporter snooping around I might take it to him. I was afraid he might have slipped past the patrolmen."

"We don't need it tonight," he said. "Can I come in?"

She stood there feeling a little aggrieved now that she knew he wasn't a threat. That Rafe was here.

"How long have you been back in the States?"

"I got in this afternoon, right about the time the baby story broke," he said.

"And you came here? But not straight here," she

said. "It doesn't take that long to get here and I know you've got a helicopter."

"Can we do this inside?" he asked.

She felt the need in him to get his own way but she wasn't threatened by him at all. She stepped back and he walked in, closing the door and leaning back against it. First thing he did was take the bat and drop it on the floor. Then he lifted her off her feet with his hands on her waist.

"I missed you, Red," he said, lowering his mouth to hers and taking a kiss that left no doubt that he wasn't going to walk away from her. She had no idea what he thought their future would be, but she realized as she wrapped her arms around his shoulders that she wanted him by her side.

Rafe took his first deep breath since he'd stepped off the plane in Miami. He was with Em, and right now that was enough. His family, who had always been his stalwart supporters, weren't really there for him now. He tucked that away for further analysis later. He knew it was important, but right now he needed to figure out this threat and convince Emily that his plan to move forward was the best one.

"I thought coming home to you was going to be the first peace I've felt in a few days," he said as he lifted his head and stepped back from her.

"I didn't realize you were coming back to me," she said.

"Are you kidding me? I've been calling you every day. What else did you think that meant?"

She bit her lower lip, reaching behind him to bolt

the door before picking up her baseball bat and leaning it against the wall. "I didn't know."

She walked down the hallway lit only by little nightlights plugged into the wall sockets, and he followed her.

All this time he'd thought he was courting her...wait a minute. Was that what he'd been doing?

Yes.

No matter how he'd tried to rationalize it, that was exactly what he'd been doing.

"That's my bad. I was trying to be cool and see if you liked me," he said as he entered her living room. The television projected a soft blue glow into the room and he noted the opened container of frozen yogurt on the coffee table.

She sat in the chair that he had fond memories of making love to her in, with her legs curled under her body. With a quick economical movement she reached over and flicked on the light on the side table.

"I think we both know I *like* you," she said.

He sat down on the ottoman in front of her and put his hands on the arms of the chair. "I'm not talking about lust. I'm talking about whether you like me for the man I am. I don't think I did much but show off the last time I was in Key West. Trying to catch your eye and show you I wasn't like all the other men in the bar."

"You did that," she said softly. "If that was you showing off, you did it very well."

He winked at her. "After all this time I do know how to present a good image."

"It worked. So is that what you were doing in Alma with the people? I saw some of the press coverage from your trip. It looks like you were falling in love with the country and the people."

"You're talking about the blonde, right?" He laughed softly when she frowned and shook her head in denial. "Her family is nuts. They want her to marry the next king. She's not…real. It's not like when I'm with you," he said. Dita was a beautiful woman, but all the scheming with her mother made him edgy. And it was impossible to think of anything other than getting away from her.

"So what do you want from me?" Emily asked.

There it was. The million-dollar question. He had been debating it for so long and still had no answer. "Right now, I need to figure out how the media found out you were pregnant."

She nodded. "The easy stuff first."

It was interesting that she thought finding the source of the leak was going to be easy. "How is that the easy stuff? Do you know who broke the story?"

"Let's just say I have some suspicions, and if that little weasel is at the coffee shop tomorrow morning I intend to confirm them," she said. "I pretty much caught some guy eavesdropping on me when you and I were talking on the phone the other day. And yesterday…I had really bad bout of morning sickness at the coffee shop and Snoopy was right there talking to me about you. Seems odd, right?"

Rafe didn't like the idea that Emily had been targeted. How had the reporter been alerted to her presence? The community in Key West was a close-knit one and Rafe couldn't for the life of him imagine any of them talking about Emily.

It must have been someone who knew him. He remembered the way she'd sneaked into his penthouse. Maybe that was where the reporter had picked up the thread of the story. Maybe he'd followed her.

Hell, he had no idea.

He rubbed the back of his neck. He was tired.

"You're not confronting anyone," he said. "I'll go tomorrow and take care of it."

She put her hand on his chest and shoved him back so she could get up from the chair. Standing next to him, she put her hands on her hips and arched one eyebrow at him.

"One—you're not the boss of me. Sorry, I'm just not going to take orders. Two—that rat bastard played me and I want to make sure that doesn't happen again," she said. "So I'll take care of it."

It was late and he was tired of being pulled in too many directions, so perhaps that was why he let his temper slip as he stood up, towering over her. He put his hands on her shoulders and realized all he wanted to do was protect her, and that was the one thing that Emily didn't seem to want from him.

"Dammit, woman. I'm trying to keep you safe. I don't want any of this dirty press to affect you. I need to know that you aren't harmed by it."

"Why?" she asked. "Because you think I can't handle it?"

"Hell, Red. You can handle anything. I am doing this because I care about you and if anything hurt you I wouldn't be able to live with it."

Nine

Rafe pulled her to him and slammed his mouth down on hers, backing her up against the wall. The moment their mouths met his anger died. It felt like too long since he'd held her in his arms. She did that thing with her tongue where she twirled it around his, and he instantly got hard.

He cupped her butt and flexed his fingers, lifting her up until he could rub his erection right over the center of her body. She was naked under her shirt, and he liked the feel of her cool buttocks in his hands. She moved against him and he feathered his finger in a circle around the small of her back. She moaned and arched against him before tunneling her fingers into his hair and holding him to her while she plundered his mouth.

There was too much pent-up emotion between them.

They'd been in the same room together three times and each time it hadn't been enough. He wanted her. The way she got to him was unlike anything else he'd ever experienced, and his gut was starting to say he wouldn't find it with anyone else.

He sank to the floor when she sucked his bottom lip between her teeth and bit him lightly. Once he was on the floor, he pushed his hands up her back, felt the way her body arched over his. He rubbed his hand up her delicate spine, finding the sensitive nerves at the back of her neck, tracing a pattern over the skin of her nape.

She pulled back and looked up at him. Her lips were swollen, her face slightly flushed pink, making her freckles more prominent. Her eyes were brilliant in the dim light and he realized he'd never seen anything more beautiful.

He wanted her so much at this moment he couldn't think of anything but getting inside her.

"The other night was a pale imitation of this," she said, her husky voice turning him on.

"Damned straight," he said. He pulled her shirt up over her body and tossed it aside.

He set her back on his thighs as he stretched his legs out and held her there so he could look at her. He took in her breasts, which were slightly larger since her pregnancy, and those darker, fuller nipples. He lightly caressed them, running his finger over first one, then the other. She reached between them and pushed his T-shirt up his body.

He let go of her to rip it off and toss it carelessly to the side. She put her fingers on his pectorals and he flexed them. She sighed and traced her finger around each of his nipples before leaning forward to nip each of them in turn.

He brought his hands back to her breasts, but she took one of them and drew it slowly down the side of her body. He reached around behind her and grabbed her ass, bringing her closer. She rocked her pelvis over the ridge of his erection where it strained against the front of his jeans.

He brought one of his arms up behind her and held her with his hand on the back of her neck as he lowered his head and kissed his way down her neck to her shoulder blade. There was a large strawberry birthmark on her left shoulder and he kissed it, laving it with his tongue before he nibbled his way lower. He dropped small kisses around the full globe of her breast and then moved lower to the underside, biting lightly at the spot where her breast rested against her chest.

She moaned his name and rocked against him as she gripped his sides, trying to bring him closer to her. But he held her where she was. He wasn't ready to let her have free rein over his body. She'd been tormenting him for days with her conversations and the little pieces of her soul that she shared with him almost as if they were an afterthought.

He had her in his arms, but she was hard to hold. So hard to keep. And he was determined that he would keep her.

He sucked at the smooth skin between her breasts and then moved on to her other breast. This one was slightly smaller than its mate. He wanted to know everything about her, to know all these details instead of just being satisfied with sex. He needed more than the physical from her this time. He wanted to lay her completely bare so that maybe he'd have the answers that he'd been seeking.

He brought one of his hands up and slowly drew his finger in circles around her areola. He felt the texture of her nipple changing as it tightened under his finger and then he rubbed his finger back and forth against it until she leaned forward, catching the lobe of his ear between her teeth and biting down hard.

He lifted his head to look into her blue eyes. He swore he could see the same desire in her eyes to get rid of all the questions and doubts that remained between them. But he knew he might just be projecting what he wanted to see. He needed something from her that he couldn't define.

She swiped her tongue around the rim of his ear and he got even harder. Uncomfortable now, he reached between their bodies, distracted by the feel of her wet sex against the back of his fingers. He turned his hand and palmed her. He liked the feel of her springy curls as he rotated his palm against her.

She arched her back and shifted against him. He teased the opening of her body with his finger and then slowly pushed it up into her. She tightened around him. And he felt as if he were going to explode. He wanted to feel her naked flesh against him.

Though he did like her naked on his lap while he was still clothed. He pulled back and looked down at her, wanting to keep this moment in his mind forever.

He used his thumb to find her clit. He tapped it lightly and then made a small circle. She responded instantly. He felt the minute tightening of her body around his finger as he continued to rub his thumb in a circle over her center.

He lowered his mouth to her breast and took her nipple between his lips, swirling his tongue over it and then sucking. Her hands were on his shoulders, nails digging into them as she rocked against his hand. She arched her shoulders and pulled her breast from his mouth.

Their eyes met and all the things he'd been afraid to say seemed to hover in the air around them. He opened his mouth and she leaned forward and kissed him.

She started to rock more quickly. She sucked his tongue deep into her mouth and plunged it back and forth to the same rhythm of his finger inside her body. Her thighs tightened around his hand and he pulled his mouth from hers.

"Come for me," he said, whispering the words against her ear.

Her hips moved more frantically and he added a second finger inside her body as she cried out his name. She thrust her hips rapidly against him and then she shuddered and fell forward, resting her head on his shoulder. Her breath was warm against his neck as she reached her hand down between them and unzipped his jeans.

Her touch through the opening of his pants almost made him come. He felt a drop leak out of him and slowly pulled his hand from her body and got to his feet, lifting her up into his arms. He didn't want this to end too quickly

He carried her down the small hallway and into her bedroom, setting her down on her feet next to the bed. She had wrapped one arm around his shoulder, holding on to him and idly toying with the hair at the back of his neck, while her other arm was awkwardly wedged between them, her hand wrapped around his length.

She stroked him up and down, her finger swirling over the top of him. His hips jerked forward and no matter how much his mind said that he was going to take this slowly, his body had different plans.

He let her body slide down his. She moaned as her hardened nipples rubbed over his chest, and he closed his eyes as he felt the dampness of her core against the front of his boxers.

He stepped back and shoved his pants and underwear down his legs and then nudged her forward until she fell back on the bed. Her legs sprawled apart slightly, her hair fanning out around her head, one brilliant dark red curl falling over her shoulder. She had her hands on the top of her thighs and she watched him with hungry eyes.

He wanted to say something profound because the emotions he felt for her welled up inside him, but instead all he could think about was touching and tasting every inch of her.

"Are you just going to stand there and stare at me?" she asked, a tinge of wry amusement visible on her face.

"I'm debating where to start. Every time we've been together I want to make it last...I haven't had the chance to taste you or to explore every one of those lovely freckles of yours."

"There's plenty of time for that later. I want you now," she said.

Her words lanced through him and his erection jumped. He shook his head. Every time he thought he had the upper hand with Emily she did something to remind him that he was putty in her hands. Now and always.

She reached for his length, circling him with her thumb and forefinger at the root. She slowly drew her hand up, closing the circle of her fingers around him as she did so. Involuntarily he thrust closer to her and she smiled up at him as a drop of precome glistened on the tip of his erection. She swiped her finger over it and then brought it to her mouth.

He groaned and crawled up over her body, and then put his hands on her hips and forced her to move back on the bed. He took her hands in his and drew them up over her head as he settled his hips between hers and the tip of his erection found the moist center of her body.

He drew his hips back and then thrust forward again, entering her slowly. She arched underneath him and yet still he resisted the urge to plunge his way all the way home. She turned her hands under his, laced their fingers together and looked up at him.

"Take me," she said.

He nodded as he drove himself hilt-deep into her body. She sighed and arched against him again and he started to thrust in and out, taking them both closer and closer to the edge. He pulled his hand free of hers and drew it down her side as he rocked back and forth. Going deeper each time and taking them higher and higher.

She ran her finger down his back and he jerked his hips forward as he came. Then he felt her legs tighten around his hips and heard her calling his name as she climaxed.

He kept driving into her until she bit him softly on

the shoulder and sighed. She turned her head to face him and he saw the completion on her face. He found her lips with his and gave her a soft, gentle kiss.

Rafe wanted to believe that everything was okay between them but he knew that sex hadn't made it so. From the beginning their bond had been strong and physical. That created its own sort of problems. He wanted to just keep making love to her and pretending that was enough, but he knew it wasn't. And there were things he had to say that she might not want to hear.

But for this moment he wanted to just hold her, look up at the moon and pretend that everything was okay.

Emily woke up in the middle of the night having to go to the bathroom. This was something that had only started in the last week. She had read in one of her prenatal books that things like this were only the beginning.

Rafe was cuddled behind her and propped himself up on an elbow as she climbed from the bed. "You okay?" he asked.

"Yes. Be right back."

He fell back down on the pillow and she knew he was tired. They'd resolved nothing except that they still wanted each other. But she felt as if this time they'd done more than just have sex. Rafe meant more to her than any other guy she'd ever dated, and she acknowledged that it had nothing to do with the fact that he was the father of her child—and yet at the same time had everything to do with that.

He made her feel more alive than anyone else ever had, and that was dangerous. She didn't want to rely on him. He could sleep in her bed and come to her bar.

Hell, he could even be involved with their baby, but she didn't want to care for him.

She washed her hands and leaned forward to look at herself in the mirror.

"Don't fall for him," she warned herself. But she sort of already knew that it was too late.

That falling for Rafe was a foregone conclusion now.

He'd come to her in the middle of the night. Wanted to defend her. Everyone knew she could take care of herself, but he still wanted to protect her.

That made her feel so safe. So cherished.

Things that had never mattered to her before tonight.

She shook her head.

He had to want something. There had to be a reason he was here tonight. She wanted it to be for her, but maybe it was about the baby. Now that the world knew about their child, the decisions they'd been making together took on a different quality. Whatever he did could impact his people back in Alma.

She knew that. She wanted it to not matter, but she knew it did.

And she also was very aware that she wasn't cut out to be a queen or consort or whatever the hell they had in Alma.

Maybe that was why he was here.

She left the bathroom and stood in the doorway leading back into the bedroom, watching him as he lay sleeping, his big, strong, sexy body taking up too much of her bed, his face relaxed in sleep. He didn't seem as if he had an agenda. He didn't act as if there were some reason he was in her bed other than that he wanted to be there.

But she knew there had to be more.

She lived in the real world, and stained glass mermaid aside, Rafe had always been very real with her. . When they'd spent their one weekend together, he'd made it clear that would be it. As had she. And when she'd barged in on him in Miami and told him she was pregnant he hadn't pretended they were suddenly a couple.

"I thought you got lost, Red."

She thought she did, too. The first time she'd looked into his hazel eyes.

"I almost did. Why are you here, Rafe?" she asked.

"Come back to bed," he said.

She walked over and sat on the edge of the bed, but he lifted the sheets and gestured for her to come closer. She wanted to. She started to lie down in the curve of his body but stopped herself.

"I need some answers. So far all we've done is establish what we both already knew. We want each other. We have some kind of lust that won't be denied. But I need some answers."

"Okay."

"Okay?"

"Sure. Ask your questions," he said, sitting up and propping his back on the headboard. "I figured we'd do this in the morning."

"I don't think I can sleep until I know if you are going to take my child from me."

She hadn't meant to say it that way. But it was 3:00 a.m. and her guard was down. Her fears were all around her. Rafe was a powerful man before she even factored in the fact that he was about to become the ruler of a foreign land.

"Hell. No. I'm not going to take our child from you,"

he said. "Why would you think I'd do that? I'm not an asshole."

She swallowed hard. "I know you aren't. But we both know I'm not the kind of woman your family has been hoping you'll marry. And now that the world knows I'm carrying the king of Alma's child, I think the stakes have changed."

He reached for her. Took her hand in his and brought it to his mouth. He dropped a warm kiss in the center of her palm before placing her hand on his chest right over his heart.

"I haven't changed, Red. I'm still the man you know. I'm not going to let anything change me."

She wanted to believe him. But the monarchy was bigger than Rafe, whether he wanted to admit it or not.

He tugged her off balance and into his arms. Rolling until she was tucked underneath him. He kissed her long and slow, and she felt her fears for the future disappearing slowly.

In his embrace she felt as if things would work out, but she feared that was false hope until she knew how he felt about her. Until she had some promises... But she'd never had a man make her promises. Never wanted them until now. Until Rafe. She needed something from him, but she was afraid to admit that even to herself.

How the hell was she going to tell him that she wanted him to be by her side? Not because of the baby, but because she needed him.

She tipped her head, closing her eyes and pretending that she had the answers she needed. But she knew that things were even more complicated now than they had been before.

Ten

Rafe woke with the sun, since he was still on European time, and left Emily sleeping quietly in her bed. Last night he'd almost lost her. He still wasn't sure he'd said the right thing or even done enough to keep her. But today he intended to change all of that.

He went out to his car and retrieved the bag that Jose had packed and brought it into the house. He scanned the street while he did so, but saw no reporters hanging around, which was reassuring. As were the two cop cars parked at each end of her street. There was no foot traffic on her block today either.

He found eggs and the fixings for an omelet in Emily's fridge and set to making breakfast for her. His hands were sweating when he put it all on the breakfast tray he'd found in her pantry. He dashed outside to pick a hibiscus from the flowering bush in her backyard and put it in a small teacup with some water. Then he patted his pocket to make sure the ring hadn't disappeared and walked back to her bedroom.

With any other woman this kind of gesture might be enough to make her swoon. But Rafe suspected it might not be enough with Red.

She was still asleep on her side with his pillow tucked up against her. She looked small and vulnerable as she slept. During the day she was a virago, constantly moving and challenging everything in her path. But like this it was easy to see she wasn't as invincible as she wanted the world to believe. Feeling like a voyeur, he put the tray on her dresser and snapped a quick photo of her with his iPhone.

Then he walked over to the bed and sat down next to her. He was tempted to slide back under the sheets with her. Make love to her again, but sex was tearing away layers that he usually used to insulate himself against women. And he couldn't afford to let Emily any closer to him than she already was.

Love was a fairy tale, one he wasn't too sure existed. He'd seen what his father had done for love and how that had torn their entire family apart.

"Em…"

"Um…"

"Wake up, sleepyhead."

She blinked up at him and shoved her hand through her thick red hair, pushing it back off her face. She sat up, ran her tongue over her teeth and then looked at him. "Aren't you chipper in the morning."

He was. He'd always been a morning person, but he sensed that she wasn't and decided silence was the better part of valor. "I'm still on a different time zone. I brought you coffee."

"I can only have decaf," she said.

"That's what I made since it was on the counter next to your machine," he said.

"Thank you," she said, reaching for the mug. Blowing on the surface of the hot liquid before taking a sip, she closed her eyes, seeming to savor it as that first swallow went down.

He felt himself stir and shook his head.

Really. Was there nothing she could do that wouldn't turn him on?

"You haven't tried the omelet yet," he said as he knelt on the bed and settled the tray over her lap.

"No. For trying to protect me. For doing this," she said. "I'm just not the kind of woman men usually do this kind of thing for."

"Yes, you are," he said.

She wrinkled her brow as she stared over at him. He took off the lid that he'd used to cover her plate so it wouldn't get cold and smiled over at her.

"Are you arguing with me?"

"Yeah, I am. I made you breakfast in bed, so clearly you are the right type. The other guys in your life haven't measured up."

She put her coffee on the tray and leaned over to kiss him. It was a little clumsy and tasted of sleepy woman and coffee. He wanted more but she pulled back.

"You're saying all the right things this morning."

"I try. How's your stomach?" he asked. "I didn't even think about your morning sickness."

"I'm not sure I can eat too much, but the coffee seems okay right now."

"That's good. I had Jose get me a bunch of books on pregnancy but haven't had a chance to read them yet," he said.

He wanted to know what was going to be happening to her so he could anticipate her needs. Make everything easier for her.

They shared the breakfast he made and then he set the tray to the side and lay next to her on the bed. "Do you have to work today?"

"No. Do you?"

"No. I'm supposed to lie low," he said. And make everything with Emily right in the eyes of the world. But that part was still better left unspoken for now.

"Good. What do you want to do?"

"Well…"

He pulled her into his arms and then rolled over, bracing his body on top of hers. He put his hand on her stomach and dropped a quick kiss there before looking up at her. He worked his free hand into the pocket of his pants and pulled out the ring box.

"I'm hoping that you'll agree to marry me, Red."

He put the ring box on her stomach and then opened it up so she could see the thin band with the pear-shaped diamond. He'd chosen the band lined with aquamarine because that stone reminded him of her eyes. He shifted to his side, knelt next to her and stared down into her heart-shaped face. "I hope you'll say yes."

She stared up at him for a long moment and he had the feeling she wasn't going to say yes. What had he done wrong? He'd made the big romantic gesture; he'd purchased a ring that reminded him of her.

He was being a good guy. Doing everything by the book of romance. He'd seen his sister reading fairy tales and *Cosmo* so he knew that he had to come across as modern and thoughtful but also deliver on all Emily's secret dreams.

It was a big ask of a man who was used to women falling for him. Especially after the time he'd spent on Alma with Dita and her ilk fawning over him.

"What did I do wrong?"

"Nothing," she said. "I like the ring and the breakfast, but I like my mermaid, too."

He processed that.

The mermaid had been a stroke of genius. Well, really it had been the gesture of a man who missed his woman.

"Doesn't matter if you wear the ring, you're mine."

"I'm yours?"

"We both know it. There isn't a wannabe debutante in all the world who can compare to you, Red."

She gave him a haughty look and then ruined it by laughing. "I know it."

"What about you?"

"Huh?"

"Is there anyone else in your life?"

"Would I be with you if there was?" she asked. "I like you way more than I should, Rafael. Your life is literally worlds away from here but I can't help letting you into my house and my bed. I'm just trying to keep us both from making a mistake."

Maybe he could convince her to say yes. This was the opening he needed. "It's not a mistake. Trust me. Together, we can take on anything."

"For now. But what happens when the newness of being lovers wears off and we have a baby who doesn't

sleep through the night? And you have to run a kingdom?"

He saw where she was coming from. And realized
the fears she had stemmed from the fact that she didn't
know him. Didn't realize how unstoppable he was once
he made his mind up.

"I said I'd give you time to get to know me, and
once you do, you will know that isn't going to be an
issue," he said.

Frankly this shocked her. Rafe didn't strike her as
all that traditional. And she knew that he was still trying to figure out the next few months of his life. She
wasn't going to be his lifesaver. His safety valve. And
that's what this felt like.

"No." The little girl who never had a mom and a dad
desperately wanted her to say yes. But she'd learned
long ago that the things she wanted most were the ones
that made her make the dumbest decisions. And marriage wasn't something to be entered into lightly. Rafe
was going to be king. He should have a wife who was
in it for the long haul.

He was going to have to do a lot of work to make
the monarchy stick in Alma. *Alma*. She wasn't even
sure where it was. Maybe she should have looked that
up on the internet instead of ogling pictures of Rafe as
he toured the island nation. But she hadn't.

"No?" he asked. "Red, think this through."

"I can't marry you," she said. She could, but it
wasn't under these circumstances. If he'd asked her
the first time she'd shown up on his doorstep pregnant
she might have said yes. But too much had happened
since then and she couldn't trust his motives.

They knew each other so much better now than they had a mere two weeks earlier, but still not well enough. Or from her perspective, maybe too well. She wanted that man who sent her the stained glass to fall down on his knees and beg her to marry him.

That wasn't going to happen. Rafe liked her. He wanted her but he didn't love her.

"Are you asking me because I'm pregnant?" she asked at last.

He rolled off the bed and got to his feet. He put his hands on his lean hips and stood there as if he could will her to change her mind. She wished he'd put a shirt on, because his bare chest was a tempting distraction.

But not enough of one that she'd say yes to this. She knew if she said yes she'd want him to love her. Why? She'd been fine with lust until this moment, and now she wanted professions of deep emotion from him. Emotion she wasn't prepared to admit she felt for him.

They didn't love each other. She had never thought she was one of those women who needed it, but in her heart she knew she did. She wasn't as practical as she'd expected to be when it came to Rafe. He was arguing that they'd be stronger together, and she thought if they loved each other then he might be right. But a couple who married for the sake of a child? That seemed like a steep hill to climb.

Maybe it was because her mother had never compromised and married that Emily felt so strongly about this. But she couldn't help it. She wasn't going to marry him for any reason. Unless he fell in love with her and proved it in some way that would convince her. She liked him. She cared about him and she had no intention of isolating him from his child. But marriage?

No. Definitely not.

"Partly. I'm traditional, Red. You know that. I want our baby to have my name. And to know who I am. We can do that so much better together," he said. He scrubbed one hand over his eyes and then sat down on the edge of the bed with his back toward her. "Every child needs a mom and a dad. Didn't you miss having a dad?"

"I did," she said. "But I found my way without one. And Harry's sort of filled the role for me. It's all I needed."

"I don't want our kid to have a relationship with some future boyfriend of yours," he said.

"Don't. Don't think of any of that. We are going to get to know each other. We will figure this out."

She crawled over to him and wrapped her arms around his shoulders, leaning her head on his chest to look at him. "Marriage like this isn't a solution. We'd have to be more businesslike and we aren't. The way you get to me…it's all I can do to remind myself every day that you belong on the throne of Alma and I have no place by your side."

He covered her hands with his and clasped them to his chest. "You might."

She shook her head and slid around on the bed next to him. He was so serious, this man of hers. "Is that why you are asking me?"

"Yes. I care for you, Emily," he said. "I want what's best for you and our child. And if you are my fiancée I can protect you from the media. I can bring the full force of the Montoro name and reputation to bear against these people. I can do it now, but they will just glom onto the fact that I'm not marrying you or taking you to Alma. Being my fiancée will make every-thing easier."

She felt the sincerity in his words. Understood that he was willing to tie his life to hers to keep her safe. But for how long? Because she knew that she didn't want to leave Key West, and there was no way he could rule from here.

"I can't."

"Don't say no. Think about it. Let's see if I can change your mind," he said.

She had no doubt that he could. If she spent time with him and fell any deeper for him then she'd say yes. She'd exchange her life for his. And she knew her-self well enough to know that she'd be angry with that.

"How?"

"Let's date and get to know each other. In a few weeks I'll ask you again," he said.

"How will we do that? Do I have to fly to Alma?"

"No. I'm in Miami to wrap up a few business deals. So while I'm here let's date."

"Okay. But what if the answer is still no. What then?" she asked.

"I'm pretty determined it won't be," he said. "And I've never lost a challenge."

"Never?"

"Nope. I'm not afraid to do whatever I have to in order to win you over."

She believed him but she also knew this decision wasn't his alone. "What about your family?"

"Leave them to me. I'd like you to come to Miami Beach next week, stay at my place and meet everyone who's here with me at a dinner. Would you do that?"

She pursed her lips but then nodded. "What day? I'll have to check my schedule at the bar."

"I was hoping for Friday night. But I know that's one of your busiest nights and this relationship isn't all about me. So you tell me which day works for you," he said.

She reached for her phone on the nightstand and checked her work schedule. Harry was going to transition her to the daytime shift starting next week since her pregnancy had really started showing.

She texted Beau, the other bartender, to see if he'd fill in for her on Friday and Saturday. He was always looking for more money and immediately responded that he could.

"Friday is fine," she said.

"Great. Now what should we do today?" he asked.

"I have a few ideas," she said. "But you're going to need swim trunks."

"I packed for a couple of days. I'm good."

The beach that Emily took him to later that afternoon was deserted and well off the beaten path. They had to carry the paddleboard from her car through a stand of mangroves to the water's edge. There were cicadas chirping and the smell of salt water mixed with ripe vegetation. It was so Florida.

The heat beat down on his back and he wore a baseball cap and large sunglasses to protect his face from the sun. Emily had surprised him by giving him a lecture about the dangers of skin cancer even to someone with his olive complexion. So he'd donned her SPF 50 sun cream and the hat even though he never burned.

Her mothering had charmed him. And it was mothering. She'd kind of ensured he had the cream on and taken her time rubbing it on his back, which had led them back to the bedroom. Hence the late start at the beach.

She'd also packed a cooler of fruit juice, sandwiches and veggies. He'd seldom—okay, never —taken a day like this. It was a Monday. He should be in Miami getting ready for the weekly management meeting where he should be discussing the new shipping deal and getting all the routes worked out for their customers, but truth be told he wouldn't trade this for anything.

The way his family had reacted when they'd landed had worried Rafe. He had the sinking feeling in his gut that they were going to make him choose between Emily and their baby and the throne. And as usual when he got his back up that meant he got stubborn. He wasn't too sure he wanted the throne, but he wasn't about to let his family force him out of it.

He had the Coleman cooler in one hand and the paddleboard under his other arm. She'd said she could help carry stuff but he'd said no. He found that he liked making gallant gestures. This morning when she'd turned down his proposal, he'd realized she hadn't had a lot of men doing that for her. And he was determined to convince her that he was the right guy for her.

On that front, he wasn't backing down.

"This spot looks good. We can leave the cooler here. Actually," she said with a blush, "we could have left it in the car. It's not that far to walk back for a snack."

"Then why did I carry it down here?"

She crossed her arms over her chest and gave him a chagrined look. "Because you were so stubborn about me helping carry the board. I hate being bossed."

"You mentioned that. But this isn't bossing, it's pampering. Like when you insisted I wear sunscreen."

She started to argue but then stuck her tongue out at him. "You're right. But don't make a habit of it."

He threw his head back and laughed. She kept him on his toes no matter how much he didn't want to admit it. He liked the challenge of being with her.

"So you've never been on a paddleboard before?" she asked.

"Nope. Never even surfed. I am scuba certified though. Want to do that instead?"

"Yes but the water around here isn't that deep. Snorkeling would be better. We could do that tonight. I know a gorgeous place where we can go at sunset. In fact, if my mom doesn't mind, we can take her boat," she said.

"I'd like to meet your mom," he said.

She got really still. "Why?"

"Because she's your mom," Rafe said. "Why else?"

"Don't try to get her on your side with this engagement thing, okay?"

He put the board on the sand and walked over to her, putting his finger under her chin and tipping her head back so he could see her eyes under the bill of her baseball cap. "When you say yes—and I'm betting you eventually do—it will be because you've decided you want to marry me. Not because I pressured you into saying yes. Got it?"

She punched him playfully in the shoulder and ran down toward the waterline. "I've got it. Get that board and come on, Your Majesty. It's time for your first lesson."

Rafe followed her to the water and they spent the

next thirty minutes with her showing him how to get his balance on the board. Finally Emily decided he could take a turn rowing and he got about two strokes in before he fell into the warm Atlantic Ocean.

He glanced at the shore to find her standing there laughing.

"I bet it wasn't easy for you at first," he said as he swam back to shore with the board.

"I don't remember. I've been on the water since before I could walk," she said.

"So you grew up here?"

"Since I was three, so I think that counts, doesn't it?"

"Pretty much. I was born in Coral Gables and grew up there," he said.

"Florida native."

"Well, just my generation," he said.

He looked at her and the future suddenly didn't seem as nebulous as it always had. The future was real and it was staring back at him with red hair and blue eyes. And that made Alma seem farther away than ever.

"Why don't you stand on the end of my board and look studly and I'll take you on a tour of this inlet?" she asked.

"Studly?"

"Yeah. Oh, is that an insult to your masculinity?" she teased. "I figured after that dunking you gave yourself you might like to play it safe."

He rushed her, scooping her up in his arms and carrying her into the water. "I never play it safe, Red. And I'm not the only one who's going to get a dunking."

He fell backward into the water, keeping her in his arms and drenching them both. She swiveled in his arms and when they both surfaced she kissed him. One kiss led to another and Rafe realized he was having the best afternoon of his life.

He told himself it was just the relief at being away from the pressures of leading Alma and Montoro Enterprises, but his heart said his future was tied to this woman.

Eleven

Emily had felt more at ease staring down a belligerent drunk at Shady Harry's than she did standing in the formal dining room of the Montoros' Coral Gables mansion holding a tonic water with lime in one hand. Rafael III had turned his back on her when she entered the room with Rafe, who had been called away by Jose. He'd seemed reluctant to leave her but she'd urged him to go. She was rethinking that opinion now.

Juan Carlos looked less than pleased to actually meet her and the PR guy Geoff had muttered under his breath that she was no style icon. Well, who was? She was a real person. She wasn't going to apologize for who she was.

Tia Isabella had been feeling well enough to be up with the family. She and her nurse were in one corner with Rafe's sister Bella. Tia Isabella was in a wheelchair and her hands and head kept shaking because of her advanced Parkinson's. When her nurse invited Emily over to join the women, she was grateful. Isabella had beautiful white hair and was the only one to smile at Emily and make her feel truly welcome.

"Hello, Emily," Bella said, coming up behind her and putting her arm around her.

"Bella right? Or should I call you Lady Bella?"

"Just Bella is fine. You look like you are about to bolt."

"I am."

"Well, don't. I've never seen Rafe like this before."

"Like what?"

"Unsettled."

"That's good. He's too sure he knows it all," Emily said.

Bella laughed and Emily noticed that her brothers smiled at the sound. "Rafe mentioned going out on your mother's boat…Is it a yacht?"

Emily realized that Bella was really in a different world. "No. She's a marine biologist. Her boat is like the station wagon of the sea."

"Did you grow up on it? Like Jacques Cousteau's family?"

"No. She had a grant that enabled her to return to Key West every night," Emily said.

"Sounds fascinating."

They were called to dinner and Rafe rejoined her. "How'd it go?"

"Most of your family hate me. If they could make me disappear they would," she said.

"They don't hate you," Rafe said.

"Don't lie to me," she retorted.

"Well, it's not you. It's the fact that I am putting our family's return to Alma and the throne in a very delicate state. No one, not even me, wants that."

Emily wanted to apologize but she couldn't. She wasn't sorry she was having his baby or that she'd gotten to know him. But she was sorry that they'd met now when his life wasn't his own. And when his family would never approve of her.

The next two weeks were busy and though Rafe would be happy to stop flying back and forth between Key West and Miami, he enjoyed every second he spent with Emily.

Tonight he was cruising toward the setting sun with Jessica, Harry and Emily. His first meeting with Emily's mom had been tense but ever since Emily had wrapped her arm around his waist and given her mom a stubborn look, Jessica had been sort of friendly toward him. Harry on the other hand looked as if he was going to need more than a stern look from Emily.

If he didn't know that they were going night diving, he'd have been worried.

"Beer?" Harry asked, walking up to him where he sat on a padded bench at the stern of the boat.

"Nah, I'm good."

Harry sat down next to him and took a sip of his Corona. Emily and her mom were at the helm of the boat talking and laughing as they got out of the no-wake zone. Suddenly Jessica hit the throttle and they were flying full speed across the ocean.

As the wind buffeted Rafe, Harry leaned forward, shouting a little to be heard over the noise. "What are your plans with our girl?"

"None of your business," Rafe shouted back. "No disrespect but you and I both know she'll skin us alive if we discuss it behind her back."

Harry threw his head back and gave a great shout of laughter. The other man was big and solid, but no taller than Rafe. And he'd noticed over the past couple weeks how Harry watched out for Emily as no other adult in her life had.

Her mom, though sweet and loving toward Emily, spent most of her time thinking about her research and reapplying for grants. Her entire world was the ocean and the creatures in it.

It had been startling to realize that in essence Emily had raised herself. That was probably why she was so tough, so feisty and so damned independent. She had a lifetime of doing things on her own. How the hell was he going to convince her that she needed him by her side?

But he understood why the arguments he'd been making hadn't worked. What was it that she needed? The one thing she couldn't give herself, he suspected, was the key to bringing her around.

His phone buzzed. He'd hoped they'd be out of range but no such luck. He looked down and saw he had received a text from Geoff Standings once again asking again if he could run with their release announcing Rafe's engagement to Emily.

He texted back no and then shut his phone off. His family didn't get how delicate the situation was and thought that he could order her to marry him.

As if.

"Just know if you hurt her, bud, I'm coming after you," Harry said with that slightly maniacal grin of his.

"That's the last thing I want to do," Rafe said loudly.

Jessica killed the engines and his words sort of echoed around the boat as everything went quiet.

"What's the last thing you want to do?" Emily said, coming over and sitting on his lap. She wrapped her arm around his shoulders and reached over to take Harry's beer. "No drinking and diving, Harry. That's dangerous."

"It was one beer, kiddo. And barely that," Harry said, getting up and going over to Jessica.

"What is the last thing you'd do?" she asked Rafe when they were alone. He heard the sounds of Jessica and Harry getting the scuba gear ready behind them.

"Hurt you," he said, looking down into her pretty blue eyes.

"No promises, remember?" she said, standing up.

He grabbed her wrist, keeping her by his side as he had a sudden flash of insight into what it was she needed but was afraid to ask for. She needed promises and she needed them to be kept.

"I'm making this one, Red. And I'm keeping it," he said.

"What about Alma and your family?" she asked.

"What about them? That has nothing to do with you and me."

She snorted and shook her head. "It has everything to do with us. I'm complicating things. I think we both know that dinner with your family didn't go very well because of it. They think…heck, I have no idea what they think. But they don't like me much."

He wondered if that were true. He believed his family didn't feel one way or another about Emily. It was him they were frustrated with. They needed him to make her his fiancée or get her out of the picture. They needed him to clean up his act so they could continue with the coronation plans. But he wasn't playing their game.

"It's me they're pissed at," he said. "I'm sure they will like you once they get to know you."

She gave him an incredulous look. "I thought you were going to be a king of Alma, not fairy-tale land."

He laughed. "I am."

"You two done flirting?" Harry called, interrupting their argument. "Ready to do some diving?"

"Yes, we are, Harry," Emily said, walking over and getting her gear on.

Rafe followed her, wishing things were as simple as flirting. But nothing with her ever was.

He joined her family and went over the side of the boat after they'd put the diver down flag in the water. He noticed that everyone scattered in their own direction.

He followed close by Emily's side and reached for her hand, linking them together. She looked at him for a moment, her face not very clear behind the glass of her scuba mask, and then led him through the underwater world. She pointed out different species of fish and coral, and caught up in the natural beauty of his surroundings, he forgot his troubles. There was something very peaceful about snorkeling. But when they surfaced, he knew that nothing had changed in their world.

But he felt strongly that he and Emily had crossed a bridge into new territory.

"That was nice," she said, treading water next to him.

"Yes, it was. Exactly what I need after a day full of

meetings and demands," he said as they took off their tanks and put them in the boat.

"What is?"

Time with the woman he loved.

Shock held him in place as he realized that he did love her.

Versailles was the most famous Cuban restaurant in Miami. Hell, probably the world. Rafe had a night away from his family planned for himself and Emily. And grabbing Cuban sandwiches at his favorite restaurant was exactly the right sort of tone he wanted to set.

He needed Emily to accept his proposal, but pressuring her wasn't the way to get the job done. So he'd been as smooth as he could be, trying not to pressure her into making a decision that he needed from her. And the sooner, the better.

Every day she waited just made his family more anxious. At first it was just the inner circle of his father, brother and cousin, but now his more distant relatives—even his ill Tia Isabella—were asking him when he was going to announce his engagement.

He suspected Tia Isabella was being egged on by his cousin Juan Carlos, the one who wanted the family's return to the throne of Alma to be…triumphant. Not mired in scandal.

Rafe got that.

He'd even had a meeting with Montoro Enterprises' board of directors today. They had been pretty threatening; the upshot was, if he screwed up things in Alma he might not be CEO for much longer.

But the more his family pushed, the less he responded. None of that mattered tonight. The dinner with Emily hadn't gone well. And they'd called a "family" meeting to discuss the matter tomorrow.

Tonight he was going to seduce the hell out of Emily and secure her as his fiancée and then go into the meeting with his family he had scheduled for tomorrow and take control of the situation.

Waiting on Emily, waiting on his family—he felt shackled on all sides. He couldn't take action the way he needed to so that he could move forward.

He and Emily were seated against the wall in the glass-and-mirrored main room of the restaurant. All around him he heard people talking in Spanish. The Cuban dialect was different from the Castilian Spanish that many of the people of Alma used. Cuban Spanish was much more familiar to him.

"So what's on the agenda tonight?" Emily said after they had placed their order.

"Dinner, dancing and then I'll show you the harbor from my rooftop patio. I think you will be impressed."

"I'm never not impressed by you, Rafe."

"Thank you. Perhaps I should ask you that question again?"

She shook her head and her face got a little pinched. "Please don't. Can we have tonight and just be Emily and Rafe, not the future king and his errant pregnant lover?"

He realized that she was facing a different kind of pressure. She'd agreed to come to Miami for a few days after a group of paparazzi had staked out Shady Harry's in Key West. It was either take the security offered by staying in his penthouse or go out on the boat with her mother.

He was pleased she'd chosen to come to him. He

felt as if they had gotten so much closer over the last few weeks together.

"Yes, we can," he said.

"Great. So tell me why you picked this restaurant. I know it's famous and all that, but I wouldn't expect you to be a regular here."

He leaned back in the chair. "Well, the food is the best. You can't find a better Cuban sandwich anywhere in the city. But when I was younger, about ten or so, our mom used to bring Gabe, Bella and me here for dinners on the nights when our dad was in one of his moods and ranting all over the place. And later it was the first place she took us when we got Gabe back."

"Where'd he go?" Emily asked.

"In his early twenties, he was kidnapped while working for our South American division. He ultimately escaped. When we got him back, Mom packed us all up and brought us here. I always associate this place with happy times."

"Where is your mom?" she asked.

"She's remarried and pretty much enjoying her life now that she's out from under the burden of her marriage to our father."

"Do you see her at all?"

"I don't see her very often. But we text. It's enough for me," he said.

She nodded. "It's like that with my mom. I know other people have these crazy-close relationships with their parents but that was never us. She raised me to think for myself and do things for myself."

"Same," Rafe said. "My father gave me the legacy... that sort of feeling of pride in being a Montoro, and my mom gave me the strength to stand on my own while I carry out my version of what that means."

Emily reached across the table and linked their hands together. "I wonder what we will give our baby?"

"Probably everything we never had and always wanted," Rafe said.

Their food arrived and their conversation drifted to lighter topics like bands and books and movies. Everything but the one thing Rafe wanted to discuss. But she'd asked for time, for an evening where they were like every other young couple out on a date.

And he struggled to give it to her. This felt like a game she was playing, and if he wasn't so sure of her confusion about what to do with him, he'd demand an answer. But he knew she wasn't acting maliciously. She was pregnant by a man she hadn't intended to get to know better. The fact that they liked each other as much as they did was fate.

Fate.

Was that what this was?

They weren't like everyone else. They never were going to be. And the fact that Emily wanted them to be didn't make him feel confident for their future together. It started a niggling bit of doubt in the seat of his soul where he'd been confident until now that he could have it all. The throne, his child and Emily by his side.

The rhythm of Little Havana pulsed around them as they walked up Calle Ocho. Rafe reached out and grabbed her hand, lacing their fingers together. Tonight they were pretending that nothing else existed.

But she was aware of the reporters who had followed them from Rafe's South Beach penthouse and were now probably taking photos of them. She wore a Carolina Herrera dress she'd found in a vintage shop earlier in the week. It was a cocktail number in turquoise that hugged her curves on top and had a plunging neckline that gave way to a full skirt that masked her small baby bump.

Everything had been different between her and Rafe since earlier in the week when he'd come diving with her in Key West.

She couldn't put her finger on it, but she knew a lot of it had to do with the new feelings she had for him. It was silly to call it anything but love. Except that she wasn't too sure what love was.

Her mom and she had a relationship based on mutual respect and caring. She could count on one hand the times her mom had told her she loved her. It wasn't that Emily felt unlovable before this; it was just that she struggled to believe these feelings were real.

"Have you been here before?" he asked as they approached the club.

"Little Havana?" she asked.

He nodded.

"Yes. This club—no. I'm not usually on the celebrity radar…though in this dress, I bet I could get in without you tonight."

"You might be able to," Rafe agreed. "The owner and I went to school together."

"The hottie baseball player?"

"He's married. And you're spoken for," Rafe said.

"Am I?"

"You are. We could make it official. I've been carrying your ring around in my pocket."

"Not tonight," she said. She was closer to saying

yes. The more time they spent together, the more she realized that being his wife was...well, exactly what she wanted.

"Prepare to be amazed," he said. "They pulled out all the stops with this club."

Emily's breath caught as they were waved past the line of waiting guests and through the grand entrance. The Chihuly chandelier in the lobby was exquisite. But then when wasn't a Chihuly glamorous?

The club was divided into several different areas. The main floor in front of the stage was a huge dance area surrounded by high-stooled tables and cozy booths set in darkened alcoves. On the second floor, where they were headed tonight, was a mezzanine that overlooked the main club and featured a Latin-inspired dance floor. The hottest Latin groups performed there. Regular people and celebrities mingled, brought together by the sexy samba beats of the music.

"Rafael! Hey, dude," said a tall, broad-shouldered man coming over to them. "Do I have to genuflect now?"

Rafe grabbed the man's hand and did that guy hug that was part shoulder bump, part slap on the back before they stepped apart. "Only you do."

The other man shook his head. "I'm going to pass on that. Why don't you introduce me to your lovely lady?"

"Emily Fielding," Rafe said. "Eric Rubio. He owns this place."

Emily held her hand out to Eric, who took it in his, winked at Rafe and then kissed it. Emily laughed at the easy camaraderie between the two men. As they made their way upstairs to the dance club, she real-

ized that this was the first time she'd seen Rafe so relaxed in Miami.

Emily suspected it was because he was away from
the Montoros and the decisions they wanted from him.
She knew that she felt the pressure, and it wasn't even
directed at her.

She should just say yes to his proposal. She wanted
to make everything easier for him, and her taking her
time and trying to figure out what she felt for him and
if he would always be there when she needed him to
be was just making everything harder for Rafe.

Eric left them as the music started, and Rafe held his
hand out to her and led her to the dance floor.

They spent the night dancing to salsa music, their
bodies brushing against each other, fanning the flames
of the desire that was always there between them.

She wished for a moment they could go back to the
people they'd been when they'd first met. Just two lusty
twentysomethings instead of a man and woman who
knew too much about each other.

"You okay?" Rafe asked.

She nodded, but as she looked into those hazel eyes
of his she realized she'd probably never be just okay
again. All the debating in her mind about whether she
loved him or not had been another diversion.

She went up on tiptoe and kissed him, pouring the
emotions that she was too scared to admit to into that
embrace. His hands skimmed down her sides to her
hips and he held her pressed close to him. It felt as if
everything dropped away but the two of them.

"Let's get out of here," Rafe said, taking her hand
and leading her out the door.

Twelve

Emily wasn't having a good morning. When Rafe's alarm went off, she sprang out of bed and ran to his bathroom to throw up. The morning sickness, which had been waning, was back with a vengeance today. But then she was still in the first trimester. It had seemed as if months had passed, but in reality it was only four weeks since she'd confronted Rafe here in his penthouse. Ten weeks since she'd gotten pregnant.

Yet her entire world had changed.

She suspected it was partially nerves, since Rafe had a big meeting with his family this morning. One that she wasn't invited to attend. He hadn't said much but it had put a damper on their evening once they'd gotten home and he'd finally read all the texts from his cousin and brother reminding him about the meeting. She thought of her little family and how her mom was never one to pressure her into making a decision. But knew she was comparing apples and oranges. Rafe was in line to become king of Alma. There was nothing in Fielding family history that even came close to that.

Both of them knew that this time of dating and getting to know each other was over. She'd overheard a very tense conversation between Rafe and his cousin Juan Carlos last night that didn't sound too promising. She rinsed her mouth out and splashed some water on her face, looking up in the mirror to see Rafe standing there. Simply watching her.

"You okay?" he asked, a gentle smile on his face. He wore only a pair of boxer briefs and she was struck again by how handsome he was. How much she loved every inch of his strong muscled body. "I didn't know what to do. I hate that you get sick in the mornings."

"Yes," she said, taking a hand towel and drying her face. "How are you?"

"I'm fine," he said. "Will you accompany me to the office? We can take the helicopter back to Key West after my meetings are over."

She nodded. "Sounds great."

"I need to shower and shave," he said.

There was an awkwardness between them this morning that hadn't been there in a long time. She wondered if he'd changed his mind about marrying her. Wondered if he wished that he'd just paid her off when she'd come here to tell him that she was pregnant. She just hoped that he didn't regret coming to Key West and Shady Harry's bar and spending that first weekend with her. But the man she'd come to know was now hidden away behind his official Montoro facade.

She knew his attitude had everything to do with his

family. He seemed angry and a little bit hurt. And she was scared. For the first time she faced the very real possibility that she might be losing him.

She thought it telling that he hadn't asked her again to marry him this morning. She assumed the time for that had passed. Maybe he wasn't in the mood to pacify his family anymore.

He turned the large shower on and she watched him get into it. For a long minute she stood there before the pain she felt radiating from him made her move.

She undressed and got into the shower cubicle with him. He was facing the wall with his face turned upward to the spray and she just wrapped her arms around him and put her face between his shoulder blades.

She held him to her, trying to give him her strength and that love she hadn't found the words to express yet. Even in her own heart and head.

He turned around, put his hands on her waist and brought his mouth down on hers. She felt the desperation in the embrace, the feeling that after this moment everything would change. He caressed her back, his palms settling on her butt as he pulled her closer to him, anchoring her body and his together.

She kissed him back, wrapped her legs around his hips and trusted that he'd hold her. And he did. He took a step forward and she felt the cold marble wall at her back. Then Rafe adjusted his hips and thrust up into her.

He filled her completely and just stayed still for a moment while her body adjusted to having him inside her. She ran her hands up and down his back, pushing her tongue deep into his mouth. She needed more and the way he was rocking into her sent sparks of sensation up her body.

He palmed her breasts and broke the kiss, lowering his head to take one of her nipples in his mouth. His strong sucking made everything inside her clench. She felt the first waves of her orgasm roll through her.

She grabbed his shoulders and arched her back to try to take him deeper and he started thrusting harder and faster into her. His mouth found hers again; he tangled his hand in her hair and pulled her head back as he thrust deeper into her.

She dug her nails into his shoulders, felt her body driving toward climax again and moaned deep in her throat as a second, deeper orgasm rolled through her. Rafe ripped his mouth from hers and made a feral sound as he thrust his hips forward and came inside her.

He turned and leaned against the wall. She rested her head on his shoulder as her pulse slowly returned to normal. She let her legs slide down his and stood there in his arms. He didn't let her go. Just kept stroking her back and not saying a word.

She realized she was crying and really didn't understand why. Maybe it was because she had the answer to the question about her love for him. It was true and deep. And she understood that now because she was willing to walk away from him if that was what it took for him to have all he wanted.

Jose was waiting in Rafe's office when they got to the headquarters of Montoro Enterprises. His trusty assistant had a cup of decaf coffee waiting for Emily and a Red Bull for Rafe. He also had a file that needed Rafe's attention before he went into the meeting.

"Jose, I've heard there is a sculpture garden in the building," Emily said, as Rafe skimmed his papers. She was dressed in a scoop-neck blouse, a pair of white denim capris and two-inch platform sandals. She'd left her hair down to curl over her shoulders.

Rafe thought she looked beautiful, but there was a hint of vulnerability to her. One that had been there since she'd dashed to the bathroom from their bed this morning. Nothing he'd done had taken it away. And that was a horrible feeling for a man to know he wasn't able to protect his woman.

"There is the Montoro collection and exhibit. It's on the third floor. Would you like me to show you to it?" Jose asked.

"If Rafe doesn't need you," she said.

"I'm good," Rafe said. Emily gave him a little wave and then walked out of the room with Jose.

The papers that Jose had given him to review showed him the main points of the new constitution of Alma. And he noticed that the part Jose had high-lighted dealt with royal marriage. Since they were just reestablishing the monarchy, the rules were strict. Of course, existing marriages would be honored. In cases of divorce, the marriage must be annulled, which was why Rafe's father couldn't inherit the throne. The final stipulation was that the only suitable matches for a single heir to the throne were members of other royal families or the European nobility.

But since Rafe had yet to assume the throne, and this was still a new, untested document, there might still be room to maneuver. Or at least that was what Rafe hoped.

Rafe walked into the boardroom to find Gabe already there.

"I've been trying to get in touch with you all morning," Gabe said.

"Sorry. I had to turn the phone off. I needed time to think," Rafe said.

"Well, I'm the one that the family elected to talk to you. Juan Carlos has been on the phone with the prime minister and the court advisors. They are insistent that we have a scandal-free transition back to the monarchy."

Rafe shoved his hands deep into his pockets and strove for the calm he'd always had when dealing with delicate business situations. And this was the most delicate merger of his entire life. He had to keep calm and not lose his temper.

"Thanks."

"Thanks. That's it? You're losing control of the situation and that's not like you," Gabe said.

"You think I don't know that? Emily is still trying to figure out if marrying me is a good idea. She's got morning sickness and looks more vulnerable every time I see her. The entire family desperately wants me to make this right and for once, Gabe, I truly have no idea how I'm going to do it."

Gabe clapped his hand on Rafe's shoulder. "You always make things work. I've seen you pull off deals that everyone else thought were lost."

Rafe nodded. He wished it were that easy. But from the first, this entire situation had too much emotion in it. There was Tia Isabella and her emotional plea for them to consider the offer from the Alma government to return to the throne. His father's bitter disappointment that he couldn't be the next king and his determination that his eldest son and namesake would be. All of it reeked of emotion, not common sense.

His chest felt tight and for once he needed that legendary coolness he was known for.

The rest of his family trickled in. Juan Carlos led the way. His expression read loud and clear: Rafe needed to act like a monarch and not a jet-setter.

Bella gave him a sad sort of smile as she came in. And his father's glare was icy to say the least. Gabe was sort of in Rafe's corner but he knew his brother didn't want to have to give up his lifestyle if Rafe abdicated.

Right now, he knew that was the only way for them to get him out of the picture.

After his family, the Alma delegation filed in. They had their lawyer and PR agent with them and quickly sat down on one side of the big walnut boardroom table.

His family settled in on the other side and Rafe took his customary seat at the head of the table.

"Rafael, has the girl agreed to marry you?" his father asked without preamble.

"We're not even sure he can marry her without the approval of this board," one of the members of the Alma delegation said.

"I think he should be allowed to marry. Look at the surge of popularity in the British monarchy after William and Kate tied the knot," Bella said with a wink at Rafe.

He gave his little sister a smile.

"A royal wedding would be grand. But we need to settle the subject of her being a commoner first."

"Did she say yes?" his father asked again. "If she's accepted then there is nothing more for this committee to consider. He's a Montoro and she's carrying an heir. The heir to the throne. I think that if he's engaged before the coronation that should be good enough for your council."

It was the first time Rafe could remember his father being on his side. Rafe was grateful to have his family's support for once in this situation.

"We can all appreciate that, Uncle Rafael," Juan Carlos said. "But Rafe has already let our family down and not just with the baby scandal. He's been very cavalier toward royal protocol and taking over the throne."

All of the voices at the table rose as everyone kept arguing their points until Rafe stood up and walked out of the room. He needed to come back to them when he'd made his decision and no sooner. Because they were going to keep fighting and tearing into each other, and in the end they'd tear him and Emily apart if he let them.

Emily wandered through the sculpture garden, admiring the eclectic collection. Famous sculptures stood next to pieces by unknown artists that reflected the Montoro taste.

As much as she'd enjoyed the few days she'd spent in Miami with Rafe, she was ready to go back to Key West. She'd be happy to grab her baseball bat and get rid of the reporters who'd been hanging around Key West hoping for a glimpse of her and then go back to normal.

She'd heard that life changed when a woman got pregnant, but this was more than she could deal with. She wanted things to work out for her and Rafe. For his family to just let her continue to try to figure out if marriage was a good idea or not.

"Emily?"

"Over here," she said, standing up from the bench where she'd been sitting and walking up the path toward Rafe's voice.

One look at his face and the turmoil of his expression and her heart sank. There was no way she could keep doing this to herself or to him. She knew in her heart that she would always love him, but she wasn't going to move to Alma. It hadn't taken more than a night in Miami to remind her how much she loved living in Key West.

"What'd they say?"

"They are still arguing about everything."

"Like what?"

"Whether I can I marry you, whether a royal wedding would be the PR coup of the year, whether I'm an embarrassment," he said.

"You're not an embarrassment," she said, taking a deep breath.

"My cousin Juan Carlos would disagree with you on that score. But none of that matters. I know I promised you time to make a decision but I do need your answer now, Red. Will you marry me? Be my partner on the throne in Alma?"

She bit her lower lip. Hesitating as she warred between what she knew was right for Rafe and what she'd started to believe she could have for herself. But he'd nailed it when he said they weren't sure he could marry her. She wouldn't be the reason he was ostracized from his family. She wouldn't be the reason he had to give up being king.

Her stomach roiled and she was afraid she was going to be sick again, but then realized it was nerves, not morning sickness. She took another deep breath.

Rafe cursed and gave her a hard look.

"Seriously?"

"I can't marry you," she said. "While I'm sure that Alma is a lovely place, I can't imagine living there."

"It is lovely. You can have your own bar and do whatever you like once you are there."

"We both know that's not true. And I can't ask you to choose between me and the throne. I won't be the reason you aren't king, and there is a very real possibility of that happening. You'd resent me."

He shoved his hands in his hair and turned away from her.

She knew she'd made the right choice, but it hurt way more than she expected. "I know you'll support our child, but I'll be okay raising him or her on my own. I think I'll be good at that."

"I bet you do," he said, turning back around to face her. "No one there to interfere with any of your decisions."

"Don't get like that with me, Rafe. You know this is the only smart decision."

He stalked over to her and she realized he was truly mad at her. She'd done the noble thing. She was sacrificing her love and her dream of a family for him.

"I only know that you've hesitated from the moment you learned about our baby to involve me in your life. You keep pushing me away. I have given you space and tried to let you have the time you needed to see that we should be together. I know I seem angry. Hell, I am angry, but I really feel like you are making a mistake."

"And I know that you are. There is no world where you and I get to be together and raise this baby as we want to. I don't want our child to be raised with a bunch of rules on how to behave. You know that would happen. And I'm not good at conforming to them myself. It would be a constant headache."

"You're not going to change your mind, are you?"

"No."

"Fine. Go ahead and leave. You're good at being on your own. You said your mother let you be independent, but it's more likely that you pushed her away so you'd feel nice and safe with only yourself to be concerned over."

His words were mean and cut her to the core.

"You're just a spoiled man who can't handle the fact that he's not going to get his way in all things. That's what this is about. Not me or the baby, but you and your pride. They said you can't have me and the throne so you're trying to shove that down their throats. And to what end?" she demanded.

"Spoiled? You wrote the book on that, Red. I think you're describing yourself and not me. Normal couples, the ones you're always going on about, trust each other, depend on each other. And have each other's backs. They don't give themselves halfway to a relationship to try to keep from getting hurt the way you do. You don't care about anything or anyone other than yourself."

"Well, if that's how you feel I'm surprised you asked me to marry you."

"As you said, I just wanted to have it all. Make you

mine for some ulterior motive. Never because I cared about you or wanted a family of my own."

She was too angry to listen as she stormed past him out of the sculpture garden and out of his life. But later she'd remember his words and cry.

Because at the end of the day, all she really wanted was to have a family with him.

Thirteen

Rafe watched Emily go and he was so angry that he didn't even contemplate going after her. Instead he thought sarcastically that at least his family would be happy. They wouldn't have to worry about him marrying a commoner any more.

But he needed time to calm down before he walked back into the boardroom, or he had the feeling he'd say something he regretted. He'd always been the one who was in control. Calm when he needed to be. Decisive. A man of action.

But then Emily stormed into his life and no matter what decisions he made he still couldn't achieve the results he needed. He remembered how he'd felt on the boat in Key West when he'd looked over at Emily and realized he loved her. He'd been so focused on everything else that the love part seemed to have gotten lost.

His mom had told him when she left to never compromise with himself, because once that happened true happiness would never be his own. As a young adult he'd taken that to mean that he should live by his moral compass and not make business deals that were underhanded. But since meeting Emily he had the feeling that his mom had meant that sometimes making the right decision in society's eyes would be the wrong choice for the person he was.

He stood up and walked slowly back to the boardroom. He opened the door to find everyone still sitting around the table, but they were no longer all talking at once. Rafe knew that they had settled something while he'd been gone and he realized as king his choices were never going to be his own. He was always going to have to compromise and go to the committee before he could do anything.

"Good, you're back," Juan Carlos said.

"I am. What have you all decided?" Rafe asked as he walked to the head of the table and took his seat. "I think you should know that Emily and I will not be marrying."

"See, this just underscores my point," one of the officials from Alma said. "He can't control his personal life. He's a PR liability."

PR liability? He'd always played by the rules. He had a double degree in business management and geology—because of Montoro Enterprises' interests in oil—and he'd always known that without a good understanding of where they got their product he wouldn't be able to lead the company.

He'd worked hard for his family to build up the company so that there was no fear that this generation or the ones that followed would ever want for anything, and this was the thanks he got.

"A liability?" he asked. "Do you all feel this way?"

Juan Carlos nodded; Bella looked down at her fingers; his father just tightened his jaw. Gabe wouldn't make eye contact with him. Screw them. But he knew he was angry in general. He'd tried to please everyone—his family, the Alma delegation, Emily—and ended up not doing a good job of it for anyone.

He stood up and walked out of the boardroom and straight to his office. Jose was waiting there as always. "What do you need, sir?"

"I need to get to Key West. I'm afraid the chopper might not be a good option," Rafe said. He didn't want to take the company helicopter in case his services were no longer needed as CEO. "Can you have my car brought around?"

"Right away."

"Jose?"

"Yes, sir?"

"You've been a great assistant," Rafe said. "I'm not sure what is going to be happening at Montoro Enterprises. Please know that I will always have room for you on my staff wherever I am."

"Yes, sir."

Jose didn't ask any further questions and Rafe was grateful. He really didn't know how to explain anything other than that.

There was a knock on the door and he looked up to see Gabriel standing there. "Damn, I've never seen a man say so much with just a look."

Rafe shook his head as he finished gathering personal effects from his desk.

"There wasn't really anything else to say. I mean when your entire family thinks you've let them down, that's a horrible place to be."

Gabriel came farther into the room and leaned his hip against the desk. "You haven't let me down. I've never seen you so…alive as you've been in the last few weeks. I think that's because of Emily. If you can have her and be happy, you should go for it. That is what you're doing, right?"

"Yes," Rafe said. It had felt wrong to just let her walk away and now that he knew there really was no pleasing everyone, he was going to take care of himself and Emily first. He loved her and he was determined to convince her of it.

"Are you abdicating?"

"I am."

Gabriel cursed.

"I can't be king of Alma when my heart is here. I guess it never felt right to me being a monarch. I'm not aristocrat material."

"I'm sure as hell not either, but I think this means I'm going to have to clean up my act."

"I probably didn't make things any easier for you," Rafe admitted. "But you are a good man, Gabriel. I think you will make a very good king."

"Truly?"

"Yes. Better than me."

"No, I know you're lying. I'm going to pretend you're not. But I'm happy you have found someone."

"Don't be happy yet. She's stubborn and ticked off. I think it's going to take me a while to make her come around."

Gabe smiled at him. "I'm confident you're just the man to do that."

Rafe was, too.

He wished Gabe luck with his royal predicament and left Miami without talking to anyone else. Traffic wasn't too heavy in the midafternoon, but the drive was a long one and left Rafe time to think.

Deciding he wanted Emily was all well and good, but he knew he had his work cut out convincing her that she still wanted him.

Emily arrived in Key West just in time to shower and get dressed for work. It was a typical day in late June. There were too many tourists in town and she knew that she was cranky.

She started her shift with attitude. The first kid who presented her with a fake ID got it confiscated, then had a stern lecture from her before she had him escorted out of the bar.

The waitress and other bartender were all giving her a wide berth, which suited her. She didn't want to talk. She didn't want to think. She simply wanted to forget everything that happened today, get through her shift and then get home.

Harry had looked at her once or twice and made as if he was going to come over and talk to her, but she shut him down with one hand in the air that told him she wasn't ready to talk. Tonight she had no idea whether she would ever be ready to talk about Rafe and the baby or anything.

Tonight all she needed to worry about was mixing drinks and keeping the tourists happy. She didn't even have to worry about reporters sniffing around anymore. Cara had told her this afternoon that another suspicious reporter had shown his face over at the coffee shop one more time. Cara and a few other locals had explained that he wasn't welcome in Key West anymore and told him to get the hell out of town.

It made Emily feel really good to know that these people had her back. She was home. This was where she and her child would live the rest of their lives together.

They would be fine. She knew that they would. It didn't matter that her heart was breaking right now. And that someday she might have to answer uncomfortable questions about where her baby's father was.

For tonight she was doing what she was good at. Rafe had accused her of being too self-sufficient and now she knew she couldn't deny it. She did get her guard up and isolate herself when things got uncomfortable.

Even when faced with love. But there was no way she was going to be the reason Rafael Montoro IV didn't become king of Alma. His great-grandfather Rafael I had been king when the family fled. She knew how important it was to the people of Alma and to the Montoros that Rafe sit on the throne.

Another kid came up to the bar and she gave him a hard stare. He looked as though he was eighteen if he was a day. "Kid, think twice before you place your order."

"What are you talking about, honey? I need a tube of LandShark for that table over there."

"Let's see your ID," she said, ready to rip him a new one.

But he pulled out his real ID and it showed he was

nineteen. Off by two years. "I can't serve you beer, Alfred."

"It's for my dad and his buddies," Alfred said. "Dad, you're going to have to come over here."

Alfred's dad came over and got the beers and the rest of the night settled into a routine. This was going to be her life.

This was what she'd chosen. She could have been with Rafe wherever he was…but she'd chosen the safety of the only home she'd ever known over him. Not because she loved Key West so much but because it was safer to love a place than a man.

Key West wasn't going to leave her.

Rafe could.

"Why don't you take a break?" Harry said. "I've got some conch fritters on my desk and a nice fruit salad."

It was really a nice gesture from Harry. His way of saying that he was there for her. She walked over to him and gave him a hug. He hugged her back.

"You okay, kiddo?"

"I screwed up."

"Want to talk about it?"

She shook her head. "I think I'll start crying and maybe never stop."

"Go eat your dinner. That will make you feel better."

She went into Harry's office and found not only dinner waiting but Rafe.

Her breath caught and her heart felt as if it skipped a beat. She wanted to believe he was here for her, but what man would give up a throne for a woman like her?

"What are you doing here?" she asked. So afraid of his answer but she had to know.

"I abdicated."

"Oh, Rafe. Are you sure?"

"Very," he said, getting up and coming over to her. "I can't rule a country when my heart is somewhere else."

"Your heart?" This was more than she'd hoped for. She had dreamed that he'd come for her but she'd never let herself believe it. She wasn't the kind of woman who a man like Rafe would give up everything for.

Yet she knew now that she was. She could see it in his hazel eyes and his wide grin. Only love made a person grin like that. She knew because she was grinning the same way.

"I love you, Red. I've never met another person who completes me the way you do. I know that sounds cheesy, but I'm new to this kind of thing."

She shook her head. "You can't abdicate. I don't want to be the reason you gave up the throne—"

"You aren't the only reason I abdicated, Em. My time in Alma was constraining. I didn't like having to follow all the rules or answer to a committee. That's not my way. I want to focus on you and our child. And I can't rule without you by my side. Plus, it wasn't really a choice when it came down to picking between you and Alma. You were miles ahead."

"Really?" she asked. "Miles?"

"Yes," he said, getting down on one knee in front of her. "Will you marry me?"

She got down on her knees in front of him and wrapped her arms around him. "I love you so much. I'm sorry for all the mean things I said today."

"Me, too," he said. "I think I knew even as you walked out that I was never going to be king of Alma. I didn't want it, especially given the way I needed you. So are you going to be Mrs. Rafael Montoro IV?"

"Yes."

He took the ring box from his pocket and put it on her finger.

"You should know that there is some question as to whether I will remain CEO of Montoro Enterprises…I might buy you that restaurant you were talking about after all."

"We can see about that. Am I dreaming this? Are you really here?"

"I am."

She still couldn't believe it. She was just so happy to have Rafe in her arms and to know that he was going to be hers. She put her hands on his jaw and kissed him with all the love she'd been afraid to admit she felt for him. He held her close and whispered softly that he was never letting her go again.

There was a knock on the door and Rafe got to his feet, lifting her up, too. "You better eat your dinner."

She went over to the desk and sat down to her meal while Rafe opened the door. It was Harry. The two men exchanged a look before Harry smiled at her.

"Everything better now?" he asked.

She nodded. "I'm engaged."

Harry let out a whoop. "Drinks on the house. And you can take the rest of the night off."

Fourteen

The moon shone brightly down, warming them as Rafe led her toward the hammock in her backyard. The grass path under her feet was soft.

He stopped, turned her around and drew her into his arms from behind. His head rested on her shoulder and his big hands spanned her waist. She stood still, feeling the heat of his body against hers.

They fit perfectly together, which was something she'd rarely experienced in real life before Rafe. There was something about him that made everything sweeter. But this was a dream. She found it hard to believe that she'd found a man she could trust with her heart and soul. But he was that man. She could just let go of everything and enjoy it. But a part of her was afraid to.

He turned her in his arms and she let him. He kept

his hands at her waist and when she was facing him she was struck again by how he was quite a bit taller than she was. He gave her a half smile before he leaned in closer.

"You have a very tempting mouth," he said.

"I don't... Thank you?"

He gave a small laugh. "You are very welcome. It was one of the first things I noticed about you when you told me to wait in line at the bar. But I knew that you wanted something more from me."

"What?"

"You seemed to be begging me to kiss you," he said.

"Perhaps I was," she admitted.

His mouth was firm on hers as he took his time kissing her. He rubbed his lips back and forth over hers lightly until her mouth parted and she felt the humid warmth of his exhalation. He tasted so...delicious, she thought. She wanted more and opened her mouth wider to invite him closer.

She thrust her tongue into his mouth. He closed his teeth carefully over her tongue and sucked on her. She shivered and went up on her tiptoes to get closer to him.

His taste was addicting and she wanted more. Yes, she thought, she wanted much more of him, not just his kisses.

She put her hands on his shoulders and then higher on his close-cropped hair and rubbed her hands over his skull. He was hers now. Something that she could finally admit she'd wanted from the moment they met.

For a moment she felt a niggling doubt... There was something she should remember, but he tasted so good that she didn't want to think. She just wanted to experience him.

His hands moved over her shoulders, his fingers tracing a delicate pattern over the globes of her breasts. He moved them back and forth until the very tip of his finger dipped beneath the material of her top and reached lower, brushing over the edge of her nipple.

Exquisite shivers racked her body as his finger continued to move over her. He found the zipper at the left side of her top and slowly lowered it. Once it was fully down and the material fell away to the ground, he took her wrists in his hands and stepped back.

She was proud of her body and the changes that pregnancy had wrought in it. She could tell he was, too. His gaze started at the top of her head and moved down her neck and chest to her nipped-in waist.

He wrapped his hands around her waist and drew her to him, lifting her. "Wrap your legs around me."

She did and was immediately surrounded by him. With his hands on her butt and his mouth on her breasts, he sucked her gently, nibbling at her nipples as he massaged her backside. When he took her nipple into his mouth she felt everything inside her tighten and her center grow moist.

Then she felt as if she was falling and soon found herself lying on the hammock while he knelt over her. His mouth...she couldn't even think. She could only feel the sensations that were washing over her as he continued to focus on her breasts.

One of his heavy thighs parted her legs and then he was between them. She felt the ridge of his erection rubbing against her pleasure center and she shifted against him to increase the sensation.

She wanted to touch him, had to hold him to her as his mouth moved from her breast down her sternum and to her belly button. He looked up at her and for a moment when their eyes met there was something almost reverent in his eyes.

"My fiancée," he said. "Finally you and the baby are officially mine."

"Yes, we are."

He lowered his head and nibbled at the skin of her belly, his tongue tracing the indentation of her belly button. Each time he dipped his tongue into her it felt as if her clit tingled. She shifted her hips to rub against him and he answered her with a thrust of his own hips.

His mouth moved lower on her, his hands moving to the waistband of her jeans and undoing the button and then slowly lowering the zipper. She felt the warmth of his breath on her lower belly and then the edge of his tongue as he traced the skin revealed by the open zipper.

The feel of his five o'clock shadow against her was soft and smooth. She moaned a little, afraid to say his name and wake from this dream where he was hers. She thought she'd learned everything she needed to about Rafe, but it seemed there was still more for her to experience.

"Lift your hips," he said.

She planted her feet on the hammock and did as he asked. She felt him draw her jeans over her hips and down her thighs. She was left wearing the tiny black thong she'd put on this morning.

He palmed her through the panties and she squirmed on the hammock. She wanted more.

He gave it to her. He placed his hand on her most intimate flesh and then his mouth as he drew her underwear down by pulling with his teeth. His hands kept moving over her stomach and thighs until she was completely naked and bare underneath him. Then he leaned back on his knees and just stared down at her.

"You are exquisite," he said.

His voice was low and husky and made her blood flow heavier in her veins. Everything about this man seemed to make her hotter and hornier than she'd ever been before.

"It's you," she said in a raspy voice. "You are the one who is making me…"

"I am making you," he said. "And I'm not going to be happy until you come harder than you ever have before."

She shuddered at the impact of his words. He spoke against her skin so that she felt them all the way through her body.

"This is the one thing I should have done when you came to my penthouse in South Beach."

"Sex? Um, we did that."

"I should have taken you to bed and kept you there until you agreed to never leave me."

He parted her with the thumb and forefinger of his left hand and she felt the air against her most intimate flesh, followed by the brush of his tongue. It was so soft and wet, and she squirmed wanting—no, needing—more from him.

He scraped his teeth over her and she almost came right then, but he lifted his head and smiled up at her. By this time she knew her lover well enough to know that he liked to draw out the experience.

She gripped his shoulders as he teased her with his mouth and then tunneled her fingers through his hair, holding him closer to her as she lifted her hips. He moaned against her and the sound tickled her clit and sent chills racing through her body.

He traced the opening of her body with his other hand, those large deft fingers making her squirm against him. Her breasts felt full and her nipples were tight as he pushed just the tip of his finger inside her.

The first ripples of her orgasm started to pulse through her, but he pulled back, lifting his head and moving down her body and nibbling at the flesh of her legs. She was aching for him. Needed more of what he had been giving her.

"Rafe..."

"Yes?" he asked, lightly stroking her lower belly and then moving both hands to her breasts and cupping them.

"I need more."

"You will get it," he said.

"Now."

He shook his head. "That's not the way to get what you want."

She was shivering with the need to come. She had played these kinds of games before, but her head wasn't in it. She just wanted his big body moving over hers. She wanted him inside her. She reached between their bodies and stroked him through his pants, and then slowly lowered the tab of his zipper. But he caught her wrist and drew her hand up above her head.

"That's not what I had in mind," he said.

"But you are what I want."

"Good," he said, lowering his body over hers so the soft fabric of his shirt brushed her breasts and stomach before she felt the masculine hardness of his muscles underneath. Then his thigh was between her legs, moving slowly against her engorged flesh, and she wanted to scream as everything in her tightened just a little bit more.

But it wasn't enough. She writhed against him but he just slowed his touch so that the sensations were even more intense than before. He shifted again and she felt the warmth of his breath against her mound. She opened her eyes to look down at him and this time she knew she saw something different. But she couldn't process it because his mouth was on her.

Each sweep of his tongue against her clit drove her higher and higher as everything in her body tightened, waiting for the touch that would push her over the edge. She shifted her legs around his head, felt the brush of his silky smooth hair against her inner thighs, felt his finger at the opening of her body once again and then the delicate biting of his teeth against her pleasure bud as he plunged that finger deep inside her. She screamed his name as his mouth moved over her.

Her hips jerked forward and her nipples tightened. She felt the moisture between her legs and his finger pushing hard against her G-spot. She was shivering and her entire body was convulsing, but he didn't lift his head. He kept sucking on her and driving her harder and harder until she came again, screaming with her orgasm as stars danced behind her eyelids.

She reached down to claw at his shoulders as pleasure rolled over her. It was more than she could process and she had to close her eyes again. She reached for Rafe, needing some sort of comfort after that storm of pleasure.

He pulled her into his arms and rocked her back and forth. "Now I feel that we are engaged. That you and I are going to be okay no matter what else happens in the world."

She shivered at his words and knew that she'd found the one man she'd never realized she'd been searching for. A man who could be her partner and respect her independence. The kind of man who'd be a good father and build a family with her.

"I've been meaning to ask you something," she said.

"What is it?"

"What did you want to be as a little boy? I never got to ask you," she said. She wondered about the man he'd become. Would his dreams have been to be a sports star or business tycoon? Well, he'd become that. Surely, he hadn't wanted to be king.

"I wanted to be your man," he said.

She punched him the shoulder. "Stop making fun."

"I didn't know that you would be the woman, Emily, but I always wanted a family of my own. The chance to have someone who was always by my side."

"Well, you've got that," she said, kissing him.

* * * * *

SEDUCED BY THE SPARE HEIR

ANDREA LAURENCE

To my fellow authors in the Montoros series —
Janice, Katherine, Kat, Jules and Charlene
It was a joy working with all of you. Thanks for
tolerating my 80 million questions on the loop.

And to our editor Charles —
You're awesome, as always. I look forward to
working with you again.

One

This party was lame. And it was *his* party. How could his own party be lame?

Normally parties were Gabriel Montoro's thing. Much to the chagrin of his family, he'd earned quite the reputation as "Good Time Gabriel." Music, alcohol, dim lighting, superficial conversation… He was the king of the party domain. But now that Gabriel had been tapped as the new king of Alma, everything had changed.

Gabriel gripped his flute of champagne and looked around the ballroom at his family's Coral Gables estate. Their tropical retreat seemed incredibly stuffy tonight. There wasn't a single flip-flop in the room, much less one of the feral parrots that lived on their property and flew in the occasional open door. His family had always had money, but they hadn't been pretentious.

But things had changed for the Montoro family since the tiny European island nation of Alma decided to restore their monarchy. Suddenly he was Prince Gabriel, third in line to the throne. And before he could adjust to the idea of that, his father and his older brother were taken out of the running. His parents had divorced without an annulment, making his father ineligible. Then, his ever-responsible brother abdicated and ran off with a bartender. Suddenly he was on the verge of being King Gabriel, and everyone expected him to change with the title.

This suffocating soiree was just the beginning and he knew it. Next, he'd have to trade in his South Beach penthouse for a foreign palace and his one-night stands for a queen with a pedigree. Everything from his clothes to his speech would be up for public critique by "his people." People he'd never seen, living on an island he'd only visited once. But his coronation was only a month or two away. He left for Alma in a week.

That was why they were having this party, if you could even call it that. The music was classical, the drinks were elegant and the women were wearing far too much clothing. He got a sinking feeling in his stomach when he realized this was how it was going to be from now on. Boring parties with boring people he didn't even know kissing his ass.

There were two hundred people in the room, but there were more strangers than anything else. He found that terribly ironic. People had come out of the woodwork since his brother, Rafe, abdicated and Gabriel was thrust into the spotlight. Suddenly he wasn't just the vice president of South American Operations, cast into the Southern Hemisphere where he couldn't embarrass the family; he was the hot ticket in town.

Him! Gabriel—the middle child whom no one paid any attention to, the one dismissed by his family's society friends as the bad boy, the spare heir and nothing more. Now that he was about to be king, he had strangers at every turn fighting to be his new best friends.

He hated to break it to them, but Gabriel didn't have friends. Not real ones. That required a level of trust in other people that he just didn't have. He'd learned far too young that you can't trust anyone. Even family could let you down when you need them the most.

Speak of the devil.

From across the room, his cousin Juan Carlos spied him and started in his direction. He was frowning. Nothing new there. Ever serious, Juan Carlos never seemed to have any fun. He was always having business discussions, working, being responsible. He was the kind of man who should be the king of Alma—not Gabriel. After hundreds of years, why hadn't people figured out that bloodlines were not the best indicator of leadership potential?

"You're not talking to anyone," Juan Carlos noted with a disapproving scowl as he loomed over his cousin. At several inches over six feet, he had a bad habit of hovering over people. Gabriel was never quite sure if his cousin deliberately tried to intimidate with his size or if he was unaware how much it bothered people when he did that.

Gabriel wasn't about to let his cousin's posture or his frown get to him. He tended not to worry too much about what his cousin thought, or what anyone thought, really. When it came down to it, Juan Carlos was serious enough for them both. "No one is talking to me," he corrected.

"That's because you're hiding in the corner sulking."

Gabriel scoffed at his blunt observation. "I am not sulking."

His cousin sighed and crossed his arms over his chest. "Then what would you call it?"

"Surveying my domain. That sounds kingly, right?"

Juan Carlos groaned and rolled his eyes. "Quit it. Don't even pretend you care about any of this, because I know you don't. You and I both know you'd much rather be in South Beach tonight chasing tail. Pretending otherwise is insulting to your family and insulting to your country."

Gabriel would be lying if he said the neon lights weren't beckoning him. There was nothing like the surge of alcohol through his veins and the thumping bass of music as he pressed against a woman on the dance floor. It was the only thing that could help him forget what a mess he was in, but after the drama with Rafe, he'd been on a short leash. The family couldn't take another scandal.

That didn't mean he felt like apologizing for who he was. He wasn't raised to be king. The Alman dictatorship had held strong for nearly seventy years. Who would've thought that when democracy was restored, they'd want their old royal family back? They hadn't anticipated this summons and he certainly hadn't anticipated his brother, the rightful king, would run off with a Key West bartender and send Gabriel's life into a tailspin. "I'm sorry if that offends your sensibilities, J.C., but I didn't ask to be king."

"I know you didn't ask to be king. It is plainly obvious to every person in this room that you don't want the honor. But guess what? The crown has landed in your lap and you've got to step up and grow up." Juan Carlos sipped his wine and glared at Gabriel over the rim. "And what have I told you about calling me that?" he added.

That made Gabriel smile. Annoying his cousin was one of his favorite pastimes since childhood. The smile was short-lived, though.

It wasn't the first time he'd been told to grow up. What his family failed to realize was that Gabriel had grown up a long time ago. They all liked to pretend it didn't happen, but in a dark room with thick rope cutting into his wrists, he'd left his childhood and innocence behind with his captors. If his family had wanted him to act responsibly, they should've done more to rescue him. He'd survived because of his own quick thinking and his first choice as an adult was to live the life he wanted and not care what anyone else thought about it.

Grow up, indeed. Gabriel took a large swallow of his champagne and sighed. The days of living his life as he chose were numbered. He could feel it. Soon it wouldn't just be his father and cousin trying to tell him what to do.

"Always good talking with you, cuz. Don't you have someone to schmooze?"

Juan Carlos didn't respond. Instead he turned on his heel and walked over to the dessert table. Within seconds, he was chatting with someone influential, whose name Gabriel had forgotten, over silver platters of chocolate truffles and cream puffs.

Gabriel turned away, noticing the side door that led

out to the patio and garden pavilion. Hopefully he could make it out there before someone noticed.

Glancing around quickly, he spied his father with his back to him. His sister was chatting with a group of ladies in the corner. This was his chance. He moved toward the door and surged through it as fast as he could.

Gabriel was immediately rewarded with the oppressive wave of heat that July in Miami was known for. The humid blast hit him like a tsunami after the air-conditioned comfort of the ballroom, but he didn't care. He moved away from the door and out into the dark recesses of the patio.

There were some tables and chairs set up outside in case guests wanted to come out. They were draped with linens and topped with centerpieces of candles and roses. All the seats were empty. Gabriel was certain none of the ladies were interested in getting overheated in their fancy clothes with their meticulously styled hair and makeup.

Glancing over at the far end of the semicircular patio, he spied someone looking out into the gardens. The figure was tall, but slender, with the moonlight casting a silver silhouette that highlighted the bare shoulders and silk-hugging curves. She turned her head to watch a bird fly through the trees and he was rewarded with a glimpse of the cheekbones that had made her famous.

Serafia.

The realization sent a hot spike of need down his spine and the blood sped through his veins as his heart beat double-time. Serafia Espina was his childhood crush and the fantasy woman of every red-blooded man who had ever achieved puberty. Eight years ago,

Serafia had been one of the biggest supermodels in the industry. Like all the greats, she'd been known by only her first name, strutting down catwalks in Paris, New York and Milan wearing all the finest designers' clothes.

And she'd looked damn good in them, too.

Gabriel didn't know much about what had happened, but for health reasons, Serafia had suddenly given up modeling and started her own business of some kind. But judging by the way that red dress clung to her curves, the years hadn't dulled her appeal. She could walk the catwalk right now and not miss a beat.

He hadn't spoken to Serafia in years. When his family was overthrown by the Tantaberras, they had fled to the United States and the Espinas moved to Switzerland. In the 1980s, they'd moved to Spain and their families renewed their friendship. When Gabriel and Serafia were children, their families vacationed together on the Spanish Riviera. Back then, he'd been a shy, quiet little boy of ten or eleven and she was the beautiful, unobtainable older woman. She was sixteen and he was invisible.

This was a fortunate encounter. They weren't children anymore and as the future king of their home country, he was anything but invisible. As Mel Brooks famously said, "It's good to be the king."

Serafia felt the familiar, niggling sensation of someone's eyes on her. It was something she'd become keenly attuned to working in the modeling business. Like a sixth sense, she could feel a gaze like a touch raking over her skin. Judging. Critiquing.

She turned to look behind her and found the man

of the evening standing a few feet away. Gabriel had certainly grown up a lot since she saw him last. He was looking at her the way most men did—with unmasked desire. She supposed she should be flattered to catch the eye of the future king, but he was in his twenties, just a baby. He didn't need to get involved with an older, has-been model with enough baggage to pack for a long vacation.

"Your Majesty," she replied with a polite bow of her head.

Gabriel narrowed his gaze at her. "Are you being sarcastic?" he asked.

Serafia's mouth dropped open with surprise, her response momentarily stolen. That wasn't what she was expecting him to say. "Not at all. Did it come out that way? If it did, I sincerely apologize."

Gabriel shook his head dismissively and walked toward her. He didn't look like any king she'd ever seen before. He exuded a combination of beauty and danger, like a great white shark, gliding gracefully across the stone patio in a tailored black suit and dress shirt. His tie was bloodred and his gaze was fixed on her as if she were prey.

She felt her chest tighten as he came closer and she breathed in the scent of his cologne mingling with the warm smell of the garden's exotic flowers. Her fight-or-flight instincts were at the ready, even as she felt herself get drawn closer to him.

He didn't pounce. Instead he leaned down, rested his elbows on the concrete railing and looked out into the dark recesses of the tropical foliage. "It's not you, it's me," he said. "I still haven't quite adjusted to the idea of all this royalty nonsense."

Royalty nonsense. Wow. Serafia's libido was doused with cold water at his thoughtless words. That wasn't exactly what the people of Alma wanted to hear from their new king. After the collapse of the dictatorship, restoring the monarchy seemed like the best way to stabilize the country. The wealthy Alma elite would get a little more than they bargained for with Gabriel Montoro wearing the crown. He didn't really seem to care about Alma or the monarchy. He hadn't grown up there, but neither had she. Her parents had raised her to value her heritage and her homeland, regardless.

Perhaps it was just his youth. Serafia knew how hard it was to have the spotlight on you at such a young age. She'd been discovered by a modeling agency when she was only sixteen. Whisked away from her family, she was making six figures a year when most teenagers were just getting their driver's licenses. By the time she was old enough to drink, she was a household name. The pressure was suffocating, pushing her to her personal limits and very nearly destroying her. She couldn't even imagine what it would be like to be the ruler of a country and have over a million people depending on her.

"I think you'll get used to it pretty quickly," she said, leaning her hip against the stone railing. She picked up her glass of wine and took a sip. "All that power will go to your head in no time."

Gabriel's bitter laugh was unexpected. "I doubt that. While I may be king, my family will ensure that I'm not an embarrassment to them."

"I thought a king can do what he likes."

"If that was true, my father or my brother would still be in line for the crown. In the end, even a king has a mama to answer to." Gabriel looked at her with a charming smile, running his fingers through his too-long light brown hair.

It was shaggy and unkempt, a style popular with men his age, but decidedly unkingly. The moonlight highlighted the streaks of blond that he'd probably earned on the beach. She couldn't tell here in the dark, but from the pictures she'd seen of him in the papers and online, he had the tanned skin to match. Even in his immaculate and well-tailored suit, he looked more like a famous soccer player than a king.

"And I know your mama," she noted. Señora Adela was a beautiful and fierce woman who lived and loved with passion. She'd also been one to give the lecture of a lifetime while she pulled you down the hallway by your ear. "I'd behave if I were you."

"I'll try. So, how have you been?" he asked, shifting the conversation away from his situation. "I haven't seen you since you became a famous supermodel and forgot about all of us little people."

Serafia smiled, looking for the right answer. She knew people didn't really want to know how she was doing; they were just being polite. "I've been well. I started my own consulting business since I left modeling and the work has kept me fairly busy."

"What kind of consulting?"

"Image and etiquette, mostly. I traveled so extensively as a model that I found I could help companies branch out into unfamiliar foreign markets by teaching them the customs and societal norms of the new country. Other times I help wealthy families groom their daughters into elegant ladies."

Although families mostly paid her to teach etiquette

and poise and give makeovers, she also spent a lot of time trying to teach those same girls that being pretty wasn't all they had to offer the world. It was an uphill battle and one that had earned her the label "hypocrite" more than a time or two. Sure, it was easy for a super-model to say that beauty wasn't everything.

"Do me a favor and don't mention your consulting business around my father or Juan Carlos," Gabriel said.

Serafia's dark eyebrows knit together in confusion. "Why is that? Do they have daughters in need of a makeover?" Bella certainly didn't need any help from her. The youngest Montoro was looking lovely tonight in a beaded blue gown with her golden hair in elegantly twisted curls.

Serafia had heard rumors that the Montoro heirs had been allowed to run wild in America, but from what she had seen, they were no different from the youths of any other royal family. They wanted to have fun, find love and shirk their responsibilities every now and then. Until those desires interfered with the crown, as Rafe's abdication had, there was no harm done.

Gabriel shook his head and took a large sip of his champagne. "No daughters. They've just got *me*. I wouldn't be surprised if they'd jump at the chance to have you make me over. I don't really blame them. I'm about to be the most unsuitable king ever to sit upon the throne of Alma. The bad boy...the backup plan... the worst possible choice..."

Her eyes widened with every unpleasant descrip-tion. "Is that their opinion or just your own?"

He shrugged. "I think it's everyone's opinion, in-cluding mine."

"I think you're exaggerating a little bit. I'm not sure

about what your family thinks behind closed doors, but I haven't heard anything about you being unsuitable. Everyone is surprised about Rafe abdicating, of course, but I just came from Alma and the people are very excited to have you come home and serve as their monarch."

She hadn't originally planned on visiting Alma, but she'd gotten a call from a potential client there. She was already coming to Florida to consult with a company in Orlando, so she made a stop in Alma on the way. She was glad she had. It was inspiring to see an entire country buzzing with hope for the future. She wished she saw some of that same excitement in Gabriel.

He narrowed his gaze, seemingly searching her expression for the truth in her words, but he didn't appear to find it. "That won't last long. I wouldn't be surprised if they'd start begging for the dictatorship to come back within a year of my reign beginning."

And Serafia had thought she was the only one around here with miserably low self-esteem. "The people of Alma fought long and hard to be free of the Tantaberras. You would have to be a wicked, bloodthirsty tyrant for them to wish his return. Is that what you have planned? A reign of terror for your people?"

"No. I guess that changes things," he said with a bright smile that seemed fake. "I didn't realize they had such low expectations for their king. As long as I don't decapitate all my enemies and force my subjects to cower in fear, I'll be a success! Thanks for letting me know that. I feel a lot better about the whole thing now."

Gabriel was leaving for Alma in a week, and that attitude was going to be a problem. Before she could curb her tongue, Serafia leaned in to him and plucked the champagne glass from his hand. "The citizens of Alma have been through a lot over the last seventy years. While the wealthy upper class could afford to flee, most of the people were trapped there to suffer at the hands of Tantaberra and his sons. They're finally free, some of them having waited their whole lives to wake up in the morning without the oppressive hand of a despot controlling them. These people have chosen to restore your family to the throne to help them rebuild Alma. They can probably do without your sarcasm and self-pity."

Gabriel looked at her with surprise lighting his eyes. He might not be comfortable with the authority and responsibility of being king, but he seemed shocked that she would take that tone of voice with him. She didn't care. She had lived in Spain her whole life. She wasn't one of his subjects and she wasn't about to grovel at his feet when he was being like this.

She waited for him to speak, watching as the surprise faded to heat. At first she thought it was anger building up inside him, but when his gaze flicked over her skin, she could feel her cheeks start to burn with the flush of sexual awareness. She might have been too bold and said too much, but he seemed to like it for some reason.

At last, he took a deep breath and nodded. "You're absolutely right."

That was not what she'd expected to hear at all. She had braced herself for an argument or maybe even a come-on line to change the subject, but she certainly didn't think he would agree with her. Perhaps he wasn't doomed to failure if he could see reason in her words.

She returned his glass of champagne and looked out into the garden to avoid his intense stare and hide her blush. "I apologize for being so blunt, but it needed to be said."

"No, please. Thank you. I have spent the days since my brother's announcement worried about how it will impact me and my life. I've never given full consideration to the lives of all the people in Alma and how they feel. They have suffered, miserably, for so long. They deserve a king they can be proud of. I'm just afraid I'm not that man."

"You can be," Serafia said, and as she spoke the words, she believed them. She had no real reason to be so certain about the success of the Montoro Bad Boy. She hadn't spoken to him in years and he was just a boy then. Now there were only the rumors she'd heard floating across the Atlantic—stories of womanizing, fast cars and dangerous living. But she felt the truth deep in her heart.

"It might take time and practice, but you can get there. A lesser man wouldn't give a second thought to whether he was the right person for the job. You're genuinely concerned and I think that bodes well for your future in Alma."

Gabriel looked at her and for the first time, she noticed the signs of strain lining his eyes. They didn't entirely mesh with the image that had been painted of the rebellious heir to the throne. He seemed adept at covering his worry with humor and charming smiles, but in that moment it all fell away to reveal a man genuinely concerned that he was going to fail his country. "Do you really believe that?"

Serafia reached out and covered his hand with her

own. She felt a warm prickle dance across her palm as her skin touched his. The heat of it traveled up her arm, causing goose bumps to rise across her flesh despite the oppressive Miami summer heat. His gaze remained pinned on her own, an intensity there that made her wonder if he was feeling the same thing. She was startled by her reaction, losing the words of comfort she'd intended to say, but she couldn't pull away from him.

"Yes," she finally managed to say in a hoarse whisper.

He nodded, his jaw flexing as he seemed to consider her response. After a moment, he slipped his hand out from beneath hers. Instead of pulling away, he scooped up her hand in his, lifting it as though he was going to kiss her knuckles. Her breath caught in her throat, her tongue snaking out across her suddenly dry lips.

"Serafia, can I ask you something?"

She nodded, worried that she was about to agree to something she shouldn't, but powerless to stop herself in that moment. The candlelight flickering in his eyes was intoxicating. She could barely think, barely breathe when he touched her like that.

"Will you…" He hesitated. "…help me become the kind of king Alma deserves?"

Two

Gabriel watched as Serafia's expression collapsed for a moment in disappointment before she pulled herself back together. He couldn't understand why he saw those emotions in her dark eyes. He thought she would be excited that he wanted to step up and be a better person for the job. Wasn't that what she'd just lectured him about?

Then he looked down at her hand clutched in his own, here in the candlelight, on the dark, secluded patio, and realized he had a pretty solid seduction in progress without even trying. That might be the problem. He'd been too distracted by their conversation to realize it.

He had to admit he was pleased to know she responded to him. In the back of his mind, he'd considered Serafia unobtainable, a childhood fantasy. The moment she'd turned to look at him tonight, he felt his heart stutter in his chest as if he'd been shocked by a defibrillator. Her stunning red silk gown, rubies and diamonds dangling at her throat and ears, crimson lipstick against the flawless gold of her skin…it was as though she'd walked out of a magazine spread and onto his patio.

She was poised, elegant and untouchable. And bold. With a razor-sharp tongue, she'd cut him down to size, sending a surprising surge of desire through him instead of anger. She didn't care that he was the crown prince; she was going to tell it the way it was. With everything ahead of him, he was beginning to think he needed a woman like that in his life. Gabriel was already surrounded by too many yes-men or needling family members.

Serafia was a firecracker—beautiful, alluring and capable of burning him. A woman like that didn't exist in real life, and if she did, she wouldn't want anything to do with a man like Gabriel. Or so he'd always thought. The disappointment in her dark eyes led him to believe that perhaps he was wrong about that.

He wasn't entirely sure that a haircut and a new suit would make him a better king, but he was willing to give it a try. It certainly couldn't hurt. Working with a professional image consultant would get his father and Juan Carlos off his back. And if nothing else, it would keep this beautiful, sexy woman from disappearing from his life for at least two more weeks. It sounded like a win-win for Gabriel.

"A makeover?" she said after the initial shock seemed to fade from her face. She pulled her fingers from his grasp and rubbed her hands together for a moment as if to erase his touch. Serafia didn't seem to think his plan was the perfect solution he'd envisioned. "For you?"

"Why not? That's what you do, right?"

Her nose wrinkled and her brow furrowed. "I teach teenage girls how to walk in high heels and behave themselves in various social situations."

"How is what I'm proposing any different? Obviously I don't need the lesson on heels, but I'm about to face a lot of new social situations. With the way my family has been nagging at me, there seem to be a lot of land mines ahead of me. I could use help on how I should dress and what I should say. And I think you're the right person for the job."

Serafia's dark eyes widened and she sputtered for a moment as she struggled for words to argue with him. "I thought you didn't want a makeover," she said at last.

Gabriel crossed his arms over his chest. "I didn't want my family to force me into one. There's a difference. But you've convinced me that it's needed if I'm going to be the kind of king Alma needs."

"I don't know, Gabriel." She turned back to the gardens, avoiding his gaze. She seemed very hesitant to agree to it and he wasn't sure why. She'd pretty much dressed him down and chastised him for being a self-centered brat. Her words were bold and passionate. But then, when he asked for her help, she didn't want to be the one to change him. He didn't get it. Was he a lost cause?

"Come on, Serafia. It's perfect. I need a makeover, but I don't want everyone to know it. You're a friend of the family, so no one will think twice of you traveling with me or being seen with me. No one outside of the family even needs to know why you're here. We can come up with some cover story. I've got a week to prepare before I leave for Alma and another week of welcome activities once I arrive before things start to settle down. I'm not sure I can get through all that without help. Without *your* help."

"I can't just drop everything and run to your side, Gabriel."

"I'll pay you double."

She turned back to him, a crimson frown lining her face. Even that didn't make her classic features unattractive. "I don't need the money. I have plenty of that. I don't even have to work, but I was tired of sitting around with my own thoughts."

He wasn't sure what kind of thoughts would haunt a young, successful woman like Serafia, but he didn't feel that he should ask. "Donate it all to charity, then. I don't care. It's good for your business."

"How? I'd be doing this in secret. That won't earn me any exposure for my company."

"Not directly, but having you by my side in all the pictures will get your name in the papers. After you're seen with royalty, maybe your services will be more in demand because you have connections."

Serafia sighed. She was losing this battle and she knew it.

Gabriel looked at her, suppressing a smile as he prepared to turn her own argument against her and end the fight. "If for no other reason, do it for the people of Alma. You yourself just said how much these people have suffered. Do your part and help me be the best king I can possibly be."

She tensed up and started biting her lower lip. Picking up her wineglass, she took a sip and looked out at the moon hovering over the tree line. At last, her head dropped in defeat. The long, graceful line of her neck was exposed by the one-shoulder cut of her gown and the style of her hair. The dark, thick strands were twisted up into an elegant chignon, leaving her flawless, honey-colored skin exposed.

He wanted to press a kiss to the back of her neck and wrap his arms around her waist to comfort her. His lips tingled as he imagined doing just that, but he knew that would be pushing his luck. If she agreed to work with him over the next few weeks, there might be time for kisses and caresses later. It couldn't take every hour of the day to make him suitable. But if she left now, he'd never have the chance.

Taking a deep breath, she let it out and nodded. "Okay. We start tomorrow morning. I will be here at nine for breakfast and we'll begin with table manners."

"Nine?" He winced. Most Saturday mornings, he didn't crawl out of bed until closer to noon. Of course, he wouldn't be closing down the bars tonight. If he left the family compound, they'd likely release the hounds to track him down.

"Yes," she replied, her voice taking the same tone as the nuns had used when he was in Catholic school. Serafia didn't look a thing like Sister Mary Katherine, but she had the same focused expression on her face as she looked him over. The former supermodel had faded away and he was left in the presence of his new image consultant.

"Modern kings do not stay up until the wee hours of the morning and sleep until noon. They have a country to lead, meetings to attend and servants that need a reliable schedule to properly run the household. After breakfast, you're getting a haircut." She reached out for his hand, examining his fingernails in the dim lights. "And a manicure. I'll have someone come in to do it. If we went to a salon, people would start talking."

Getting up early, plus a haircut? Gabriel self-consciously ran his fingers through the long strands of his hair. He liked it long. When it was short, he looked too much like his toe-the-line brother, CEO extraordinaire Rafe. That wasn't him. He was VP of their South American division for a reason. Since the news of Alma's return to monarchy, he'd spent most of his time in Miami, but he preferred his time spent south of the equator. Life down there was more colorful, less regimented. He didn't even mind the constant threat of danger edging into his daily routine there. Once you'd been kidnapped, beaten and held for ransom, there wasn't much else to fear.

All that would end now. A new VP would take over South American Operations and Gabriel would take a jet to Alma. He'd be ruling over a country with a million citizens and dealing with all the demands that went with it.

What had he signed himself up for?

"I wish I had my tablet with me, but I'll just have to make all my notes when I get back to my hotel. Sunday, we're going through your wardrobe and determining what you can take with you to Alma. Monday morning, I'll arrange for a private shopper to come to the house and we'll fill in the gaps."

"Now, wait a minute," he complained, holding up his hands to halt her long list of tasks. He knew he could use some polishing, but it sounded as if Serafia was preparing to gut him and build him up from scratch. "What is wrong with my clothes? This is an expensive suit."

"I'm sure it is. And if you were the owner of an exclusive nightclub in South Beach, it would be perfect, but you are Prince Gabriel, soon to be King Gabriel."

He sighed. He certainly didn't feel like royalty. He felt like a little boy being scolded for doing everything wrong. But he'd brought this pain upon himself. Spending time with his fantasy woman hadn't exactly gone to plan. It had only been minutes since he made that decision and he was already starting to regret it.

"Are you dating anyone?"

Gabriel perked up. "Why? Are you interested?" he said with the brightest, most charming smile he could conjure.

Serafia wrinkled her nose at him and shook her head. "No. I was just wondering if I needed to work with you on dealing with any sticky romantic entanglements before you leave."

That was disappointing. "I'm not big on relationships," he explained. "There are plenty of women I've seen on and off, but there shouldn't be any heartbroken women trying to follow me to Alma."

"How about pregnant bartenders?" she asked pointedly.

Gabriel chuckled. His brother's relationship drama had everyone in the family on edge. If he didn't work out, the crown would be dumped on Bella and she was only twenty-three, barely out of college. "No pregnant bartenders that I am aware of," he answered. "Or dancers or cocktail waitresses or coeds. I'm extremely careful about that kind of thing."

"You always use protection? Every time?"

Gabriel stiffened. "Do we really have to talk about my sex life?"

Serafia sighed and shook her head. "You have no real idea what you've gotten yourself into, do you? From now on, your sex life is the business of a whole country. Who you're seeing and who might be your future queen will be one of the first issues you'll tackle as king. After that, fathering heirs and continuing the Montoro bloodline will be the chief concern of each of your subjects. Every woman you're seen with is a candidate for queen. Every time your wife turns down a glass of wine or puts on a few pounds, there will be pregnancy rumors. Privacy has gone out the window for you, Gabriel."

"There's not going to be someone in the room while I *father* these heirs, is there?"

At that, Serafia smiled. "No. They have to draw the line somewhere."

That offered little comfort to Gabriel in the moment. Each step he took toward being king, the more concerned he became. He wanted to be a good leader, but the level of scrutiny in every aspect of his life was suffocating. His hair, his clothes, his sex life... He could feel the pressure crushing against his chest like a pile of stones.

Serafia pointed to a pair of chairs nearby. "Why don't we sit down for a minute. You look like you're about to pass out and these shoes are starting to pinch."

Gabriel pulled out a chair for her and took the one beside her. "I guess I just never thought about all this before. A few weeks ago, I was just a VP in my family company, someone with far-off ties to a country and a history most of us have forgotten all about. Then, boom, I'm a prince. And before I can adjust to that, I find out that I'm going to be king of the place. My life has taken a strange turn."

She nodded sympathetically. "I hate to be the one to tell you this, but it's just going to get worse. Once you're in the spotlight, your life is no longer your own. But from someone who's lived through it, know that the sooner you adjust to the idea of it, the better off you'll be."

Serafia hated to see Gabriel like this. He seemed like such a vibrant, fun-loving man, and the weight of his future was slowly crushing him like a bug. She was pushing him. Maybe more than she had to, at least at first, but he needed to know how things were going to be now. He would adjust to the crown much more easily if he understood the consequences of it.

"Is that what it was like for you? Is that why you gave up modeling?"

Serafia couldn't help the pained expression she felt crossing her face. It happened every time her old career came up. She smiled and shook her head. "That was just a part of it."

"Do you miss modeling?" he asked.

"Not at all," she said a touch too quickly, although she meant it. It wasn't the glamorous business everyone thought it was. It was harsh, and despite how many millions she made doing it and how famous she became, there were still days where she was treated like little more than a walking coat hanger. And a fat one at that. "I'm not really interested in being in the spotlight anymore. It is both a wonderful and terrifying place to live."

Gabriel nodded thoughtfully. "The runways and magazine covers suffer for your absence. I understand why you stopped after what happened to you on the runway, though. I can imagine it's scary to come that close to death without any kind of warning. I mean, to go all that time without knowing you had…what was it, exactly?"

"A congenital heart defect," she replied, the lie slipping effortlessly off her tongue after all these years.

"Yeah, that's terrifying to think your own body is just waiting to rebel against you."

Serafia stiffened and tried to nod in agreement. That would be frightening, although she really wouldn't know. Her parents had done an excellent job spreading misinformation about her very public heart attack. Why else would a perfectly healthy twenty-four-year-old woman go into cardiac failure on the runway and drop to the floor with a thousand witnesses standing by in horror?

She could think of a lot of reasons, and for her, all of them were self-inflicted. Serafia had fallen victim to an industry-endorsed eating disorder, which had spiraled out of control leading up to that day. Anorexia was a serious illness, an issue that needed more visibility in the cutthroat modeling industry, but her family wanted to keep the truth out of the papers for her own protection. At the time, she had been in no condition to argue with them on that point.

Instead the word was that she'd retired from the modeling business to get treatment for her "heart condition" and no one ever questioned it. Instead of surgeries, her actual treatment had included nearly a year of intensive rehabilitation. She had to slowly put on thirty pounds so she didn't strain her heart. Then she learned to eat properly, how to exercise correctly and most important how to recognize the signs in herself that she was slipping into bad habits again.

"Are you better now?" he asked.

That was debatable. With an eating disorder, every day was a challenge. It wasn't like being an alcoholic or a drug user, where you could avoid the substance of choice. She had to eat. Every day. She needed to exercise. Just not too much. She had to maintain her weight and not swing wildly one way or another, or she'd put too much strain on her damaged heart. But she was managing. One day at a time, she reminded herself. "Yes," she said instead. "The doctors got me all fixed up. But you're right, I couldn't face the catwalk again after that. After nearly dying, I realized I wanted to do something else with my life. I'm much happier with what I'm doing now."

"Gabriel Alejandro Montoro!" a sharp voice shouted through the doorway to the patio. It was followed by several loud steps across the stone and a moment later, the figure of his younger sister, Bella, appeared.

"There you are. Everyone has been looking for you."

Gabriel shrugged, unaffected by his sister's exasperation. "I've been right here the whole time. And since when do you get to call me by my full name? Only Mama gets to do that."

"And if Mama were here, she'd haul you back into the house by your ear."

Serafia chuckled. Her memories of Adela were spot-on. "I'm sorry to monopolize Gabriel's time," she said, hoping to draw down some of his sister's ire. "We were discussing the plans for his royal transformation."

Bella eyed Serafia suspiciously, then turned to look at Gabriel. "Good luck with that. Either way, Father wants you inside, and now. He's wanting to do some kind of toast and then he wants to see you out on the dance floor. The press wants a shot of you dancing."

Gabriel stood with a reluctant sigh, reaching out his hand to help Serafia up. "And so it begins. Would you care to join me inside?"

"Absolutely." Serafia slipped her arm through his and they walked back into the house together.

There were even more people in the room now than there were when she'd decided it was too crowded and gone outside. Nothing she could do about it, though. She stayed by his side as they cut through the crowd in search of his father. They found him standing by the bar with Gabriel's cousin, Juan Carlos.

Serafia had never had much contact with the Salazar branch of the Montoro family, but she had heard good things about Juan Carlos. He had a good head on his shoulders. He was responsible and thoughtful. To hear some people talk, he was Gabriel's polar opposite and a better choice for king. She would never tell Gabriel that, though; he had enough worries. Perhaps Juan Carlos would accept a post as the king's counsel. He would make an excellent adviser for Gabriel or royal liaison to Alma's prime minister.

"There you are," Rafael said once he spied them. "Where have you..." He paused when his gaze flicked over Serafia. "Ah. Never mind. Now I know what has occupied your time," he said with a smile.

"It's good to see you again," she said, returning his grin and leaning in to hug her father's oldest friend.

"Too long!" Rafael exclaimed. "But now that some

of us will be back in Alma, that will not be the case. Your father tells me he's considering moving back if the monarchy is stable."

"He told me that, as well." Her dad had mentioned it, but the Espina family was a little gun-shy when it came to their home country. Their quick departure from Alma in the 1940s had been a messy one. There were rumors and accusations thrown at anyone who fled before Tantaberra rose to power, and her family was not immune. Serafia knew they would move slowly on that front and some might never return. Spain was all she had ever known and she had fallen in love with Barcelona. It would take a lot to lure her away from her hacienda with beachfront views of the Mediterranean.

Rafael clapped his son on the back. "Now that you're here, I want to make a small speech, do a toast, and then maybe you can take a spin around the dance floor and encourage others to join you. The party is getting dull."

Gabriel nodded and Juan Carlos went over to silence the band and bring Rafael the microphone. The music stopped as Rafael stepped onto the riser with the band and raised his hand to get the crowd's attention. He had such a commanding presence; the whole room went deathly silent in a moment. He would've made a good king, too. Alma's archaic succession laws needed to be changed.

"Ladies and gentlemen," Rafael began. "I want to thank all of you for coming here tonight. Our family has waited seventy years for a night like this, when we could finally see the monarchy restored to Alma. With it, we hope to see peace, prosperity and hope restored for the people of Alma, as well. I'm thrilled to be able to stand up here and join all of you in wishing my son and future king, Prince Gabriel, all the success in the world as he returns to our homeland."

Several of the people in the crowd cheered and applauded Rafael's statement. Gabriel stood stiff at Serafia's side, his jaw tight and his muscles tense. He didn't seem to be as excited as everyone else. After their discussion outside, she understood his hesitation. Still clinging to his arm, she squeezed it reassuringly and smiled at him.

"I ask everyone here to raise their glass to the future king of Alma, Gabriel the First! Long live the king!"

"Long live the king!" everyone shouted as they held up their glasses and took a sip. Serafia raised her glass as well, drinking the last of her wine.

"Now I would like to ask Gabriel to step out onto the dance floor and show us a few moves. Everyone, please, join us."

"Looks like I have to ask a lady to join me on the dance floor." Gabriel leaned in closer to her, a sly smile curling his full lips. "Have your doctors cleared you for vigorous physical activity?"

Serafia smiled at Gabriel and nodded. "Oh yes, I've got a clean bill of health. I could go all night on the dance floor if you can keep up with me."

Gabriel took her hand and led her out into the center of the room. As the band started playing an upbeat salsa tune, his hand went to her waist and tugged her body tight against his. "Is that a challenge?" he asked.

The contact of his hard body against hers sent a shock wave through her system that she had little time to recover from. He was no longer the mop-topped little boy she remembered running up and down the beach with his kite. Now his green eyes glittered with attraction and a flash of danger. And he *was* dangerous. She might not have finished high school, but she read enough history to know that getting involved with a king never ended well.

Before she could answer him they started moving in time with the music. It had been a long time since she'd danced, but the movement came easily with his strong lead. She almost seemed to float across the wooden floors, the rhythm of the music pulsing through their bodies. The crowds and the cameras around them faded away as they moved as one.

Soon other couples joined them on the dance floor and she didn't feel so exposed. The people around her made her feel better about the prying eyes, but being in Gabriel's arms was still a precarious place to be. The way he held her, the way he looked at her… The next two weeks were going to be a challenge to her patience and her self-control. Gabriel wanted more from her than just a makeover, and when he held her, she felt the same way. She never should've accepted the job, and she knew that now.

This was no teenage girl or Spanish businessman she was dealing with here. Gabriel Montoro was a sexy, rebellious handful and if she wasn't careful, she was going to get in way over her head.

Three

"You're late. Again."

That wasn't anything Gabriel didn't already know. After the last few days he'd had, he wasn't really in the mood to hear it. He'd signed himself up for this nightmare, but he was almost to the point where he'd pay Serafia more to leave him alone than to stay. He was used to the constant criticism of his family, but for whatever reason, Serafia's critical comments grated on him. He just didn't want a woman like her pointing out his faults. He wanted her nibbling on his ear. Unfortunately critiquing him was her job.

"Thanks for the information," he snapped. "When I'm king, I will have you named the official court time-keeper."

He expected her to respond with a smart comment, but instead she turned on her heel and walked across the room. She returned a moment later with a velvet-covered tray in her hands. Laid across it were four different styles of watches.

"One of these, actually, will be the official court timekeeper. I had them brought over from a local jeweler for you to choose the one you like."

His cell phone chimed and he looked down at the screen to avoid the display of watches in front of him. It was a text from a woman he'd gone out with a few weeks ago: a brunette named Carla. He opted to ignore it. He'd been getting a lot of those texts lately and he couldn't do anything about them now that he was on house arrest. What would he say, anyway? "Sorry, love, I've got to fly to a country you've never heard of and be king"?

Slipping the phone back into his pocket, he sighed when he realized the tray of watches was still there, waiting on him. *Watches.* Gabriel hated watches. He didn't wear one, ever. And why did he need to with the clock on his cell phone? "I don't need a watch."

Her resolve didn't waver. "You say that, and yet I've noticed punctuality seems to be a problem for you."

Was she an image consultant or a drill sergeant? "It's not a problem for me. I'm fine. It seems to be more of a problem for you."

Serafia's pink lips tightened as she seemed to fight a frown. "Please choose one."

"I told you, I'm not going to wear a watch." Gabriel couldn't stand the feel of something on his wrists. He'd worn watches all through high school and college, but after his abduction, he gave them all away. Even the nicest watches reminded him of the restraints he'd worn for too long. In an instant, he was back in that cold, dark basement and he never ever wanted to go back to that place.

"There's a Ferragamo, a Patek Philippe and two Rolexes. How can you turn your nose up at a Rolex?" Serafia reached down and plucked one off the tray. "Try this on. It's steel and yellow gold, so it will coordinate nicely with whatever you might be wearing. The faceplate is surrounded by pave diamonds and there are diamonds on the hours. I think it will really look elegant—"

Gabriel didn't move fast enough and before he knew what she had planned, he felt the cold steel of the metal at his wrist. His whole body tensed in an instant. On reflex, he hissed and jerked away from her. He was instantly transported back to Venezuela and the dark, claustrophobic room he was held in for almost a week. He could smell the mildew and filth, the air stale and thick with humidity.

"I said no!" he shouted without intending to. His eyes flew open, taking in the open, airy bedroom. He drew in a deep breath of air scented with hibiscus flowers and felt the tension fade from his shoulders. Looking at Serafia, he immediately regretted his reaction. There was fear as real as his own reflected in her dark eyes. "I'm sorry to yell," he said, but it was too late. The damage was done.

She shied away from him, turning her back and carrying the hundred thousand dollars' worth of watches back to the desk. She didn't speak again until she returned, more composed. It was amazing how she always seemed so put together. He could rattle her for a moment, but she always seemed to snap right back.

That was one skill he could use, but she hadn't taught him that yet.

She crossed her arms over her chest and looked at him. "What was all that about?"

Gabriel didn't like talking about his abduction. And his family had done a good job keeping the story out of the media. "I...I just don't like to wear a watch. I don't like the feel of anything around my wrists." He didn't want to elaborate. She already looked at him as if he was flawed. She had no idea how truly flawed he was. He was broken.

Serafia sighed, searching his face for answers he wasn't going to give her. "Okay, fine. No watch." She picked up her tablet and tapped through a few screens. "Your first public event in Alma will be a party hosted by Patrick Rowling. We need to get you fitted for your formal attire."

Patrick Rowling. Gabriel had heard his father and brother talking about the man, but he hadn't paid any attention. "Who is Patrick Rowling?"

"He's one of the richest men in Alma. He's British, actually, but when oil was discovered in Alma, his drilling company led the charge. He owns and operates almost all the oil platforms and refineries in the country. He's a very powerful and influential man. This party will be your first introduction to Alman society. Forging a solid relationship with the Rowlings will help secure a strong foothold for the monarchy."

Gabriel would be king, but somehow he got the feeling that he would be the one kissing Patrick's ring and not the other way around. He was already dreading this party and he didn't know anything about it.

"Now, this is a formal event, so custom dictates that you should wear ceremonial dress."

Serafia swung open the door of the armoire and pulled out a navy military uniform that looked like something out of an old oil painting in a museum. It looked stiff and itchy and he had absolutely no interest in wearing it.

"All right, now," he complained. "I've been a really good sport about most of this makeover stuff, but this is going too far." Gabriel frowned at Serafia as she held up the ridiculous-looking suit. "I let you cut my hair, give me a facial, a manicure, a pedicure and all other kinds of cures. You've given half my wardrobe to charity and spent thousands of dollars of my own money on suits no man under sixty would want to wear. I've tried to keep my mouth shut and go with it. But that... that outfit is ridiculous."

Serafia's eyes grew wider the longer he complained. "It's the ceremonial dress of the king!" she argued.

Of course it was. "It's got ropes and tassels and a damn baby-blue sash. I'm going to look like Prince Charming at the ball."

Serafia frowned. "That's the point, Gabriel. You are going to be *Su Majestad el Rey Don Gabriel I.* That's what kings wear."

"Maybe in the 1940s when my great-grandfather was the king. It's old-fashioned. Outdated."

"It's not for every day. It's for events like coronations, weddings and formal events like this party at the Rowling Estate. The rest of the time you'll wear normal clothes."

"Normal clothes you picked out," he noted. Not much better in his estimation.

Serafia sighed and returned the suit to the armoire. When she shut the door, she slumped against it in a posture of defeat. Closing her eyes, she pinched the bridge of her nose between her fingers. "We leave for Alma in two days and we have so much to cover. At this rate, we're never going to get it all done. You hired me, Gabriel. Why are you fighting me on every little thing?"

He didn't think he was fighting her on everything. The watch issue was nonnegotiable, but they'd gotten that unpleasantness out of the way. The clothing was just a hard pill for him to swallow. "I'm not intentionally trying to make your job more difficult. It just seems to be a gift I have."

Serafia rolled her eyes. "So it seems. Admittedly, you appear to enjoy getting me all spun up. I've seen you smile through my irritation."

Gabriel had to admit that was true. There was something about the flush of irritation that made Serafia even that much more beautiful, if it was possible. In his mind, he imagined the same would hold true when she was screaming out in passion, clawing at the sheets. The woman who had sashayed down the runway all those years ago had nothing on the vision in his mind as he thought of her at night.

And he had. Since the night on the patio, he'd lain alone in bed every night thinking about her. He hadn't intended to. Serafia was a fantasy from his younger years; the image of her in a bikini was the background of his first computer. It had been a long time since he'd had a crush on Serafia, and yet those desires had rushed back at the first sight of her.

It was probably his family-imposed curfew. The day his brother abdicated, he was practically dragged from his penthouse to the family compound. He'd gone weeks with no clubs, no bars, no socializing with friends at parties. His every move was watched and that meant he was on the verge of his longest dry spell since he broke the seal on his manhood.

It didn't really matter, though, at least where Serafia was concerned. He could've bedded a woman this morning and he would still want her the way he always had wanted her.

"Yes," he admitted at last. "I get pleasure from watching you spin."

"Why? Are you a sadist?"

Gabriel smiled wide and took a few steps closer to her. "Not at all. It might be cliché to say it, but, Serafia, you are even more beautiful when you're angry."

Serafia rejected the flicker of disbelief in the back of her mind and silenced the denial on her lips. As her therapist had trained her, she identified the negative thoughts and reframed them. She was a healthy, attractive woman. Gabriel found her eye-catching and it wasn't her place to question his opinion of her. "Thank you," she said. "But please don't spend the rest of our time together trying to annoy me. You might find I'm more attractive, but it's emotionally exhausting."

Gabriel took another step toward her, closing in on her personal space. With her back pressed against the oak armoire, she had no place to go or escape. A part of her didn't really want to escape, anyway. Not when he looked at her like that.

His dark green eyes pinned her in place, and her breath froze in her lungs. He wasn't just trying to flatter her with his words. He did want her. It was very obvious. But it wasn't going to happen for an abundance of reasons that started with his being the future king and ended with his being a notorious playboy. Even dismissing everything in between, it was a bad idea. Serafia had no interest in kings or playboys.

"Well, I'll do my best, but I do so enjoy the flush of rose across your cheeks and the sparkle of emotion in your dark eyes. My gaze is drawn to the tension along the line of your graceful neck and the rise and fall of your breasts as you breathe harder." He took another step closer. Now he could touch her if he chose. "If you don't want me to make you angry anymore, I could think of another way to get the same reaction that would be more...*pleasurable* for us both."

Serafia couldn't help the soft gasp that escaped her lips at his bold words. For a moment, she wanted to reach out for him and pull him hard against her. Every nerve in her body was buzzing from his closeness to her. She could feel the heat of his body radiating through the thin silk of her blouse. Her skin flushed and tightened in response.

One palm reached out and made contact with the polished oak at her back. He leaned in and his cologne— one of the few things she hadn't changed—teased at her nose with sandalwood and leather. The combination was intoxicating and dangerous. She could feel herself slipping into an abyss she had no business in. She needed to stop this before it went too far. Serafia was first and foremost a professional.

"I'm not sleeping with you," she blurted out.

Gabriel's mouth dropped open in mock outrage. "Miss Espina, I'm shocked."

Serafia chuckled softly, the laughter her only release

for everything building up inside her. She arched one eyebrow at him. "Shocked that I would be so blunt or shocked that I'm turning you down?"

At that, he smiled and she felt her knees start to soften beneath her. Much more of that and she'd be a puddle in her Manolos.

"Shocked that you would think that was all I wanted from you."

Serafia crossed her arms over her chest. She barely had room for the movement with Gabriel so close. She needed the barrier. She didn't believe a word he said. "What exactly were you suggesting, then?"

His jewel-green gaze dropped down to the cleavage her movement had enhanced. She was clutching herself so tightly that she was on the verge of spilling out of her top. She relaxed, removing some, if not all of the distraction.

"I'm feeling a little caged up. I was going to suggest a jog around the compound followed by a dip in the swimming pool," he said.

"Sure you were," she replied with a disbelieving tone. "You look like a man who's hard up for a good run."

He smiled and she felt a part deep inside her clench with need. Desire had not been very high on Serafia's priority list for a very long time. She was frustrated at how easily Gabriel could push her body's needs to the top of the list.

"The king's health and well-being should be at the forefront of the minds of the Alman people. Long live the king, right?"

"Long live the king," she responded, albeit unenthusiastically.

"So, how about that run?"

The way he looked at her, the way he leaned into her, it felt as if he was asking for more than just a run. But she answered the question at hand and tried to ignore her body's response to his query. "First, you need your ceremonial dress tailored. It will take a couple days to get it back and we need it before we leave. Then you can run if you like."

"And what about you? Don't you need a little rush of endorphins? A little…release?"

"I exercised when I got up this morning," she replied. And she had. Every morning when she woke up, she did exactly forty-five minutes on her elliptical machine. No more, no less, doctor's orders. Her treadmill at home was gathering dust, since running was out of the question unless her life was in danger.

His gaze raked over her, making every inch of her body aware of his heavy appraisal before he made a sucking sound with his tongue and shook his head. "Pity."

He dropped his arm and took a step back, allowing her lungs to fill with fresh oxygen that wasn't tainted with his scent. It helped clear her head of the fog that had settled in when he was so close.

The persistent chirp of his cell phone drew his attention away and for that, Serafia was grateful. Apparently Gabriel's harem of women were lonely without him. Since they'd begun this process four days ago, he averaged a text or two an hour. Most of the time he didn't respond, but that didn't stop the messages from coming in. She didn't care about what he'd been involved in, but she couldn't help noticing all the different names on the screen.

Carla, Francesca, Kimi, Ronnie, Anita, Lisa, Tammy, Jessica, Emily, Sara…it was as if his phone was spinning through a massive Rolodex of names. His little digital black book would be ungainly if it were in print.

"I'm going to go see if the tailor has arrived," she said as he put the phone away again. "Do you think you can fight off all your lovers long enough to get this jacket fitted properly?"

Gabriel narrowed his eyes at her and slipped his phone into his pocket. "You sound jealous."

Maybe a little. But that was none of his concern. She would deal with it accordingly. "Not jealous," she corrected. "I'm concerned."

He frowned at her then. "You sound like my father. Why would you be concerned with my love life?"

"It's like I told you that first night, Gabriel. Your life is no longer your own. Not your relationships or your free time or even your body. You can't drive your sports cars around like a Formula One driver and put the king's health at risk. You can't party every night with a different woman and put the future of your country in the hands of a bastard you father with some girl you barely remember. You can't waste the realm's money on the hedonistic pleasures you've built your whole life on."

"From what I learned in school, that's what most kings do, actually."

"Maybe four hundred years ago, but not anymore. If King Henry the Eighth had to deal with the modern press, things would've ended very differently for him and all his poor wives."

"So you're saying it's all about appearances? I have

to be squeaky clean on the outside to keep the press and the people happy?"

"It's bigger than that. Your recklessness is indicative of an emotional disconnect. That's what worries me. You need to prepare yourself for the marriage that is just around the corner for you. You may not even have met the woman yet, but I guarantee you'll be married before the first year of your reign comes to an end. That means no more skirt chasing. You have to take this seriously. You have to really connect with someone, and I don't see that coming easily to you."

"You don't think I can connect with someone?" He seemed insulted by her insinuation.

"Relationships—*real relationships*—are hard. Love and trust and honesty are difficult to maintain. I've only been around here for a few days, but I haven't seen you interact with a single person on a sincere level. You have no real relationships, not even with your family."

"I have real relationships," he argued, but even as he spoke the words, she sensed a question in his voice.

"Name one. If something huge happened in your life, who would you run to with the news? If you had a secret, who would you confide in?"

There was an extended silence as he thought about the answer to her question. There would be a quicker response for almost anyone else she asked this question of. A mother, a brother, a best friend, a buddy from college… Gabriel had no answer. It was both sad and disconcerting. Why did he keep everyone at arm's length?

"I have plenty of friends and family. Since I've been announced as the future king, they've been coming out of the woodwork. I don't know what you're talking about."

"I'm talking about having a person in your life who you can tell anything, good or bad. Someone to confide in. I don't think Jessica or Tammy is the right answer. But I also don't think Rafe or Bella are, either. Everyone needs a person like that in their lives. I feel like there are people who would be there for you, but you won't let them in. I feel a resistance, a buffer there, even with your own family, and I don't know what it's about. What I do know is that you need to learn to let those walls down or this week will be nothing compared to the next year."

"I figured the opposite would be true," he replied at last. "When you're the king, everyone wants something from you. You can't trust anyone. Your marriage is arranged, your closest advisers jockeying for their own pet projects. I would've thought that keeping my distance would be an asset in that kind of environment."

"Maybe you're right," she admitted with a sad shrug. "I certainly would've been more prepared for the world of modeling if I'd gone in believing that everyone wanted something from me and that I couldn't trust them. But I think everyone, even a king, needs someone."

"Believe me, it's easier this way," he said. "If you don't trust anyone, they can't betray you and you'll never be disappointed."

There was an honesty in his words that she hadn't heard in anything else he'd said when they were together. That worried her. Someone, at some point, had damaged Gabriel. She knew it shouldn't be her concern, but she couldn't help wondering what had happened and how she could help.

The people of Alma—Serafia included—wanted

more from their king than Gabriel was willing to give them. He hadn't even been crowned king yet and she worried this was going to be a mistake. No amount of haircuts or fancy clothes could fix the break deep inside of him.

He had to do that himself.

Four

Two days later, Gabriel stepped onto a private jet and left the life he knew behind him. They flew overnight, his father, Rafael, sleeping in the bedroom of the plane as he and Serafia slept in fully reclining leather chairs. It was a quiet flight without a lot of conversation once they finished their dinners and dimmed the cabin lights.

Gabriel slept soundly, and when he awoke, they were thirty minutes out from landing in his new country. He'd only been there once before with Rafe on a whirlwind tour, but when he got off the plane this time, he was supposed to be their leader.

"You need to get dressed," Serafia said beside him. "Your suit is hanging up in the bathroom."

He hadn't heard her get up, but she had changed her clothes, refreshed her makeup and styled her thick,

dark hair into a bun. For the next week, she was publically filling the role of his social secretary while privately coaching him through all the events. She was
dressed for the part in a ladies' taupe suit. The blazer
was well tailored and didn't look boxy, and the sheath
dress beneath it was fitted and came down just to her
knee, showcasing her long and shapely calves.

It was elegant, but Gabriel found himself longing
for the clingy red silk gown from their first night together. In this outfit, she completely faded into the
background. He supposed that was the idea, but he
didn't like it. Serafia might not care for the spotlight,
but she was born to be in it.

He went to the bathroom, getting ready and changing into the navy suit she'd hung out for him. She'd
paired it with a lighter blue shirt and a plain blue tie.
It was a sophisticated look, she'd argued, but it seemed
boring to him. It made him want to wear crazy socks,
but he wouldn't. She'd already laid out a pair of navy
socks for him.

By the time he came back out, his father had emerged
from the bedroom and the pilot was announcing their
descent into Del Sol, the capital of Alma.

"The press will be waiting for you when we arrive.
They've arranged for a carpet to be laid out and your
royal guards will be there for crowd control. They've
already secured the area and screened all the attendees.
Your press secretary, Señor Vega, briefed everyone on
appropriate questions, so things should go smoothly.
I will exit the plane first and make sure everything is
okay," Serafia explained. "Then Señor Montoro, and
then you're last. Wait until the carpet is clear. Take your
time so everyone can get their photos."

Gabriel nodded, taking in her constant stream of instructions as he had done all week. She was a font of information.

"Don't forget to smile. Wave. It should just be the press, so no need to greet anyone in the crowd. No speeches, no interviews. Just smile and wave."

The wheels of the jet touched down and suddenly everything became very real. Gabriel looked out the window. Beyond the airport, he could see the great rock hills that rose on the horizon, their gray stone peppered with evergreens. Closer to Del Sol was a smaller hill topped with some kind of ancient fortress. Climbing up the incline were whitewashed buildings clustered together with clay tile roofs.

Ahead, clear blue skies with palm trees led the way toward the beach. His last trip here with his brother had been all business, so he had no idea what kinds of beaches they had in Alma, but he prayed they were at least halfway as nice as the ones in Miami. He was already feeling pangs of homesickness.

The plane stopped and the engines turned off. The small crew unlocked and extended the staircase. Serafia gathered up her bag and her tablet. "Smile and wave," she said one last time before disappearing down the stairs.

His father followed her a moment later and then it was Gabriel's turn. His heart started pounding in his rib cage. His lungs could barely take in enough air, his chest was so tight. Once he stepped out of this plane, he was a coronation away from being *Su Majestad el Rey Don Gabriel I.* It was a terrifying prospect, but he pushed himself up out of his seat anyway.

Taking a deep breath, he stepped into the doorway.

He was momentarily blinded by the sun. He paused for a moment to adjust, a smile on his face and his arm raised in greeting. He slowly made his way down the stairs, careful not to fall and make the worst possible impression. By the time he reached the bottom, he could look out into the crowd of photographers. There were about fifty of them gathered with cameras and video crews.

To the left and right of the stairs were two large gentlemen in military suits similar to the one Serafia had recently had tailored for him. In addition to their shiny brass buttons and collections of metals, they wore earpieces with cords that disappeared under their collars. He hadn't really given the idea of his personal security much thought until now.

The men bowed, and after he nodded to them both, they walked two paces behind Gabriel as he made his way down the carpet. At the end of the path, he could see his father and Serafia waiting for him with a man he presumed was his press secretary. Serafia had an exaggerated smile like a stage mom, reminding him to smile and wave.

He was almost to the end when a man with a video crew charged to the edge of the barricade and shouted to him. "Gabriel! How do you feel about your brother's abdication? Did you know he had a child on the way?"

The bold question startled him.

"Rafe made his choice. I don't blame him for his decision." Serafia had told him he wasn't to answer questions, but he was thrown off guard with a film crew pointing the camera right in his face.

"What about the child?" the man pressed.

He felt a protectiveness build up inside him, his fists

curling tight at his side. "I was unaware of the seriousness of his relationship with Ms. Fielding, but the matter of their child is their business, and I must insist that
you respect their privacy."

"Have you chosen a queen yet?" Another reporter
shouted before he could take another step. From there,
it was a rapid fire he couldn't escape.

"Will she be a citizen of Alma or a member of a European royal family to strengthen trade agreements?"

"Did you leave a lover behind in America?"

Gabriel felt his throat close. He didn't know how
to even begin addressing these questions, but he was
certain his required smile had faded.

"Please!" Serafia shouted, stepping in front of him
and holding her hands up to the camera. "He's been in
Del Sol for five minutes. Let's allow Don Gabriel to get
settled in and perhaps coroneted before we start worrying about the line of succession, shall we?"

She took his arm and with a forceful tug, led him
down the rug and inside the terminal. From there, security ushered them quickly out a side door to a black
SUV with Alma's flag flying on each corner of the
hood.

The door had barely shut before the convoy was on
the road. The inside of the vehicle was quiet. He was
stunned by the turn of events. Serafia was stiff beside him.

"What the hell was that?" his father finally asked.

"I didn't realize—" Gabriel began to defend himself
to his father, but he realized he was looking at Serafia
with eye daggers.

"You said there were to be no questions," Rafael
snapped. "Why wasn't the press properly briefed?"

"They were," she argued, her spine lengthening in defiance. "Hector assured me that they were told Gabriel wasn't answering questions, but to tell them they can't ask is suppression of free press. No matter what they're told, reporters will ask questions in the hopes they can catch someone off guard and get an answer that will provide a juicy headline."

"Unacceptable."

Serafia sighed angrily. "I can assure you that I will work with Hector to have the offending reporters identified and will see to it that their press privileges are suspended."

"Gabriel should've been briefed. If you knew the press might push him for questions, he should've been better prepared. That's your job."

"I'm an image consultant, not his press secretary. What kind of briefing does he need to walk down a rug and wave? I suggest that when we arrive at the palace, we arrange to meet with Hector immediately. He'll need to be able to handle those sorts of things better in the future. There are more public appearances this week. We can't risk that happening again. I'm sorry that—"

"Stop," Gabriel said. He'd grown angrier with every apologetic word out of her mouth. There was no reason for her to ask for forgiveness. "You've done nothing wrong, Serafia. I apologize for my father's harsh, inappropriate tone. I should've anticipated they would ask questions like that. I will be more prepared next time. End of discussion. For now, let's just focus on getting settled in and prepared for our next event."

His father's sharp gaze raked over him as he spoke, the older man's tan Mediterranean complexion mottled with red. He was clearly angry his son had shut him down, but that was too bad. The balance of power had shifted in the family. The moment Gabriel stepped off that plane, he was in charge. They weren't in Miami anymore where his father ruled over the family with an iron fist.

They were in Alma now and Gabriel was going to be the king. His father had ruined his chance to be the boss when he divorced Gabriel's mother without an annulment, so he'd better get used to the way things were going to be now. Gabriel was no longer the useless middle son who could be berated or ignored.

Gabriel was going to be king.

"It's beautiful," Serafia said as they entered the main room of the palace.

El Castillo del Arena was the official royal residence in Del Sol. Looking like a giant sandcastle, hence its name, it sat on a fortified wall overlooking the bay. The early Arabian influences on the architecture were evident everywhere you looked, from the arches to the intricate mosaic tile work. The inner courtyards had gardens that made a cool escape from the sun with lush trees, fountains and blooming flowers in every direction.

Clearly it wasn't as grand a palace as it had once been: the Persian rugs had threadbare corners and the upholstery on the furniture was worn and dirty. Seventy years in the hands of a dictatorship had made their mark, but it still had the grand design and details of its former glory. It wouldn't take long to restore the palace.

Few people had been allowed in under the Tantaberras. It was a pity. The grand rooms with the arched ceilings were begging for a royal event with all the elite of Alma in attendance.

From the expression on his face, Gabriel wasn't as impressed. Since the heated discussion in the car, he'd been quiet. She thought that when Señor Montoro skipped the tour and asked to be shown to his rooms so he could nap Gabriel would perk up, but he didn't. Now he silently took it all in as they followed his personal steward, Ernesto, on a tour through the palace.

"These are the king's private chambers," Ernesto said as he opened the double doors to reveal the expansive room.

There was a king-size bed in the center of the room with a massive four-poster frame. It was draped in red fabric with a dozen red and gold pillows scattered across the bed. Large tapestries hung on the walls, and a Moroccan rug covered the stone floors.

"Your bath and closet are through those doors," Ernesto continued.

She watched as Gabriel looked around, a slightly pained expression on his face. "It's awfully dark in here," he complained. "It's like a cave or an underground cellar. Are there only those two windows?"

Ernesto looked at the two arched windows crafted of stained glass and nodded. "Yes, Your Majesty."

She watched Gabriel tense at the use of the formal title. "I'm not king yet, Ernesto. You can just call me Gabriel."

The man's eyes grew wide. "I would rather not, Your Grace. You're still the crown prince."

"I suppose." Gabriel sighed and fixed his gaze on a set of double doors on the other side of the room. "Where do those doors go to?"

Ernesto, lean and dark-complexioned, moved quickly to the doors and opened them. "Through here are the queen's rooms. And beyond it are chambers for her ladies-in-waiting, although the rooms may be better suited in these times as an office or a nursery. The rooms haven't really been used since your great-grandmother, Queen Anna Maria, fled Alma."

Gabriel frowned. "The queen doesn't share a room with the king?"

"She may. Traditionally, having her own space allowed her to pursue more feminine activities with her ladies such as sewing or reading without interfering with the running of the state."

"It's like I've gone back in time," Gabriel grumbled, and ran his fingers through his hair in exasperation.

"The staff is still working on restoring and modernizing the palace. Perhaps Your Majesty would prefer to spend some time prior to the coronation at Playa del Onda. It's a more modern estate, built for the royal family to vacation at the beach in the summers. It's lovely, with floor-to-ceiling windows that overlook the sea and bright, open rooms."

For the first time since they'd arrived, Serafia noticed Gabriel perk up. "How far is it from here?"

"It's about an hour's drive along the coastal highway, but you won't mind a minute of it. The views are exquisite. I can call ahead to the staff there and let them know you'll be coming if you'd like."

Gabriel considered his options for a moment and finally turned to look at Serafia. "I know we'll be coming back to Del Sol for a lot of activities this week, but I think I'd like to stay out there while I can. Care to continue our work at the beach?" he asked.

She nodded. The location wasn't important to her, but she could tell it mattered to him. He seemed to have a tense, almost claustrophobic reaction to his own quarters, despite the room being massive in scale with tall, arched ceilings. If he could relax, he would absorb more information. She could accommodate the extended drive times in their schedule.

"Then let's do that. My father will be staying here, but Señorita Espina and I will be going to Playa del Onda. We'll be staying there for the next week. I'll return as we start preparing for the coronation."

"Very good. I'll arrange for your transportation."

"Ernesto?"

The steward paused. "Yes, Your Majesty?"

"See if you can arrange for a convertible with a GPS. I'd like to drive myself to the compound and enjoy the sun and sea air on the way."

"Drive yourself?" Ernesto seemed stumped for a moment, but then immediately shook off his concerns. It wasn't his place to question the king's requests. "Yes, Your Grace." He turned and disappeared down the hallway.

"They're not going to know what to do with a king like you," Serafia said.

"Me, neither," Gabriel noted dryly. "But maybe if we spend a couple days at the beach, we can all be better prepared for my official return to the palace."

They walked out of the king's chambers and down the winding staircase to the main hall. Within minutes, they were greeted by the royal guard, who reported that they already had a car waiting for him outside. They would be following in the black SUV that brought him there.

Gabriel didn't argue. Instead they walked out into the courtyard. A cherry-red Peugeot convertible was parked there. "Whose car is this?" he asked as an attendant opened the door for Serafia to get in.

"It is Señor Ernesto's car, Your Majesty."

"What will he drive while I have it?"

"One of the royal fleet." The attendant pointed to an area with several vehicles parked there. "He is happy to let you borrow it. The address of the beach compound is already entered in the system, Your Majesty."

Gabriel took the keys, slipped out of his suit coat and got in beside her. He waited until the guard had assembled in the SUV behind them; then he started the car and they headed toward the gates.

Once they slipped beyond the fortress walls, Serafia noticed Gabriel's posture relax. It was as if a weight had been lifted from his shoulders. She couldn't help feeling the same way. Ernesto had been right: the view was amazing. Once they escaped Del Sol and started climbing up the mountain, everything changed. The winding coastal road showcased wide vistas with bright blue skies, turquoise waters and ships along the shoreline.

With the sun warming her skin and the ocean air whipping the strands of her hair around her face, she felt herself relax for the first time since she'd left Barcelona. Although the Atlantic islands were different from her Mediterranean hacienda, it felt as if she were back there, the place where she felt the most at home, and safe.

"Are you hungry?" he asked.

"Yes." They'd had croissants and juice on the plane, but it was past lunchtime now and she was starving.

Gabriel nodded. A mile up the road, he slowed and

pulled off at a small, hole-in-the-wall restaurant over-looking the sea. A moment later, the royal guard pulled up beside them and lowered a window.

"Is there a problem, Your Majesty?" the one with the slicked-back brown hair who was driving the SUV asked.

"I'm hungry. Have you two had lunch?"

The two guards looked at each other in confusion and the driver turned back to him. "No, we haven't."

"Is this place any good?" he asked.

"I have eaten here many times, but in my opinion, it isn't fit for the king."

Gabriel looked at her and smiled widely. "Perfect. I'm starving. Let's all grab something to eat."

The two of them waited outside with the younger blond guard as the other went inside to make sure the restaurant was secure. It wasn't big enough to house much more than a tiny kitchen and a few tables on the veranda.

When they got the all-clear, a small, slow-moving old woman greeted them as they came in and gave them their choice of tables outside. As Gabriel had insisted they eat as well, the guards took a table near the door to watch anyone coming in or out, allowing him and Serafia privacy while they dined.

The menu was limited, but the royal guard with the dark hair named Jorge recommended the *calde-reta de langosta*. It was a seasonal lobster stew with tomatoes, onions, garlic and peppers, served with thin slices of bread.

They all ordered the caldereta and Serafia was not disappointed. Normally she gave great care and thought into every bite she put in her mouth, but the stew was too amazing to worry about it. The lobster was soft and buttery in texture, while spicy in flavor thanks to the peppers. The bread soaked up the broth perfectly and helped carry the large pieces of lobster to her mouth without her wearing most of it on her pale taupe suit.

"This is wonderful," she said, when she was more than halfway finished with her stew. "Thank you for stopping."

"I was getting cranky," Gabriel said. He glanced over the railing at the sparking blue sea below them. "If I can be cranky looking at a view like this, I've got to be hungry."

"I would've thought the incident this morning had more to do with it than hunger."

"This morning was nothing and my father wanted to make it into something. I have enough to worry about without him making you uncomfortable. You've gone out of your way to help me through this. You've tolerated my bad moods and my childish behavior. I think I will be a better king for what you've done, so I should be thanking you, not criticizing you."

Serafia was stunned by his thoughtful words. He seemed to be almost a different person since they'd arrived in Alma. Or at least since the moment he'd stood up to his father. He had seemed to grow taller in that moment, physically stronger even, as he sat in the vehicle. Perhaps he truly was gaining the confidence he needed to rule Alma.

"Thank you," she said. "I appreciate that. And I appreciate you standing up for me this morning. The look on your father's face when you put an end to the discussion was priceless, really."

Gabriel looked at her with a wry grin. "It was good,

wasn't it? It's the first time I've stood up to him in my whole life and I'm glad I did."

"Is he always like that?"

Gabriel sipped his sparkling water and nodded. "Nothing was ever good enough for my father, but especially me. I could never understand it growing up. I did everything right, everything he wanted me to do. I went to school where he wanted me to go, took the position at the company he wanted me to have. I let him banish me to South American Operations. After everything that happened there, I almost got the feeling he was disappointed I came back. I've never understood why."

"After everything that happened there?" Gabriel seemed to be alluding to some incident she was unaware of. "What happened?"

With a sigh, he popped the last of his bread in his mouth and shook his head. "It doesn't matter. What matters is that I learned some valuable lessons. First, that you have to be careful who you can trust. And second, that I'm a grown man who can live and do however I please. These last few years my behavior has just been written off by my family as reckless and selfish, but it's been good for me. If my father doesn't approve of me either way, I should do whatever I want to, right?"

Serafia suppressed her frown. How had she not seen how wounded he was before now? The cracks in his facade were starting to show and they made her wonder what had turned the obedient middle son into the rebellious, distant one. He didn't want to talk about it and she understood. She had dark secrets of her own, but she couldn't help wondering if his past and its effect on him might hinder his leadership in Alma.

"I never wanted to be king, but now that I'm here, I think this might work out. My father may still disagree with what I do and how, but now I don't have to listen to it any longer." Abruptly standing, he pulled some euros from his wallet and threw them down on the table to cover everyone's lunch tab. Serafia got up as well, placing her napkin on the table.

"Let's get back on the road."

Five

"You look very handsome tonight."

Serafia stood at Gabriel's side and looked over the railing at the crowd below. There was a sea of people there, all dressed in their finest tuxedos and gowns. A string quartet was in the corner, filling the large space with a soothing background melody. It was a glittering display of marble floors, towering flower arrangements and twinkling crystal chandeliers. Patrick Rowling spared no expense when it came to his home or the parties he hosted there.

They had arrived at the Rowling mansion via a side door and were escorted upstairs to wait in Patrick's library so Gabriel could make a grand entrance. To their right was an elaborate marble staircase that twisted its way into the center of the ballroom. It just begged for a king to stroll down with a regal air.

Regal was not the vibe she was getting from Gabriel.
Her compliment seemed to unnerve him. He shifted uncomfortably under her scrutiny, although there was no
reason for him to be nervous. The ceremonial dress had
been tailored beautifully and despite his complaints, he
looked noble, powerful and very appropriate for a party
like this. He had come a long way in the last week and
she'd felt a swell of pride in her chest when he stepped
out of his bedroom in full regalia earlier.

"I still feel like Prince Charming at the ball. And
from the look of the crowd here tonight, all the eligible young maidens have come to land a king for a
husband."

"I did notice that," she admitted. There were a lot of
young women at the party, all painted and coiffed to
the max. Decked out in an array of eye-catching jewel-
tone silks and satins, they were like parading peacocks
among the dark tuxedos. If Serafia had to guess, she'd
say that millions of dollars had been laid out tonight in
the hopes that they might catch the future king's eye.

She had gone the opposite route. Her gown was
a very soft pink, almost a blush color. The organza
ruching wrapped around her body, dotted with tiny
crystals and beads. While sedate in color, it still had
a few scandalous details like a plunging V-cut neckline and a slit on the side that almost reached the top
of her thigh. She wanted to look as if she belonged, but
she didn't want to stand out. She wasn't here to enjoy
a party; she was here to help Gabriel get through his
first real event in Alma.

"It certainly looks like you have your pick of ladies
here tonight."

"Do I?"

Serafia turned to look at him and was surprised to see the serious way he was looking at her. He had the same heated intensity in his eyes he'd had the day he pinned her against the armoire. What exactly did he mean by that? She couldn't possibly be his pick when there were so many younger, more attractive women in the room tonight. "I…uh…" She hesitated. "I…think you've got a lot to choose from and a long night ahead of you. Don't make a decision too quickly. Keep your options open."

Gabriel sighed and turned away to look at the crowd. "I'll try."

A man in a tuxedo approached them on the landing and bowed to Gabriel. "If Your Majesty is ready, I'll cue the musicians to announce your arrival."

"Yes, I suppose it's time."

"May I escort you downstairs, Señorita Espina?"

"Yes, thank you." She took the man's arm and turned back to Gabriel. "I'll see you downstairs after the guests have all been presented."

"You're not going down with me?"

Serafia chuckled. "This is like the arrival at the airport, but without the pushy reporters. You need to have your moment. Alone." She wouldn't make many new girlfriends tonight if she showed up on the king's arm and beat them all to the punch.

"Good luck," she said, giving him a wink before carefully descending the staircase and joining the crowd. She parted with her escort, finding a spot at the edge of the room near one of the royal guards to watch Gabriel's entrance.

The orchestra started playing Alma's national anthem. The bustling crowd immediately grew silent and everyone turned their gaze to the flag hanging from the second-floor railing. When the last note died out, Gabriel appeared at the top of the stairs looking as much like a king as a man raised to have the position.

"His Royal Highness, El Príncipe Gabriel, the future El Rey Don Gabriel the First of Alma."

The crowd applauded as he came down the stairs. The air in the room was electric with excitement. Gabriel didn't fully appreciate how important this was for the people of Alma. They were free, and his arrival was the living, breathing evidence of that freedom. People bowed and curtseyed as he passed.

"Oh my God, he's so handsome. I didn't think it was possible, but he's even more attractive than Rafe."

Serafia turned to see a young woman and her mother standing nearby. The woman was maybe twenty-three and she was in a sapphire-blue gown that looked amazing with her golden skin and flaxen hair. Her mother was an older carbon copy in a more sedate silver gown. They were both dripping with diamonds, but the twinkle in their eyes sparkled even brighter as they looked at Gabriel.

"Oh, Dita," the mother gushed. "He's perfect for you. This is your big chance tonight. You look absolutely flawless, better than any of the other girls here." She looked around the room, scanning the competition again. Her gaze lit on Serafia for only a moment, then moved on as though she were an insignificant presence. Apparently the woman didn't read *Vogue*, or she would realize she was standing beside a former supermodel.

Serafia recognized *her*, however. At the mention of her daughter's name, she realized the mother was Felicia Gomez. The Gomez family was one of the richest in Alma, although unlike the Rowlings, they were natives like the Espinas. Many of the wealthier families had fled Alma when Tantaberra came to power, but the Gomez family had stayed.

Serafia had never met them, but she had heard her mother talk about them from time to time. It was rarely flattering. She got the impression that they were fair-weather friend types who worked hard to ingratiate themselves with whoever was in power. She didn't know what they had to do to maintain their money and lands under the dictatorship, but she was certain it was a price the Espinas wouldn't have paid.

It would not surprise her mother at all to know they were here on the hunt for a rich husband. With the dictatorship dissolved, they had to put themselves in a good position with the new royal family, and what better way than to marry into it? Serafia took a step closer to listen in as Felicia continued her instructions to Dita.

"When we're introduced to the king, remember everything I've told you. You've got to make a good impression on him. Be coquettish, but not too aggressive. Make eye contact, but don't hold it for too long. Make him come to you and then you'll have him like putty in your hands. It worked on your father. It will work on him. You deserve to be queen, always remember that."

Serafia tried not to chuckle. She was certain a similar conversation was taking place all over the room. There were easily thirty bright-eyed girls here with their parents. All were after the same prize. Serafia might be the only single woman in the room who wasn't on the hunt. She had no interest in competing with a bunch of little girls for Gabriel's attention.

When Gabriel reached the bottom of the stairs, he

was greeted by his father and Patrick Rowling. They escorted him over to a raised dais on the far side of the room. They took their seats there and the crowd gathered for a receiving line. Everyone was excited for their chance to be introduced to the new king.

Serafia took advantage of the distraction to go to the empty bar. She got glasses of wine for them both, hugging the edge of the room to deliver the drink to Gabriel. As she got close, Patrick was introducing his sons, William and James, to Gabriel and his father. Will was Patrick's heir apparent to the oil and real estate empire they'd built. James, like Gabriel, was the second son, the spare heir, even though he was born only minutes after his twin brother.

Neither of the men looked particularly happy to be here tonight. Even then, they seemed more comfortable than Gabriel. He kept cycling between a stiff regal pose, a slightly slumped-over bored stance and a fidgety anxious carriage that made it obvious to Serafia that he was very uncomfortable. Perhaps a glass of wine would be enough to relax him without loosening his tongue too much.

Out of the corner of her eye, Serafia spied one of the party's many servers. The petite girl with chin-length black hair was lurking along the edge of the room, her gaze focused fully on the Rowling brothers as they greeted the king.

It took a moment, but Serafia was finally able to wave her over. As a model, she was used to towering over people, but the server was probably close to five feet tall, a little pixie of a thing with sparkling dark eyes that immediately caught Serafia's attention. On her immaculately pressed black shirt, she wore a small brass nametag that read *Catalina*.

"Yes, ma'am?"

"Would you please take this wine to Prince Gabriel?" Serafia placed the wine on her tray.

Catalina took a deep breath and nodded. "Of course," she said, immediately departing. Well trained, she waited until Will and James were escorted away, slipping over quietly to deliver the drink, then disappearing so quickly that some people might not have even seen her.

Gabriel took a heavy sip of the wine, searching Serafia out in the crowd. When his gaze lit on her, Serafia felt a chill run down her spine. Goose bumps rose across her bare arms, making her rub them self-consciously. He winked at her, and before she could prompt him to smile, he broke out his practiced grin and turned to the next family being presented.

Serafia had to admit she was pleased with the results of her work. In only a week, they had managed to smooth over his rough edges and mold him into a man fit to be royalty. As she watched him interact with the Gomez family and the young and beautiful Dita, she couldn't help the pang of jealousy inside her.

Perhaps she had done too good a job. She had polished away all the reasons she needed to stay far, far away from Gabriel Montoro.

Gabriel was exhausted. All he'd done for the last hour was get introduced to people, but he was done. He was tired of smiling, tired of greeting people. It wasn't as if he was going to be able to remember a single name once each person turned away and the next was presented.

Unfortunately there were hours left in the night. Now started the dancing and the mingling. With the formalities out of the way, people would seek him out for more casual discussions. The ladies would expect him to solicit a dance or two.

He did none of those things. Instead he sought out another glass a wine and a few bites from the buffet of canapés and fresh fruits. He was hoping to find Serafia, who had disappeared at some point, but instead his father cornered him at the baked brie.

"What do you think of William?"

William? Gabriel went through the two hundred names he'd just heard and drew a blank.

"William Rowling, Patrick's oldest son," Rafael clarified, seemingly irritated with Gabriel for dismissing the Rowlings so easily.

"Oh," Gabriel said, taking a sip of wine. He refrained from mentioning to his father that he couldn't tell the two brothers apart. That would just agitate him. "He seemed very nice. Why? Are you trying to fix me up with him? He's really not my type, Dad."

"Gabriel," Rafael said in a warning tone. "I was thinking about him and Bella."

Gabriel tried not to frown at his father. All this royalty nonsense was going to his father's head if he thought he could start arranging marriages and no one would question it. "I think Bella would have a great deal more to say on the subject than I would."

"Rowling is the most powerful businessman in Alma. Combining our families would strengthen our position here, both financially and socially. If he had a daughter I'd be shoving her under your nose, too."

"Dad, it's a marriage, not a business merger."

"Same difference. I had a similar arrangement with your mother and now our company is in the Fortune 500."

"*And* you're divorced," Gabriel added. Their mother was living happily on another continent and had been since Bella turned eighteen and she had fulfilled her obligation to Rafael and the children. That was just what Bella would want for her own marriage, Gabriel was sure. Turning from his father, he scanned the crowd again.

"Who are you looking for?" Rafael pressed.

"Serafia."

Rafael popped a shrimp into his mouth and chewed it with a sour expression. "Don't get too dependent on her, Gabriel. She's just here through the end of the week. You've got to learn to stand on your own without her."

Gabriel was taken aback by his father's words. What did he care as long as Gabriel parroted all the right words and did all the right things? "I'm not dependent on her. I simply enjoy her company and I'm finding this party tedious without her."

"Yes, well, don't get too involved on that front, either. If you're bored, I suggest you focus on the ladies here tonight. Take Dita Gomez or Mariella Sanchez for a spin around the dance floor and see if you feel differently."

"And what if I want to take Serafia for a spin around the dance floor, Father? Stop treating her like she's just an employee. The Espinas are just as important a noble family in Alma as any of these others."

His father stiffened and the red blotchiness Gabriel had seen so often lately started climbing up his neck.

"Now is not the time to discuss things like this," he hissed in a low voice. "Now is the time to mingle with your new countrymen and start your search for a suitable queen. We will talk about the Espina family later. Now go mingle!" he demanded.

Gabriel didn't bother arguing with him. If mingling meant he could get away from his father for a while, he'd do it gladly. Perhaps he'd find where Serafia was hiding in the process. With a nod, he set aside his plate and ventured out into the crowd. Every few feet he was stopped by someone and engaged in polite banter. How did he like Alma so far? Did the weather suit him? Had he had the opportunity to enjoy the beaches or any of the local culture?

He was halfway through one of these discussions when he spied Serafia over the man's shoulder. She was standing across the room chatting with a gentleman whose name he had immediately forgotten when they were introduced in the receiving line.

Gabriel had seen a lot of beautiful women tonight, but he just couldn't understand how his father could think that any of them could hold a candle to Serafia. She was breathtaking, catwalk perfection. Sure, she wasn't as rail-thin as she had been in her modeling days, but the pounds had just softened the angles and filled out the curves that her gown clung to. The pale pink of her dress was like soft rose petals scattered across her olive complexion. It was a delicate, romantic color, unlike all the bold look-at-me dresses the other women were wearing.

Serafia didn't need that for men to look at her, at least for Gabriel to look at her. He had a hard time looking anywhere else. Her silky black hair was loose tonight in shiny curls that fell over her shoulders and down her back. She wore very little jewelry—just a pair of pink sapphire studs at her ears—but between the beads of her dress and the glitter of her delicate pink lipstick, she seemed to sparkle from head to toe.

He felt his mouth go dry as he imagined her leaving a trail of glittering pink lipstick down his bare stomach. He wanted to pull her body hard against his and bury his fingers in the inky black silk of her hair. For all he cared, this party and these people could disappear. He wanted to be alone with Serafia and not for etiquette lessons or strategy discussions.

He hadn't given much thought to the man she was speaking to, but when he laid a hand on Serafia's upper arm, Gabriel felt his blood pressure spike with jealousy. Quickly excusing himself from the conversation he'd been ignoring, he moved through the room, arriving at her side in an instant.

Serafia's eyes widened at his sudden arrival. She took a step back, introducing him to the man she was speaking to. "Your Majesty, may I reintroduce you to Tomás Padillo? He owns Padillo Vineyards, where we'll be taking a tour tomorrow afternoon. I was just telling him how much you've enjoyed the Manto Negro from his winery since you arrived."

"Ah yes," Gabriel replied with a nod of recognition. He held up his glass. "Is this a vintage of yours, as well?"

"Yes, Your Majesty, that's my award-winning Chardonnay. I'm honored to have you drink it and looking forward to hosting your visit with us tomorrow."

The man seemed harmless enough; then again, Ga-

briel didn't see a ring on the man's hand. He didn't intend to leave Serafia alone with him.

"I'm looking forward to it, as well. May I steal away
Miss Espina?" he asked.

"Of course, Your Majesty."

Gabriel nodded and scooped up Serafia's arm into
his own. He led her away into a quiet corner behind
the staircase where they could talk.

"Is everything going all right?" she asked.

Gabriel nodded. "I think so. My dad is pressuring
me to mingle with the ladies, but I haven't gotten that
far yet."

Serafia sighed and patted his forearm. "You've done
your fair share of wooing ladies, Gabriel. This shouldn't
be very difficult for you."

"That was different," he argued. "Picking up a
woman at a nightclub for a little fun is nothing like
shopping for a wife. It feels more like a hunt anyway,
except I'm the fox. I'm surprised one of the hounds
hasn't ferretted me out from our hiding place by now.
Would you stay with me for a while?"

"Not while you dance!"

"Of course not. But go around with me while I mingle for a while. I think I'll be more comfortable that
way. You might remember people's names."

"Gabriel, you need to be able to—"

"Please…" he said, looking into her eyes with his
most pathetic expression.

"Okay, but you have to promise me you will ask no
fewer than two ladies to dance tonight. No moms or
grandmothers, either. Eligible, single women of marrying age. And not me, either," she seemed to add for
good measure.

"If I dance with two women who meet your criteria, would you be willing to dance with me just for fun?"

Serafia gave him a stern look, but the smile that teased at the corners of her full lips gave her away. "Maybe. But you've got to put in a good effort out there. You're looking for a queen, remember. If you don't find a good one, your father will do it for you, like poor Bella."

"You've heard about that?" Gabriel asked.

"Yes. I overheard Patrick discussing the idea of it with Will."

"How'd he take it?"

"About as well as Bella would, I expect. But my point is that you need to get out there and make that decision yourself."

"Fair enough." Offering her his arm, he led them back into the main area of the room. As they slipped through the crowd, he leaned down to whisper in her ear, "Who would you choose for me? Where should I start?"

Serafia looked thoughtfully around the room, her gaze falling on a buxom, almost chubby redhead whose fiery hair was in direct contrast to her personality. She was a shy wallflower of a girl who had barely met his gaze when they were introduced.

"Start with Helena Ruiz. Her family is in the seafood business and they provide almost all the fresh fish and shellfish to the area and to parts of Spain and Portugal, as well. And," she added, "unlike the others, she seems to be *reluctantly* hunting for a husband. She reminds me very much of a lot of the girls I work with in my business. Choosing her first might be good for her social standing and her self-esteem."

Gabriel was pleased with Serafia's choice and her reasoning behind it. It was one of the things about her that really stuck with him. She wasn't just concerned about making over his outside, but his inside, as well. In their training sessions, they'd discussed charities he'd like to support and causes he wanted to rally behind as king. Parliament and the prime minister would draft and enforce the laws of Alma, but as king, he would have a major influence over the hearts and minds of the people. He had a platform, so he needed to be prepared to have a cause.

In such a short time, Serafia had not just made over his wardrobe. She had made over his soul. He felt like a better person, a person more deserving of a woman like her. He'd never felt that way before in his entire life. He'd always been second to Rafe, not good enough in his father's eyes. His mother had recognized the value in him, but even she couldn't sway his father's opinion.

Since he returned home from Venezuela after the kidnapping, he'd been a different man. He'd stopped seeking everyone's approval, especially his father's. With his mother traveling the world and unable to call him on it, he'd settled happily into his devil-may-care lifestyle. It had suited him well and no one had questioned the change in him. But Serafia had. She had the ability to see through all his crap, and it made him think that perhaps he could open up to her, really trust her, unlike so many others in his life.

As he left her side and approached the doe-eyed Helena, he knew Serafia had made the right choice. The bright, genuine smile on the girl's face and the pinched, jealous expressions of some of the other girls proved that much. He led her out onto the dance floor for the first official dance of the evening. Helena was nearly trembling in his arms, but he reassured her with a smile and a wink.

Serafia made him want to be a better man. She helped him become a better man. He could think of no other woman who should be at his side but her. And he would tell her that.

Tonight.

Six

"Okay," a voice announced over Serafia's shoulder. "I have met your requirements."

She turned to find Gabriel standing behind her. She'd been expecting his arrival. It had been nearly two hours since she sent him out onto the dance floor with Helena Ruiz. He had danced with her and at least five other ladies Serafina had chosen for him. Her inner spiteful streak had led her not to choose Dita as one of the dance partners. She wasn't entirely sure if it was because she knew the Gomezes were disingenuous, or if it was because the idea of him dancing and potentially falling for the statuesque beauty made her blood boil.

"You have," she said with a pleased smile. "You've more than met them. You've exceeded them. Well done, Your Majesty. Any pique your interest?"

Gabriel arched an eyebrow at her and held out his hand. "Join me on the dance floor and I'll tell you."

There were quite a few pairs dancing now, so the two of them would not stand out as much as they would have earlier. Deciding there was no harm in it—and she had promised—she took his hand and followed him out into the center of the dance floor.

Gabriel slipped his arm around her waist and cupped her hand with his own. For the first twenty seconds or so of the dance, she found she could hardly breathe. Her bare skin sizzled where they touched, and her heart was racing in her chest. Fortunately Gabriel was a strong lead and she didn't have to think too much about her feet. She simply followed him across the floor and focused internally on suppressing the physical reaction she had to his touch.

"So, find any chemistry out on the dance floor?" she asked, desperate for a distraction.

"Not until now," he said, his green gaze burrowing into her own.

"Gabriel," she scolded, but he shook his head as though he wasn't having any of that.

"Don't start. I've had enough of the reasons why I can't have what I want. I don't really care. All I know is that I want you."

The power of his words struck her like a wave and she struggled to argue against it. "No, you don't."

"Are you honestly going to stand there and tell me you know my feelings better than I do?"

She shook her head, focusing her gaze on the golden ropes at his shoulder instead of the intensity in his eyes. "You might want me for tonight, for one of your one-night flings, but not for your queen."

"Do we have to decide what it will be tonight?"

If she had to decide in the moment, she would say

no. She was wrapped up in the sensation of being so close to him. Her body was rebelling against her, desiring him desperately even as she argued against the very idea of it. "You aren't in Miami anymore, Gabriel. Every eye in the room is on you tonight. This feeling for me will pass and then you can focus on making a smart decision about your future. A future without me."

"Serafia, you are beautiful. You're the most stunning woman I've ever seen in real life or on a magazine cover. You're graceful, elegant, thoughtful, smart and incredibly insightful. I don't know why you find it so hard to believe that I could want you so desperately."

Desperately? Her gaze met his, her lips parting softly in surprise. His words were said with such sincerity, but she simply didn't believe a single one. She was too aware of her own faults to do that. She'd spent too many years having every aspect of her appearance ripped apart by modeling experts, their voices far louder than any of her fans' praises. And even if he could see past all her imperfections, he didn't know how broken she was. The truth of her past would send any man running. "You don't want me, Gabriel. You want your teenage fantasy from ten years ago. That person doesn't exist anymore."

She pulled away from his grasp as the music ended and made her way through the crowd of people coming on and off the dance floor. Spying a set of French doors, she opened them and slipped outside into the large courtyard of the Rowling mansion. She kept going, following a path into the gardens. It was landscaped like the formal English gardens of Patrick's homeland, so she continued on a gravel path along a long line of neatly trimmed shrubs until she came upon a clearing and a circular fountain.

She collapsed onto the stone ledge of the fountain and took a deep breath. She felt much calmer out here, away from the crush of people in the ballroom, but the sense of relief didn't last long. Not a minute later, she heard the sound of footsteps on the gravel and spied Gabriel coming toward her on the garden path.

He approached silently and sat on the edge of the fountain beside her. She expected him to immediately give her the third degree for running out on him. It was incredibly rude, after all, and she kept forgetting he was the king. People were probably inside talking about her hasty departure.

But Gabriel didn't seem to be in a hurry. He seemed to enjoy the garden as well, taking a deep breath and gazing up at the blanket of stars overhead. She did the same, relaxing as she tried to identify different constellations. Looking at the stars always made her problems seem less important, less significant. The universe was a big place.

When he finally got around to speaking, Serafia was ready to answer his questions. She was tired of hiding her illness, anyway. She might as well put it all out there, warts and all. It would likely put an end to their pointless flirtation and she could stop torturing herself with possibilities that didn't really exist.

"What was that all about in there? Really? Why is it so impossible that I would want you as you are, right now?"

"It's impossible for me to believe it because I know how seriously messed up I am, Gabriel. The truth is that I don't have a congenital heart defect and I didn't spend a year having surgeries to correct it."

Gabriel frowned at her. "Well, then, what really happened to you?"

Serafia sighed and shook her head. "No one knows the truth but my family and my doctors. My parents thought it would be easier for me if we told everyone the cover story, but that was all a lie. I had a heart attack on that runway because I had slowly and systematically tried to kill myself to be beautiful. The modeling industry is so high pressure and I couldn't stand up to it. I swallowed the lies they told me along with the prescription diet pills. I barely ate. I exercised six to eight hours a day. I abused cocaine, laxatives…anything that I thought would give me an edge and help me drop those last few pounds. My quest to be thinner, to be prettier, almost made me a very attractive corpse."

She was terrified to say the words aloud, but at the same time, it felt as if a weight was lifted from her chest. "The day I collapsed on the runway, I was five foot nine and ninety-three pounds. I was nothing but a walking skeleton and I received more compliments that morning than I ever had before. After I collapsed, I knew I had to leave the modeling industry because the environment was just too toxic. I had to spend a year in rehab and inpatient therapy for anorexia. I had to be completely reprogrammed, like I'd left some kind of cult."

Gabriel didn't recoil or react to her words. He just listened until she got it all out. "Are you better now?" he asked.

That was a difficult question to answer. Like an alcoholic, the danger of falling off the wagon was always there. "I've learned to manage. I've put so much strain on my heart that my day-to-day life is a very delicate balancing act. But for the most part, yes, the worst of it is behind me."

He sat studying her face for a few minutes. "I can't believe anyone had the audacity to tell you that you were anything but flawless. I mean, you're *Serafia*—supermodel extraordinaire, catwalk goddess and record holder for most *Vogue Italia* covers."

Once again, she started to squirm under his praise. "When you say things like that, Gabriel, it's really difficult for me to listen and even harder for me to accept. I was told for so long that I was fat and ugly and would never make it in the business. Even when I made it to the top, there's always someone there to try and knock you down. The modeling industry can be so venomous. You're never thin enough, pretty enough, talented enough, and both your competition and your customers feed you those criticisms every day. You believe something after you hear it enough times. Even all these years later, after all the therapy, there's a part of me that still believes that and thinks everything you're saying is just insincere flattery."

Gabriel reached out and covered her hand with his own. It was comforting and she was thankful for it, even as it surprised her. She expected him to finally see her flaws and run, but he didn't.

"It might be flattery, Serafia, but it's true. Every word. If I have to say it each day until you finally believe it, I will. I know how hard it can be to trust someone once that faith is abused. Once it's lost, it's almost impossible to get back, but I want to help you try."

There was a pain in his expression as he spoke. The lines deepened in his forehead with his frown. She knew something had happened to him in South

America. Perhaps now, perhaps here, after she'd told her story, he might finally tell her his. "How do you know? What happened to you, Gabriel?"

With a sigh, he sat back and looked up at the sliver of a moon overhead. "I was fresh from college and my father named me VP of South American Operations. As part of my job, I had to travel to our various shipping and trade ports in Brazil, Argentina, Venezuela and Chile. Dealing with Venezuela was controversial, but my father had decided that the country had oil and needed it shipped. Why shouldn't we profit from it instead of someone else?

"I saved Caracas for my last stop and things had gone so well in the other locations that I wasn't wary any longer by the time I arrived in Venezuela. I went down there and spent a few days getting acclimated and met with the team there. One evening, my guide and translator, Raoul, offered to take me out for an authentic Venezuelan dinner. The moment we stepped outside, a van pulled up by the curb. Raoul hit me on the back of the head with something and I blacked out. The next thing I knew, I was lying on a stinky, lumpy mattress in a cold, dark room with no windows. My wrists and ankles were tied with thick rope."

Serafia could barely believe what she was being told. How had she never heard about this before? She wanted to ask, but she didn't dare interrupt.

"When my captor finally showed up a few hours later, he told me that I was being held for ransom and as soon as my family paid them, I'd be released."

"Did they pay them?" she asked.

He avoided her gaze, swallowing hard before he spoke. "No. I was in that underground room in virtual darkness for over a week. Every day the guy would come down and bring me a jug of water and some food, but that was it. After about the sixth day alone with my thoughts, and with constant taunts from my captor that my family hadn't paid the ransom yet and must not care if I lived or died, I came to the conclusion that if I wanted out of this place, I'd have to save myself. And I decided that when I did, I was going to live the life I wanted from that moment on."

"You escaped?" Serafia asked, near breathless with suspense.

"My rusty metal bed frame was my savior. I used it to slowly cut through my bindings. It took almost all day to do it. When my captor opened the door to bring my evening meal, I was waiting for him. I leaped on him, beating his head against the concrete floor until he stopped fighting me. Once I was sure he was unconscious, I took his gun and keys, locking him in the room. It turned out he was my only guard, so I literally went up the stairs and walked out onto the busy streets of Caracas. I made my way to the US embassy, told them what had happened and I was back in Miami by sunrise."

Serafia was nearly speechless. "Did they ever catch the people responsible?"

"Raoul was arrested for his part in the conspiracy, but he was just a facilitator paid a flat fee for delivering me at a special place and time. They found my captor still locked in the room where they kept me. Anyone else who was involved got away with it. But really, in the end, I wasn't angry with them. I was angry with my family. They knew what could happen if they sent me down there."

"What did they say when you showed up at home?"

Gabriel stiffened beside her and shrugged. "They welcomed me home and then tried to pretend it never happened. But I could never forget."

It was a horrible story to hear, but suddenly so much of Gabriel's personality suddenly made sense to her. He never got close to anyone and got a lot of grief from his family for being superficial. Even Serafia had been guilty of judging him, thinking he cared more about partying than worrying about anything serious. She'd accused him of being reckless, but when they were both faced with death, they reacted differently. She became supercautious, nearly afraid to live life for fear of losing it for good. He had done the opposite: living every moment to the fullest in case it was his last. Who was she to judge him?

Serafia reached out and took his hand. She felt a surge of emotion when they touched. When she looked at him, for the first time she was able to see the sadness in his green eyes, the wariness behind the bright smile. The bad boy facade kept people away and she had fallen for it. She didn't want to keep him at arm's length any longer.

Gabriel gripped her hand in his, letting his thumb brush across her skin. It sent a shiver of awareness down her spine, urging her to lean in closer to him.

"I know that's a lot of information to process," he said. "I didn't tell it to you so you'd feel bad for me. I told you because I wanted you to understand that we're coming from a similar place. No one is perfect. We're all messed up somehow. But it's how we deal with it that matters. I'm an expert at pushing people away. You're the first woman I've ever met who had made me want to try to trust someone again. Stop thinking that you don't measure up somehow, because you're wrong."

Serafia gasped at his bold words. She couldn't hold back any longer. She lunged forward, pressing her lips against his own before she lost her nerve. It had been a long time since she had trusted herself in all the various areas of her life, and romance had fallen to the bottom of the stack. What good was she to a man in the state she was in? Especially a prince? Still, she couldn't help herself. And neither could Gabriel.

He met her kiss with equal enthusiasm. He held her face in his hands, drawing her closer and drinking her in. He groaned against her lips and then let his tongue slip along hers. His touch made her insides turn molten with need and wore away the last of her self-control.

At last, Gabriel pulled away, their rapid breaths hovering between them in the night air. "Is it too early to make our exit?" he asked.

Serafia shook her head and looked into his eyes. "I think the prince can leave whenever he wants to."

It wasn't as simple to leave as Gabriel had hoped. He'd had to make the rounds, thank Patrick for his hospitality and avoid the cutting glares of his father, but within half an hour, he and Serafia were in the back of the royal limousine on their way home to Playa del Onda.

When they climbed inside, Gabriel couldn't look away from the high slit in her pink gown and how it climbed nearly to her hip as she sat. He wanted to run his hands over that bare skin. His palms tingled with the need to reach for her, but there was a forty-five-minute drive home from the Rowling Estate.

Eyeballing the limousine's tinted partition, Gabriel called out to his driver, "We're going to need a little privacy back here, please."

"Of course, Your Majesty." In an instant, the heavily tinted glass slid up, blocking them from their driver's view and making for a more private drive home.

"What are you doing?" Serafia asked.

Gabriel turned to her, placing his hand on her knee. "I want you. Right now. I can't wait until we get back."

"We're in a car, Gabriel. The driver is right there. The royal guard are in the SUV right behind us."

"They can't see us." His hand glided higher up her leg, brushing at the sensitive skin of her inner thigh. "Whether or not the driver *hears* us is up to you."

"I don't know about this," Serafia said, biting her full bottom lip.

Gabriel brushed his fingertips along the lacy barrier of her panties, making her gasp. "You may have reformed me, but there's still a little bad boy inside me." He stroked harder, making her stiffen and close her eyes. He leaned into her, placing a searing kiss against her neck before he whispered, "Let's both be bad tonight."

He gripped one strap of her gown, easing it down her shoulder, and then dipped his head to taste her flesh, nibbling on the column of her throat, the hollow behind her ear and the round of her shoulder. He slipped one hand behind her, finding the zipper of her gown and tugging it down enough to allow her gown to slip farther and expose the round globes of her large breasts.

They were more glorious than he'd ever imagined after seeing her in bikinis and skimpy gowns on magazine covers. "So beautiful," he murmured as his gaze devoured her. They were full and heavy, tipped with tight mocha nipples that he immediately covered with his hands and then his mouth.

Serafia bit her lip hard to keep from crying out as his tongue flicked across her skin. He teased her flesh, and then sucked hard at her breast. The hand he'd kept beneath her gown continued to stroke her, finally slipping under the lacy edge of her panties to feel the moist heat of her desire hiding beneath it.

"Gabriel!" she exclaimed in a hoarse whisper.

"Just lie back and enjoy it," he replied, turning with her as she leaned back across the seat to rest on her elbows. When she shifted her hips, he was better able to slide her gown out of the way and part her thighs. He stopped touching her only long enough to slip off her panties.

When he returned, he leaned down, parted her flesh and stroked her with his tongue. Serafia squirmed and writhed against him, but he didn't let up. He wrapped his arms around her thighs to hold her steady as he teased at her sensitive flesh again and again. Gabriel waited until he had her hovering on the edge; then he slipped one finger inside her. It sent her tumbling over, gasping and whimpering as quietly as she could manage while her release rocked through her.

When at last her body stilled except for her rapid breaths, Gabriel pulled away. While she recovered, he unbuttoned his suit pants and tugged them down. Reaching into his back pocket, he pulled a condom from his wallet and slipped it over the length of him. When he turned back to Serafia, she was watching him with a twinkle of deviousness in her dark eyes.

He reached for her and tugged her into his lap, her thighs straddling him as the limousine raced down the highway. Gabriel gripped her waist as she eased down and pushed him inside her. He gritted his teeth and pressed desperate fingertips into her flesh as he fought for control. She felt amazing. When he was buried fully inside her, he held her still for a moment, then reached for her face. He pulled her forward and captured her lips with his own.

As his tongue slipped inside her mouth and stroked her, he started moving slowly beneath her. Pushing the pink organza of her gown out of the way, he gripped the curve of her rear to guide her hips. At first, their movements were deliciously slow, and he savored every pang of pleasure. As the intensity built, they moved more frantically. Serafia grasped his shoulders and threw her head back, a silent cry in her throat.

"Let go for me," Gabriel pressed. "I want to watch it happen. You're so beautiful when you come undone."

She found her release again. This time, he held her close, not just watching, but feeling the pleasurable tremors running through her body and experiencing them with her. Her inner muscles tightened around him, coaxing his own release. As she collapsed against him, he wrapped his arms around her waist and thrust into her one last time. He buried his face in her neck, growling his climax against her flushed skin.

They sat together, not moving for several minutes.

In the stillness, Gabriel was finally able to mentally catch up with everything that had happened in the last few hours.

The moment he had stepped out into the garden after her, he knew things would be different. He wasn't going to let her keep pulling away from him, and if opening up to her about his own past was what it took, he was willing to do it. She…inspired him in a way no other woman had. It wasn't just an attraction; it was more. She didn't want anything from him. Unlike the sharks circling around the Rowling ballroom, Serafia didn't need his money and she certainly didn't want to share his spotlight. He felt that she was someone he could trust, especially after she shared her own story with him. Her past was different from his but he could tell that it had scarred her in a similar way. The difference was that he didn't trust others and she didn't trust herself. But she should. And he wanted to help her with that.

It made her ever more attractive to him, if that was possible. She wasn't just the supermodel from his teenage fantasies. She was so much more. He just had to convince her of that.

"The car is slowing down," Serafia noted. She climbed from his lap and quickly started pulling herself back together.

Gabriel turned and looked out the window. They were approaching the gate to the compound. "We're home. Time to get dressed so we can go inside and I can take it all off you again."

Serafia tugged the top of her dress back up over her shoulders and looked at him. "Really?"

How silly she was to doubt him on that point. "Oh yes," Gabriel said in a tone as serious as he was capable of. "That was just to hold me over until we got home."

Seven

Serafia woke up the next morning with a small smile on her lips. Opening her eyes, she spied Gabriel's broad shoulders as he slept beside her. She rolled onto her back with a yawn and reached for her phone to check the time. It was eight-thirty, practically midday for her. She wasn't surprised, considering that Gabriel hadn't let her sleep until after three.

Flinging back the sheets, she gently slipped out of the bed so she wouldn't wake Gabriel. She snatched up a blanket off the foot of the bed, wrapped it around her naked body and walked toward the wall of French doors that led from the master bedroom onto a secluded patio that overlooked the sea.

She stepped out onto the balcony, pulling the door shut behind her. The sun was bright, warming her skin as she took in the remarkable view.

Playa del Onda was built on a sheer cliff overlooking the sea. It was perched at the apex of a crescent-shaped bay lined with sailboats and beaches that would hopefully draw tourists now that the Tantaberras had fallen. The water was an enchanting mix of blues and greens that begged you to dip a toe into it. It reminded her of her hacienda in Barcelona. Her view overlooked the Mediterranean, but the feelings it inspired in her were the same. Peacefulness. The ability to breathe. Relaxation.

She wanted to take a mug of coffee and sit out here the rest of the morning, but that just wasn't possible. The house was crawling with guards and servants. She couldn't stroll into the kitchen wearing a blanket and slip back into the prince's suite without someone noticing. Not that it was necessarily a secret to those who'd traveled back to the beach house with them last night, but she thought it was inappropriate to flaunt it.

As it was, she needed to get down the hall to her own room. Going back inside, she checked to see that Gabriel was still asleep. She had worked wonders with his transformation, but bless him, he was still a night owl.

She retrieved her gown from the floor and slipped it back on, and then slowly opened the door of his bedroom, glancing both ways down the hall to see if anyone was there. The coast was clear. She slipped out, pulling the door closed. She had taken about three steps toward her room when she heard something behind her.

"Good morning, Señorita Espina."

She turned to find the houseman, Luca, standing behind her. "Good morning, Luca," she said, self-consciously smoothing her hand over her tousled hair and trying to downplay how overdressed she was for the early morning hours.

His dark gaze traveled over her quickly, a twinkle of amusement in his eyes, but he didn't mention her appearance. "Is His Majesty still sleeping?" he asked.

"Yes, he is. But he should be getting up soon. Please wake him by ten if he hasn't roused by then."

"As you wish."

Serafia started to turn back toward her room, and then she stopped. "Please don't mention this to anyone," she said.

Luca shook his head. "Of course not, señorita. The affairs of the prince are no one's concern but the prince's. But…" He hesitated. "You should know your involvement with the prince is no secret."

Serafia looked up at him with eyes wide with panic. "What does that mean?"

He unfolded the Alma newspaper he'd been clutching in his hand and held it up for her to read. On the front page, just below the article about Gabriel's big introduction at the Rowling party, was a headline that read *"The Future Queen?"* Another article followed, speculating about a romance brewing between her and Gabriel. A grainy black-and-white photo of them kissing by the fountain accompanied the story.

With a sigh, she closed her eyes. She felt foolish for thinking she could have one moment of privacy. "Thank you for showing me this, Luca. May I take it to my room and read it?"

He folded the paper and handed it to her. "Of course."

Serafia tucked it under her arm. "Please don't mention it to the prince until I have a chance to read the article. I'll discuss it with him at breakfast."

"As you wish. I'll have Marta start preparing it."

Luca disappeared down the hallway, leaving Serafia with the newspaper clutched against her. Before anyone else saw her, she dashed down the hallway to her own room.

Throwing the paper onto the bed, she headed straight for the shower. As the steaming hot water pounded her sore muscles and washed away Gabriel's scent from her skin, her mind started to race with the implications of the article. From what little she'd read, the tone didn't seem negative. The prince and his quest for a bride would be front page news no matter who he was seen with. But that didn't do much to calm her anxiety.

She should've known better than to think that someone hadn't noticed their departure from the ballroom and followed them outside. She hadn't noticed anyone there, but with the walls of hedges and arborvitae columns, there were plenty of places to hide and spy on their painfully private moments together.

Hopefully whoever took their picture hadn't been able to hear their conversation over the sound of the nearby fountain. The photo was one thing, but she didn't want the revelations about her departure from modeling to taint Gabriel somehow.

Stepping from the shower, Serafia wrapped herself in a fluffy white towel and started combing through the thick and easily tangled strands of her hair. She rushed through the rest of her morning routine. Trying to maintain a bit of professionalism, she put her hair up in a tight bun and dressed in a dark plum pantsuit. They had another official event to attend this afternoon, so she might as well get ready and put her consultant hat back on.

After she slipped on her shoes, she reached for the paper and read through both articles on Gabriel. The first, about his introduction at the Rowling party, was extremely positive. The consensus was that he was well received and those in attendance were pleased to have such a fine man to be their future king.

The second article, about her, wasn't really bad, either. It discussed the various ladies he had danced with that night, highlighting Helena Ruiz as his first choice and Serafia as his last. Of course, there was the photo of them kissing, and then a lot of speculation about whether or not she was really his social secretary, or if it was a cover for their relationship. If they were dating, was it serious? Might she be their new queen? The few people they interviewed for the article seemed to think she'd make a good candidate for queen of Alma and would make a charming match for Gabriel.

It wasn't a horrible write-up, but she really wished she could have avoided the papers. How could he turn around and select one of the other women in Alma after this? No one wanted to be second choice and really, she wasn't in the running to be queen, despite what they might think.

Or was she?

Gabriel seemed as serious about her as he had been about anything they'd discussed so far. He'd swept her off her feet and for once, she'd gone with it and had an amazing night. She hadn't entertained second thoughts about it, but now anxiety started pooling in her stomach. She wasn't opposed to being his lover, but queen? She wasn't sure she could handle that. The only people more famous in Europe than models were the royal families. The United Kingdom's Princess Kate couldn't wear an unflattering dress or have a bad hair day without it being in the papers and commented on. Every time Prince Harry was seen with a woman, the rumors would fly.

Serafia knew what it was like. In her modeling days, it wasn't enough for everyone to critique her appearance, and they did. Her whole life was public. The cameras showed up on dates, on vacations, while she was trying to spend a day with her family. If she was dating anyone famous, the magnifying glass tripled along with the coverage. It was incredibly difficult to maintain a relationship under the microscope, much less a shred of self-esteem.

It had nearly killed her to do it, but Serafia had escaped the spotlight. Gabriel's queen would be subject to the same kind of scrutiny. The private would become painfully public, with every aspect of her life exposed. She had no intention of ever going back in front of the cameras.

Even for Gabriel. Even for the chance to be queen. She would be much happier in Barcelona, living a quiet, unexciting life. Passionless, yes, but private.

With a sigh, she folded up the paper and headed out to breakfast. By the time she reached the dining hall, Gabriel was dressed and waiting for her there. Without her standing by the closet, laying out his clothes, he'd opted for a pair of jeans and a clingy green T-shirt that matched his eyes. His hair was still wet and slicked back, his cheeks still slightly pink from his shave. He was sipping a cup of coffee and thumbing through emails on his smart phone.

"Good morning," she said as she entered the room.

She had her tablet in one hand and the newspaper in the other.

Gabriel smiled wide when he looked up at her. There was a wicked light in his eyes. "Good morning."

Serafia took a seat at the table across from him, holding off their discussion as Marta poured her a cup of coffee and returned to the kitchen to bring out their breakfast. They were three bites into their *tortilla de patatas* before she spoke about it.

"Apparently," she began, "we were not the only people out in the garden last night. Our kiss made the front page of the newspaper." She laid the paper out on the table for Gabriel to look at it.

He picked it up, reading over the article as he chewed his eggs, a thoughtful expression on his face. "I'm not surprised," he said at last, dropping the paper on the table and returning to his breakfast. He didn't seem remotely concerned.

"It doesn't bother you?" she asked.

"This isn't my first romance documented in a gossip column. Nor is it yours, I'd wager. There's nothing inflammatory about it, so why should I care? You're not a dark secret I'm trying to hide."

"The press scrutiny will be higher now. They'll question every moment we're together. We'll need to meet with your press secretary, Hector, to discuss how to handle it."

"I know how we'll handle it," he said, sipping his orange juice. "The palace will not comment on the personal life of the prince. Period. If and when I select a queen, I will announce it through the proper channels, not through some gossip column. They can speculate all they like. It doesn't concern me."

Serafia sat back in her chair. She was near speechless. That was the most tactful and diplomatic thing he could've said on the subject. Maybe her lessons were finally sinking in. "That is an excellent answer. I'll make sure Hector knows that's the official position of the palace."

After a few minutes of silent eating, Gabriel put down his fork and looked at her. "What do you think about the article? You seemed to be more concerned about it than I am. Am I missing something?"

"No, it's not the content of the article itself, so much as being in it. I've lived happily out of the spotlight for years," she explained. "Finding myself back in the papers was…unnerving to say the least."

"Do you regret last night?" he asked.

Serafia's gaze lifted to meet his. "No. But I regret not being smarter about it."

Gabriel nodded and speared a bite of tortilla with his fork. "Good. Then we can do it again."

Lord, but Gabriel was hot. He would've been much more comfortable in the jeans and T-shirt he'd started the day in, but Serafia had made him change before they left Playa del Onda. Did Serafia give no thought when she selected his wardrobe that he would be touring the countryside of Alma in July? The vineyards were beautiful, and he really was interested in everything Tomás was telling him, but it was hard to focus when he could feel his back sweating under his suit coat.

As they walked through the arbors, he turned to look at Serafia. She had her hair up in a bun off her neck. She was wearing a wide-brimmed hat and a linen shift dress in a light green that looked infinitely cooler than his own suit.

"I'm dying here," he whispered, leaning into Serafia's ear. "I'm no good to anyone if I melt into a puddle."

"We're going inside in a minute."

Gabriel sighed. "We better be or I'm going to look terrible if the press take any more photos." There was a small group invited to the vineyard today. They'd taken some shots as he arrived and as they toured the fields and sampled grapes from the vines, but they had given him some space after that. They were probably hot, too, and waiting for the group to return to the air-conditioned comfort of the building.

"Such a warm day!" Tomás declared. "Let's head inside. I'll give you a tour of the wine cave, and then we'll get to the good part and sample my wares."

Gabriel's ears perked up at the mention of a wine cellar. He was happy to go inside, but that didn't sound like a place he was interested in visiting. "Did he say 'cave'?" he asked as they trekked back up the hill to the villa.

Serafia frowned at him. "Yes. Why?"

"I don't like going underground."

"I'm sure it will be fine. Just relax," she insisted. "We really need a nice, uneventful visit today."

Gabriel snorted. She was optimistic to a fault. "Do you actually think that's ever going to happen with me as the king?"

She tipped her head up to look at him from under the wide brim of her white-and-green hat. Her nose wrinkled delicately as she said, "Probably not, but I'll keep striving for it. Before long, I'll be turning you over to your staff and going home. I hope they're prepared."

They finally reached the top of the hill and stepped through the large doors of the warehouse. Inside, they were greeted by a servant with a tray of sparkling water and a bowl with cool towels.

"Please, take a minute to cool off," Tomás said. "Have you enjoyed the tour so far?"

"It's been lovely, Tomás. There's no doubt that this is the finest vineyard in Alma," Serafia said, sipping her water.

She must not have trusted Gabriel to say the right thing. "It's a beautiful property," he chimed in. "How many acres do you have here?"

"About two hundred. It's been in my family for ten generations."

"You withstood all the political upheaval?"

Gabriel felt Serafia tense beside him. He supposed it was impolite to ask the residents of Alma how they managed to cope with the dictatorship, but he was curious. Some fled, but most made the best of it somehow.

"My great-grandfather refused to abandon his family's home. It was that simple. To survive, we supplied our finest wines to the Tantaberras and were forced to pay their heavy commercial taxes, but we survived better than others. We had a commodity he wanted."

Lucky. Gabriel sipped the last of his water and after dabbing his neck and forehead, returned the cloth to the bowl. "And now?"

Tomás smiled brightly. "Much better, Your Grace. Now we are finally able to export our wines to Europe and America. Before, we were restricted by heavy trade embargos that punished us more than the dictatorship. The free trade of the last few months has had a huge impact on our sales and profits. We were able to hire more staff and plant more grapes this year than ever before. We are prospering."

Gabriel smiled. He had nothing to do with the changes, but he was happy to see them. Serafia had impressed upon him how hard it had been on his people since the Montoros left. He was glad to see the course reverse so quickly with the Tantaberras gone.

"Are we ready to continue?"

Gabriel was not, but he followed behind Tomás, anyway. A few of the journalists joined them as they walked through the warehouse to a heavy oak door. Tomás went down first with a few others, leaving Gabriel standing at the top of the stairs with a sense of dread pooling in his stomach. His hands clutched the railing, but his feet refused to take another step.

"Go!" Serafia urged him from behind.

He could see Tomás standing at the bottom of the stairs waiting for him with a few reporters. The light was dim and the air cool. Their host had an expectant look on his face as he stood there waiting for Gabriel to follow.

Serafia nudged him in the back with her knee and he took a few steps down without really wanting to. It was only two more steps to the bottom, so he forced himself to go the rest of the way down. At the very least he needed to keep going so that the ladder would be clear for his escape. Right now Serafia, a vineyard assistant and a few other reporters were behind him.

Gabriel took a labored breath and looked around him. The room was bigger than he'd expected. The long corridor with its arched ceiling stretched on for quite a distance. Dim gold lights were spaced out down the hall, providing enough light to see the hundreds of barrels stored there.

The air was also fresher than he'd anticipated. He looked up, spying air vents that led to some type of ventilation system. At least the room didn't smell of stale bread and mildew. But it didn't need to. Gabriel's brain easily conjured those smells. Dank, musty air filled his lungs, tainted with the stench of his own waste and leftover food that was rotting in the corner of his prison.

"This is my pride and joy," Tomás said, taking a few steps down the rows of barrels. "This is a natural cave my family found on the property. It was perfect for storing our wine barrels, so we didn't have to build a separate cellar. My great-grandfather added the electrical lighting and ventilation system so we can maintain the perfect temperature and humidity for the wine."

He continued to talk, but Gabriel couldn't hear him. All he could hear was his own heartbeat pounding in his ears. There were no windows, no natural light. He hated that. He couldn't even stand his room at the palace with the dim light and cavelike conditions.

It was all too much. He could feel the walls start to close in on him. He could feel the rope chafing his ankles. Beads of perspiration that had nothing to do with heat formed on his brow and on his palms. He rubbed his hands absently against the fabric of his light gray suit, but it didn't help. They were starting to tremble.

"We have nearly five hundred barrels—"

"I have to go!" Gabriel announced, interrupting Tomás and pushing through the crowd to reach the staircase. He ignored the commotion around him, taking the steps two at a time until he reached the ground floor.

There, he could finally take a breath. Bending over, he clasped his knees and closed his eyes. He breathed slowly, willing his heart rate to drop and his muscles to unwind. He stood upright and turned when he heard the stampede of footsteps coming up the steps behind him.

"Your Majesty, are you well?" Tomás approached him, placing a cautious hand on his shoulder.

Gabriel raised his arm to dismiss his concerns. "I'm fine. I'm sorry about that. I don't do well in closed in spaces."

"I wish I had known. I would never have taken you down there. Señorita Espina didn't mention it."

"She didn't know." Not really. He'd explained about his kidnapping the night before, but he hadn't expressed how much things like small spaces or wrist watches bothered him as a result. He didn't like talking about it. To him, it felt like a weakness. Kings weren't supposed to have panic attacks. He didn't mind being flawed, but he hated for anyone, and especially Serafia, to think of him as weak.

"Gabriel, are you okay?" Serafia asked, coming to his side with concern pinching her brow.

"I just needed some air. Sorry, everyone, the heat must've gotten to me," he said more loudly to the crowd that followed him.

"I think what you need is a seat on the veranda with some wine and food to reinforce you," Tomás suggested.

They followed the crowd into the villa, but before they entered, Serafia tugged at his jacket and held him back. "What was all that about?" she asked once they were alone.

As much as he hated to tell her, he needed to. He couldn't have another incident like this. "I've developed a sort of claustrophobia since my kidnapping. I can't take small or dark spaces, especially underground ones like the room where I was kept. I have panic attacks. It's the same with watches. I can't bear the feel of things against my wrists."

Serafia sighed and brought her hand to his cheek. "Why didn't you tell me?"

Gabriel covered her hand with his own and pulled it down to his chest. When he looked into her dark brown eyes, he felt overcome with the urge to tell her whatever she wanted. He wanted to be honest with someone for the first time since he came home from Venezuela. Serafia was the one person he could trust with his secrets.

"Because I've never told anyone."

Eight

Serafia got up early the next morning, slipping from Gabriel's bed to get ready. An hour later she returned and started sifting through his clothes for the perfect outfit.

"It's seven-thirty," he groaned as he sat up in bed. His hair was tousled and as the sheets pooled around his waist, Serafia couldn't help stealing a glance at the hard muscles she'd become accustomed to touching each night. "Why are you up so early clinking wooden hangers together?"

With a sigh, she turned back to the closet. "I'm trying to figure out what you should wear today for the parade."

"I'm going to be in a parade?"

It was becoming clear to her that in the early days of working together, Gabriel had paid very little attention to what she'd said. The prime minister's office had arranged for a full week of activities and Gabriel had been briefed on them in detail while they were still in Miami. And yet each day was like a surprise for him.

After the incident at the vineyard, Serafia was afraid to know if Gabriel had a problem with parades, too. She didn't dare ask. "Yes. As we discussed in Miami," she emphasized, "they're holding a welcome parade for you this morning that will go through the capital of Del Sol."

"Are there going to be marching bands and floats or something?"

"No, it's not really that kind of parade." She pulled out a gray pin-striped suit coat. It would be too hot for his ceremonial attire and that was better saved for the coronation parade, anyway. A nice suit would be just right, she thought. Eyeing the ties, she pondered which would look best. She knew Gabriel would be more inclined to skip the tie, but that wouldn't look right. She frowned at the closet. The more she got to know Gabriel, the more she realized she was trying to force him into a box he didn't really fit in, but he was still royalty and needed to dress appropriately.

"People are just going to stand out on the sidewalk and wait for me to come by and wave? Like the pope?"

Serafia looked at him with exasperation and planted her hands on her hips. "You're going to be the king! Yes. People want to see you, even if it's just for a moment as you drive by and wave. It won't be as big as your formal coronation parade, but it gives everyone in Alma the chance to come and see you, not just the press or the rich people at Patrick Rowling's party."

"For their sake, I hope there are at least vendors out

there selling some good street food," he muttered as he climbed out of bed.

"Get in the shower," Serafia said, laying the suit out across the bed.

Gabriel came up behind her and pulled her into his arms, crushing her back against his bare body. "Wanna get in there with me?" his low voice grumbled into her ear.

Serafia felt a thrill rush through her body, but she fought the reaction. They didn't have time for this now, as much as she'd like to indulge. There were thousands of people already lining the streets in the hopes of getting a good spot to see Gabriel. She turned in his arms and kissed him, then quickly pulled away. "Sorry, but you're going it alone today," she said. "We leave in less than an hour."

She was amazed they were able to keep to their schedule, but everything went to plan. They rendezvoused with the rest of the motorcade a few miles away from the advertised route. Gabriel was transferred to a convertible where he could sit on the top of the backseats and wave to the crowd. Royal guards and Del Sol police would be driving ahead of his car and behind, with guards running alongside them.

"Remember," Serafia said as he got settled in the back of the car. "Smile, wave, be sure to turn to look at both sides of the street. People are excited to see you. Be excited to see them, too, and you'll win the hearts of your people. I'll see you at the end of the route."

"I thought you might ride with me."

Serafia shook her head. "You're Prince Gabriel, soon to be King Gabriel. As far as anyone else knows, I'm your social secretary. Social secretaries wouldn't ride along on something like this. We don't need to give the newspapers any more material to put into their gossip columns. So no, I'm not going with you. You'll do fine."

Ignoring nearly everything she'd just said, he leaned in and gave her a kiss in front of fifty witnesses. Hopefully none of them had cameras. "See you on the flip side," he said.

Serafia shook her head and climbed into another car that was driving ahead to ensure that the route was clear and to secure the end rendezvous location.

Looking out the window, she was impressed by how many people were lining the streets. Thousands of people from all over, young and old alike, had come to the capital to see Gabriel. Some held signs of welcome; others had white carnations, the official flower of Alma, to throw into the street in front of Gabriel's car. Their faces lit up with excitement and anticipation as they saw Serafia's official palace vehicle drive down the road, indicating that the new king would soon follow.

They needed a reason to smile. The Tantaberras had ruled over these people with an iron fist for too long. They deserved freedom and hope, and she sincerely believed that Gabriel could be the one to bring it to them. He wasn't the most traditional choice for a king, but he was a good man. He was caring and thoughtful. There might be a rocky start, but she could tell these people were desperate for the excitement of a new king, a new queen and the kind of royal baby countdown that the British had recently enjoyed.

Serafia spied a different sign as they neared the end of the route. A little girl was holding up a board with Gabriel's picture and her own. Across the top and bottom in blue glitter it read "We need a fairy tale romance! King Gabriel & Queen Serafia forever!"

A few feet down, another declared "We have our king, please choose Serafia as our queen!" This one was held by an older woman. A third declared "Unite the Montoros & the Espinas at last!"

Serafia sat back in her seat in surprise. Although she preferred to avoid the press in general, the tone of the earlier article about her and Gabriel had been positive. The crowd here today seemed to corroborate that. They had their king and now they wanted their fairy tale. But her? Serafia didn't need to be anyone's queen. She was done with the spotlight.

The only hitch was her growing feelings for Gabriel. She'd never planned them. If she was honest, she hadn't wanted to have feelings for him at all. And yet, over the last two weeks, he had charmed his way into her heart. She wasn't in love, but she was closer than she'd been in a very long time. Her time with Gabriel was coming to an end. Soon he would be on his own, transitioning into his role as king. Serafia planned to return to Barcelona when it was over.

But as the time ticked away, she felt herself dreading that day. What was her alternative? To stay? To let her relationship with Gabriel grow into something real? That would give the people of Alma what they wanted, but it came at too high a price. Serafia didn't want to be queen. She was done with the criticism and the magnifying glass examining her every decision and action.

The car stopped at a park and she got out, waiting with a small crew of guards and Hector Vega, who was speaking to some journalists. She found a spot in the shade where she could lean against one of the vehicles and wait for the royal motorcade. It wasn't in sight yet, so she glanced down to pull out her tablet to make some notes.

"Serafia?"

She looked up at the sound of a woman's voice and noticed Felicia Gomez and her daughter crossing the street to speak with her. The older woman had traded her ball gown for a more casual blouse and slacks, but she was wearing almost as many diamonds. She was smiling as much as her Botox would allow, but there wasn't much sincerity in the look. Dita was wearing a sundress and a fresh-faced look guaranteed to turn Gabriel's head.

Serafia swallowed her negative observations and tried to smile with more warmth than she had. "Señora Gomez, Dita. Good morning. How are you?"

"I'm well," Felicia replied, coming to stand beside her. "We came down in the hopes we'd get a chance to speak with the prince after the parade. We didn't get a lot of time at the Rowling party."

Felicia's tone was pointed, as though Serafia were the one responsible for that fact. In a way she was, she supposed. Serafia didn't want the crown, but she really didn't want the spoiled Dita to have it, either.

Instead of responding, Serafia just smiled and turned to look down the street. She could see the motorcycle cops leading the motorcade. "Here's your opportunity," she said.

Within a few minutes, all the vehicles had pulled into the park. Gabriel leaped out of the back of the convertible with athletic grace. He shook the hands of his driver and the guards who were running along with him, and then made his way over to Serafia. He was smiling as he looked at her, barely paying any attention to the Gomez women standing beside her.

"I'm starving," he said. "All that waving and smiling has worked up a hellacious appetite. I caught a whiff of something delicious on the parade route. I think it was coming from this little tapas place. I tried to remember the landmarks and I'm determined to track it down for lunch."

"That's fine, we're almost done here."

"What else do I have to do?" he asked.

Serafia shifted her gaze toward the two expectant women beside her without turning her head. Gabriel followed the movement and put on his practiced smile when he noticed who it was. She'd taught him well, it seemed. "Señora and Señorita Gomez have been waiting for you."

"Your Grace," Felicia said as both she and Dita gave a brief curtsey. "We'd hoped to have a moment of your time after the parade. The party had simply too many people for us to have a proper conversation."

That translated to: *You didn't spend enough time with my daughter and if she's going to be queen, she needs time to work her charms on you.*

"Are you hungry?" he asked.

Felicia seemed a little taken aback. "Hungry, Your Grace?"

"I was just telling Señorita Espina that I spied the most delicious-smelling tapas restaurant. It looks like a hole in the wall, but I'm anxious to try it. Would you care to join us?"

Serafia could see the conflict in Felicia's eyes. The Gomez family wasn't one to be seen at a run-down tapas restaurant. Serafia fought to hold in a twitter of laughter as she watched the older woman choose between two unpleasant fates—dining with commoners and being turned away by the prince once again. There was a pained expression on her face as she finally responded.

"That is very kind of Your Grace. We have already eaten, unfortunately. But perhaps you would give us the honor of hosting you at our home for dinner sometime soon."

"That's a very kind offer. I'll see when I can take you up on it. It was good to see you both again. Señora Gomez. Señorita Gomez," he said, tipping his head to each in turn. "Have a lovely afternoon."

At that, he smiled and put his arm around Serafia's shoulder. Together, they made their way from the disgruntled Gomez women over to his private car to track down some tasty tapas.

Serafia waited until the car door was shut and the tinted windows blocked them from sight, and then burst out laughing. "Did you see the look on her face when you invited her to go get some lunch? I nearly dislocated a rib trying not to laugh."

"Did I handle it okay?"

"You did very well. It isn't your fault she won't stoop to the level of an average person. She isn't going to give up, though. She wants you to marry Dita and she'll keep trying until you do."

Gabriel looked at her in a way that made her bones turn to melted butter. "She can *try*," he said. "But I'll be the one with the crown on my head. I make the decisions when it comes to who I date and who I'll marry."

Serafia felt her heart stutter in her chest as he spoke the words, looking intently at her. She knew in that moment that she needed to be very, very careful if she didn't want the crown of Alma on her head, as well.

The following morning, Gabriel decided he wanted to take his breakfast out on the patio overlooking the sea. The weather was beautiful, the skies were blue and the fresh sea air reminded him of home.

Sitting in the shade of the veranda, he sipped the coffee Luca brought him and watched a sailboat slip across the bay. How long had it been since he'd gone sailing? Too long. Once this coronation business was over and he could settle into being king, he intended to remedy that.

He could just picture Serafia standing on the deck, clutching the railing and watching the water as they cut through the waves. He imagined her wearing nothing but a pair of linen shorts hugging the curve of her rear and a bikini top tied around her neck. Her golden skin would darken in the sun, her long dark hair blowing in the sea breeze.

That sounded like heaven. It made him wonder if there was already a boat in the possession of the royal family. If there was, he'd ensure that they took it out for a spin as soon as possible.

As he took another sip, Luca appeared in the doorway. "Luca, do you know if we have a boat?"

"A boat, Your Grace?"

"Yes. We have a beach house. Do we have a boat?"

"Yes, there is a sailboat at the marina. The youngest Tantaberra was an avid sailor."

At the marina. Perhaps they could go out sooner than later. When he looked back at Luca, he realized he had the Alma newspaper in his hand. "Is that today's paper?" he asked.

Judging by the concerned expression on Luca's face, the latest royal coverage was not as positive as he'd hoped. He imagined the press had had a field day ragging on him about that panic attack at the vineyard. It wasn't the most kingly thing he'd done this week. He'd thought the parade went alright, though.

Gabriel frowned as he looked at Luca. "That good, eh? Should I go ahead and call Hector?"

"Señor Vega already knows, Your Grace. Ernesto called a moment ago to let me know that Señor Vega was already on his way here to speak with you."

Great. Gabriel would much rather use his spare time to get acquainted with every square inch of Serafia's body, but instead he would be discussing damage-control strategies with his high-strung press secretary. He had only met Hector a few times, and that was enough. The man consumed entirely too much caffeine. At least, Gabriel hoped he did. If the man was naturally that spun-up, he felt bad for the mother who'd had to chase him around as a toddler.

Hector made him anxious. Serafia made him calm. He knew exactly who he preferred to work with. He had to convince her to stay beyond the end of the week, be it as a paid employee or as his girlfriend.

"Let me see the damage before he gets here," Gabriel said, reaching out for the paper. "It must be bad if Hector immediately hopped in his car."

Gabriel glanced at the headlines, expecting the story to be about him, but instead he found a scathing story about the Espina family. He looked up at Luca. "Have you told Miss Espina about this, yet?"

"No, sir, but she should be down for breakfast momentarily. Would you like me to warn her?"

"No, I'll tell her."

Maybe they could have a game plan before Hector arrived and started spinning.

Turning back to the article, he started reading it in depth. Apparently, back when the coup took place in the 1940s, there were rumors about the loyalty of the Espina family. He hadn't heard that before. Surely if there had been any legitimacy to that claim, their families wouldn't have vacationed together and his father wouldn't have allowed Serafia to work with him these past few weeks.

Of course, his father had been quite curt where Serafia was concerned. He'd alluded to her family being unsuitable somehow, but Gabriel hadn't had a moment alone with his father to press him on that point. He was sure it was nothing to do with Serafia herself. Gabriel had chalked up his father's bad mood to jealousy. That was the most likely reason for his behavior since they arrived in Alma.

"Good morning." Serafia slipped out onto the patio in a pair of black capris and a sleeveless top. Her dark hair was swept up into a ponytail and she was wearing bejeweled sandals instead of dress pumps. They didn't have any official events on the calendar today, so she had apparently dressed for a more casual afternoon by the sea.

"Hector is on his way," he replied, not mincing words.

Serafia's smile faded and she slipped down into the other chair. "What happened?"

"Apparently the newspaper headlines have gone from speculating about your role as future queen to speculating about your family's role in the overthrow of the Montoros."

Serafia's eyebrows drew together in concern as she reached for the paper. "What are they talking about?" Her gaze flicked over the paper. "This is ridiculous. Our families aren't enemies and we most certainly didn't have anything do with the coup. Have they forgotten that the Espinas were driven from Alma, too? They lived in Switzerland for years until the dictatorship fell in Spain. I was born in Madrid just a few years after they left Switzerland."

Gabriel shrugged. "I am deficient in Alman history. We should probably fix that. I didn't even have a clue our families had been rivals for the throne at one point."

"That was over a hundred years ago. How is that even relevant to what's going on now?"

"It has everything to do with what's happening now," Hector Vega said, appearing in the doorway and butting into their conversation. He, too, had the newspaper under his arm. "Your family had the crown stolen away from them two hundred years ago. The Espinas and Montoros fought for years to seize control of these islands. The Montoros ended up winning and eventually the families did reconcile. They even planned to marry and combine the bloodlines.

"But," he continued ominously, "Rafael the First broke off his engagement with Rosa Espina to marry Anna Maria. There were more than a few hurt feelings about that and plenty of rumors went around during the time of the coup about the Espinas' involvement. Your whole family vanished from Alma right before everything fell apart. Some see that as suspicious."

"And now?" Serafia pressed. "I think my family has gotten over the embarrassment of a broken engagement during the last seventy years. There is no reason to suspect us of anything."

"Isn't there? With the Tantaberras gone and the Montoros returning to Alma, your family is closer to reclaiming their throne than ever before," Hector explained.

"How?" Gabriel asked. "By marrying me? That plan only works if I'm on board with it."

Hector shrugged. "That's one way to do it." He moved out onto the veranda with them, but instead of taking a chair, he started pacing back and forth across the terra-cotta tiles of the patio. "Another way is to remove the Montoros entirely. If the Montoros and the Salazars were scandalized or discredited, Senorita Espina's family would be the next in line."

Gabriel had no idea that was the case, and judging by the surprised drop of Serafia's jaw, she didn't know it, either. "But there are several of us in line. They'd have to discredit us all, not just me."

"There are fewer of you than you think. Your father and brother have already been put aside. That just leaves you, Bella and Juan Carlos. Don't think it can't be done."

"There is no way that Juan Carlos can be discredited by scandal," Gabriel insisted. "He's annoyingly perfect."

"It doesn't matter," Hector said. "That article insinuates that Serafia was deliberately planted within the royal family to undermine you from the inside."

"She's here to help me!" Gabriel shouted. He was

irritated that this stupidity had ruined a perfectly beautiful morning.

"Is she?" Hector stopped moving just long enough to look over Serafia with suspicion.

"Of course I am. How dare you suggest otherwise?" Serafia flushed bright red beneath her tanned glow.

Hector raised his hands in defeat. "Fine. Fine. But the accusations are out there. We have to figure out how we're going to address them."

"They're ridiculous," Gabriel said. "I don't even want to address the rumors. At least not yet. It could all blow over if we treat it like the unfounded gossip it is."

Hector nodded and stopped pacing long enough to take notes in the small notebook he had tucked into his breast pocket.

"I just don't understand," Serafia said. "The press was so positive toward our relationship just a day ago. What changed so quickly?"

Hector put his notebook away and turned to look out at the sea, his fingers tapping anxiously on the railing. "My guess would be that someone leaked the story to discredit Serafia."

"Why?" Gabriel asked. "What could she have done to anger someone so quickly?"

Hector's gaze ran over Serafia with his lips pressed together tightly. "She didn't do anything. My guess is that it was your doing. You rejected the daughters of all the wealthiest families at the Rowling party."

Gabriel rolled his eyes. "Even if I hadn't left that night with Serafia—which really means nothing, since she's staying here with me for work—only one woman can be chosen as queen. There were easily twenty or thirty girls there that night. How could I possibly choose without offending *someone*?"

"It bet it was Felicia Gomez," Serafia said, speaking up. "Yesterday's incident just compounded their irritation over the party. The Gomez family doesn't like to lose and as I recall, you didn't even dance with Dita that night. I imagine Felicia would see that as a major snub. Combine that with yesterday after the parade… I'm sure they ran right to the press after we left. She can't take it out on you, as king, so she focused her ire on their main competition—me."

Gabriel muffled a snort and shook his head. "They wouldn't go to this much trouble if they knew the truth."

"What's the truth?" Serafia asked.

Gabriel looked into her dark eyes with a serious expression. "They're hardly your competition."

Nine

"How, exactly, did you come up with a boat?" Serafia asked as she turned to Gabriel.

Gabriel looked up from the wheel of the yacht and grinned. After a morning of unpleasantness with Hector, he'd had Luca arrange for the boat to go out. He needed to escape, to think, and there was nothing better than the sea for that.

Marta had packed them a picnic basket so they could dine on the water. The sea was calm and the breeze was just strong enough to fill the sails and keep them from getting too hot. "Turns out it's mine," he said. "Or at least it is now. I thought it was a good day to be out on the water."

"To escape the press?" she asked.

He chuckled and shook his head. "That's just a bonus. Mainly I wanted to see you in a bikini."

Serafia smiled and held out her arms to display her mostly bare curves. She was wearing a bright blue-and-pink paisley bikini top with a pair of tiny denim shorts that made her legs look as if they went on for miles. He ached to touch them, but he needed to steer the boat.

"You got your wish," she declared.

"Indeed I did." The reality standing in front of him was even better than he'd imagined this morning.

"If they know we're out here, the paparazzi will follow us, you know."

"Then they'll get an eyeful and the pictures will leave no doubts that their seedy story made no impact on my opinion of you."

He focused on steering the boat out of the sheltered bay and into open water as she laid a beach towel down on the polished wooden deck. She slipped out of the tiny shorts and went about rubbing sunblock all over her golden skin.

Thank goodness there weren't many ships out on the water today. His eyes were so glued to her that he could've run aground or rammed another boat. He couldn't wait to find a good place to stop so he could join her on the deck.

Serafia glanced up at him and smiled. She looked beautiful and carefree for once; she'd even left her tablet behind today. Not at all like someone scheming her way into his life, he thought, as the events from the morning intruded on his admiration of her. The whole thing was just absurd. Their families might have had animosity a hundred years ago, but that wasn't the case now. The people involved in that were long dead. It didn't have a thing to do with him or Serafia.

The idea that she had been "planted" in his inner

circle to undermine him made his hands curl into fists at his side. Serafia hadn't been *planted* anywhere. He had hired her. She hadn't even suggested the idea; in fact, she'd been very reluctant to take the job. If she was here to lure him into bed, she'd certainly made it difficult. He'd worked harder on her seduction than he had in a long time.

As much as he wanted to just laugh off the story, he couldn't. It made him too angry. He wouldn't tolerate such ugly speculation, especially about Serafia or her family. He'd quietly tasked Hector with tracking down the author of the article and seeing if the source could be identified. If the Gomez family really was behind this story, they'd regret it. If they thought his snubbing Dita at the dance was a huge deal, they'd better be prepared to be shut out of his court entirely. Gabriel was able to carry grudges for a very long time. He wouldn't quickly forget about the people who tried to undermine his faith in the one person he trusted.

Everyone had seen that article. Not long after Hector left, Gabriel's father had called from Del Sol. Rafael was agitated about the whole thing, repeating what he'd said at the Rowling party about the Espinas. Since this time they weren't in public where they could be overheard, Gabriel had pushed his father for more information. Arturo Espina was one of his father's best friends. How could he turn around and be suspicious of the family?

Rafael insisted it wasn't the truth that was the problem. It was seventy years of rumors that would taint his relationship with her. If he were to go as far as to make Serafia his queen, they would forever be dogged by those same ugly stories. Everyone had seen this article and it was just the beginning. Rafael insisted he was just trying to help Gabriel avoid all that. Being king was hard enough, he reasoned, without adding unnecessary complications.

If staying away from Serafia was the only way to save his reign from rumors, innuendo and scandal, too bad. He wasn't going to let something like this drive a wedge between them.

"It's so beautiful out here," Serafia declared, pulling him from his dark thoughts.

It was beautiful. The water was an amazing mix of blues and greens; the sky was perfectly clear. Looking back to the shore, you could see the coastline dotted with marinas and tiny homes hanging on the side of the cliffs. He couldn't imagine a more amazing place to rule over.

Before too long, he would be king of this beautiful country.

From the moment he found out, he had fought the news. He'd made a bold decision to take control of his own life after his abduction, and yet somehow fate had taken away his free will once again. Most people would probably jump at the chance to be in his shoes, but all Gabriel had been able to see were all the reasons why he was a bad choice.

But now that he was here with Serafia at his side, it seemed as though things might work out. The people were welcoming and friendly. The land was beautiful and full of natural resources that would help the country bounce back from oppression. Prime Minister Rivera was a smart man and a good leader, taking the reins on the important decisions for the management of the country. The press were the press, but once he chose a queen and married, hopefully they would settle down.

Gabriel was told that he would soon sit down with his council of advisers, a group of staffers that included Hector and others. He was certain they would have lots of opinions about whom he should choose for his queen. There were geopolitical implications that even he didn't fully understand. Marrying a Spanish or Portuguese princess would be smart. Securing trade by marrying a Danish princess wouldn't hurt, either. Then there were the local wealthy citizens whose support was so important to the success of the new monarchy.

But factoring in all those things would mean he was following his head, not his heart. Gabriel wasn't exactly known for making the smart choices where women were concerned. When it came to Serafia, none of those other things mattered. The minute he saw her out on the patio in Miami, he'd wanted her. And the more he'd had of her, the more he'd wanted. He wasn't just flattering her when he told her the other women in Alma were no competition. It was the truth.

Serafia was smart, beautiful, honest, caring...everything a good queen should be. She was from an important Alman family—one with blood ties to the throne if that article could be believed. He saw more than one sign at the parade declaring the people's support for her as queen. She was a good choice on paper and a great choice in his heart.

He wasn't in love with Serafia. Not yet. But he could see the potential there. In any other scenario, he would've anticipated months or years together before they discussed love and marriage, but as king, he saw this as an entirely different animal. He was expected to make a choice and move forward. With Serafia, he had no fears that their marriage would be a stiff, arranged situation with an awkward honeymoon night. It could be the best of both worlds if they played their cards right.

He just had to get her to stay past the end of the week. If he could do that, then maybe, just maybe, she would agree to be his queen someday soon.

"This looks like a good spot. Drop the stupid anchor and get over here. I'm lonely."

Gabriel checked the depth sounder for a good location. They seemed to be in an area with a fairly level depth. He lowered and secured the two sails, slowing the boat. It took a few minutes to get the anchor lowered and set, but the boat finally came to a full stop.

He turned off any unnecessary equipment and made his way over to where Serafia was lying out. She was on her back, her inky black hair spilling across the sandy blond wood of the deck. She had her wide, dark sunglasses on, but the smile curling her lips indicated she was watching him as he admired her.

Gabriel dropped down onto the deck beside her. He slipped out of his shoes and pulled his polo shirt over his head, leaving on his swimming trunks.

Serafia sat up, grabbing her bottle of sunscreen and applying some to his back. He closed his eyes and enjoyed the feel of her hands gliding across his bare skin. After she finished his back and arms, she placed a playful dab on his nose and cheeks. "There you go."

He rubbed the last of the sunscreen into his face. "Thanks. Are you hungry?"

"Yes," she said. "After everything this morning, I couldn't stomach any breakfast."

Gabriel reached for the picnic basket and set it closer to them on the blanket. Opening it, they uncovered a container filled with assorted slices of aged Manchego and Cabrales cheeses, and cured meats like *jamón ibérico* and *cecina de León*. Smaller containers revealed olives, grapes and cherry tomatoes dressed in olive oil and sherry vinegar. A jar of quince jam, a couple fresh, sliced baguettes and a bottle of Spanish Cava rounded out the meal. His stomach started growling at the sight of it.

Serafia started unpacking the cartons, laying out the plates and utensils Marta had also included. "Ooh," she said, lifting out a package wrapped in foil. "This smells like cinnamon and sugar." She unwrapped a corner to peer inside. "Looks like fruit empanadas for dessert."

"Perfect," Gabriel said.

They scooped various items onto their plates and dug into their meals. They took their time enjoying every bite in the slow European fashion he was becoming accustomed to. In America, eating was like a pit stop in a race—to quickly refuel and get back on the track. Now, he took the time to savor the food, to really taste it while enjoying his company. He sliced bread while Serafia slathered it with jam. She fed him olives and kissed the olive oil from his lips. By the time the jars were nearly empty, they were both full and happy, lying on the deck together and gazing up at the brilliant blue sky.

Gabriel reached out beside him and felt for Serafia's hand. He wrapped his fingers through hers and felt a sense of calm and peace come over him. He didn't know what he would've done without her these last few days. In that short time, she had become such a necessary fixture in his life. He couldn't imagine her going back to Barcelona. He wanted her here by his side, holding his hand just as she was now.

"Serafia?" he asked, his voice quiet and serious.

"Yes?"

"Would you...consider staying here in Alma? With me?"

She turned to him and studied his face with her dark eyes. "You're going to be fine, Gabriel. You've improved so much. You're not going to need my help any longer."

Gabriel rolled onto his side. "I don't want you here for your help. I'm not interested in you being my employee, I want you to be my girlfriend."

Her eyes grew wide as he spoke, her teeth drawing in her bottom lip while she considered his offer. Not exactly the enthusiastic response he was hoping for.

"You don't want to stay," he noted.

Serafia sat up, pulling her hand away from his to wrap her arms around her knees. "I do and I don't. I have a life in Barcelona, Gabriel. A quiet, easy life that I love. Giving that up to come here and be with you is a big decision. Being the king's girlfriend is no quiet, easy life. I don't know if I'm ready."

Gabriel sat up beside her and put a comforting hand on her shoulder. He knew he was asking a lot of her, but he couldn't bear the idea of living in Alma without her. "You don't have to decide right now. Just think on it."

She looked at him with relief in her eyes. "Okay, I will."

* * *

After a day at sea, they'd returned to the house and taken naps. They decided to dine al fresco on the patio outside his bedroom. It was just sunset as they reconvened with glasses of wine to watch the sun sink into the sea. The sky was an amazing mix of purples, oranges and reds, all overtaken by inky blackness as the night finally fell upon Alma.

It was beautifully peaceful, but Serafia felt anything but. Despite the surroundings, the wine and the company, she couldn't get Gabriel's offer out of her mind. To stay in Alma, to be his girlfriend publically...that would change her entire life. She wasn't sure she was ready for that, even though her feelings for him grew every day.

The king didn't have a girlfriend. At least not for long. Unless something went wrong pretty quickly, being his girlfriend would mean soon being his fiancée, and then his queen. That meant she would never return home to her quiet life in Barcelona.

But was that life becoming too quiet? Had she been hiding there instead of living?

The questions still plagued her as they finished the last of the roasted chicken Marta had made for dinner. She felt pleasantly full as she eased back in her chair, a sensation she wasn't used to. She might be comfortable hiding from the world in her hacienda, but she wasn't living her life and she wasn't really getting better. She was managing her disease, controlling it almost to the point that she'd once let it control her. But in Alma, with Gabriel, the dark thoughts hadn't once crept into her mind. He was good for her. And she was good for him.

Maybe coming here was the right choice. Her heart certainly wanted to stay.

She didn't have to decide now, she reflected, and the thought soothed her nerves. To distract herself, she decided now was the right time to give Gabriel his gift. "I got you something."

Gabriel looked at her in surprise and set down his glass of wine. "Really? You didn't have to do that."

"I know. But I did it, anyway." Serafia got up and went to her room, returning a moment later with a small black box.

Gabriel accepted it and flipped open the hinged lid. She watched his face light up as he saw what was inside. "Wow!" He scooped the gift out of the box, setting it aside so he could admire his gift with both hands. "A pocket watch! That's great. Thank you."

Gabriel leaned in to give her a thank-you kiss before returning to admiring his gift. The pocket watch was a Patek Philippe, crafted with eighteen-karat yellow gold. It cost more than a nice BMW, but Serafia didn't care. She wanted to buy him something nice that she knew he didn't have. "I told you in Miami that I would find a way to get around your watch issue."

"And you've done a splendid job. It's beautiful."

"It comes with a chain so you can attach it inside your suit coat."

He nodded, running his fingertip along the shiny curve of the glass. Closing the box, he put it on the table and stood up. He approached her slowly, wrapping his arms around her waist and tugging her tight against him. "Thank you. That was an amazingly thoughtful gift."

Serafia smiled, pleased that he liked it. When she

bought it, she wasn't sure if he would see it as a further criticism of his time-management issues or if he would feel it was too old-fashioned for him. She'd known it was perfect the moment she saw it, and she was pleased to finally know that he agreed.

"I feel like I need to get you something now," he said.

"Not at all," she insisted. "After our discussions about watches earlier and realizing why you disliked them so much, I knew this was something I wanted to do for you. There's no need to reciprocate."

He stared at her lips as she spoke, but shook his head ever so slightly when she was finished. "I'll do what I like," he insisted. "If that means buying you something beautiful and sparkly, I will. If that means taking you into that bedroom and making love to you until you're hoarse, I will."

"Sounds like a challenge," she said.

When his lips met hers, the worries in her mind faded away. Serafia wrapped her arms around his neck and melted into him. The roar of the waves below was the only sound except for the pounding of her heart.

After a moment, he started backing them into the bedroom. Their lips were still pressed together as they moved across the tile to the king-size bed against the far wall. Serafia clung to him, losing herself in touching and tasting Gabriel. No matter what happened each day, she knew it was okay because she knew he would help her forget all her worries each night.

When her calves met with the bed, they stopped. Serafia tugged at his shirt, pulling it up and over his head. She ran her fingertips across his bare chest and scattered soft kisses along his collarbone. His skin was warm from a day in the sun and scented with the hand-made soaps they kept in the bathrooms here.

She felt Gabriel's fingertips on her outer thighs, slowly gathering up the fabric of her dress. Before he could pull it any higher, she turned them around so that his back was to the bed. Then she shoved, thrusting him onto the mattress, where he sprawled out and bounced.

"Are we playing rough tonight?" he asked with a laugh.

Serafia shook her head and took a few steps backward. "I just wanted you to sit back and enjoy the view."

Pushing aside her self-consciousness, she let the straps of her sundress fall from her shoulders, the soft cotton dress pooling at her feet. She coyly turned her back to him, unfastening her bra and letting it drop to the floor. With a sly glance over her shoulder at him, she slipped her thumbs beneath her cheeky lace panties and slid them down her legs. Completely nude, she turned back to face him.

Gabriel watched from the bed with a glint of appreciation in his eyes. He really, truly thought she was beautiful, and knowing this made her feel beautiful. She lifted her arms to brush the cascading waves of her hair over her shoulders, displaying her breasts and narrow waist. He swallowed hard as he watched her, his jaw tightening.

"Come here," he said.

Serafia took her time, despite his royal command. She sauntered over to the bed, crawling across the coverlet on all fours until she was hovering between his thighs. She reached for the fly of his jeans, but the moment she was within Gabriel's reach, he lunged for her.

Before she knew quite what had happened, she was on her back and the weight of Gabriel's body was pressing her into the soft mattress.

He kissed her, his mouth hard and demanding against her own. His fingertips pressed into her, just as hard. She gasped for air when he pulled away to taste her throat. His teeth grazed her delicate skin, almost as though he wanted to mark her, claim her as his own.

She wanted to be his. His alone. At least for tonight. She could feel his desire against her bare thigh, the rough denim keeping them apart. She reached between them, slipping her hand beneath his waistband to grip the length of him. He growled against her throat, leaning into her for a moment, and then reluctantly pulling away before she wore out the last of his self-control.

Slipping off the edge of the bed, he removed the last of his clothes, sheathed himself in latex and returned to his home between her thighs. Without saying a word, he drove into her, stretching her body to its limit. She cried out and clung to his back, her fingernails pressing crescents into his skin.

Their lovemaking was more frantic tonight, more passionate and intense. She wasn't sure if it was the end of their relationship looming that pushed them to a frenzy, but she happily went along for the ride. Nothing else mattered as he drove into her again and again. All she could do was give in to the pleasure, live in the moment and not let the future intrude on their night together. It wasn't hard. Within minutes he had her gasping and on the verge of unraveling.

That was when he stopped moving entirely.

Her eyes flew open, her breath ragged. "Is something wrong?" she asked.

"Stay with me," he demanded.

She wanted to. She wanted to give him her body, her heart and her soul. In that moment, she knew she already had. Despite her hesitation, despite her worries, she had fallen in love with Gabriel Montoro, future king of Alma. But was she good for him? Would she be the queen the country needed?

Those critical articles were just the first of many she was sure would surface. Rumors about her family wouldn't disappear overnight. She didn't want to bring scandal to the new monarchy. It was too new, too fragile. She couldn't risk that, even for love.

She also couldn't risk herself. Would she slip back into her old habits with the eyes of an entire country on her? It was a dangerous prospect.

But when he looked at her like that, his green eyes pleading with her, how could she say no? She wanted to stay. She wanted to be with him, to help him on his new journey. If that meant she might someday be queen and take on all the pressures and joys that entailed...so be it.

"Yes," she whispered into the darkness before she could change her mind.

Gabriel thrust hard into her and she was lost. The waves of emotions and pleasure collided inside her, making her cry out desperately. She repeated her answer again and again, encouraging him and confirming to herself that she truly meant it. She loved him and she was going to stay.

His release came quickly after hers. He groaned loud against her throat, surging into her one last time as he came undone. Serafia held him, cradling his hips between her thighs until it was over.

When he'd finally stilled, she heard him whisper almost undetectably in her ear, "Thank you."

He was grateful that she'd agreed to stay. She just hoped that would still be the case in the upcoming weeks.

Ten

Serafia should've woken up on cloud nine. She was in love, she'd agreed to stay in Alma with Gabriel and everything was perfect. And yet there was a cloud hanging over her head. It was as though she couldn't let herself breathe, couldn't let herself believe that this was really going to work between them, until after today.

Today was the last hurdle before the coronation. After today's public appearance, Gabriel would have met all the initial requirements and could settle quietly into his life at Alma while the preparation for the coronation took place. She didn't anticipate any problems today. All they had to do was make it through the tour of one of Patrick Rowling's oil platforms off the coast, but for some reason, she woke up anxious.

They got on the road after breakfast, driving the hour back into Del Sol, where they would take a helicopter out to sea. Helicopters. Better safe than sorry, she decided to get his opinion on it during their drive to the capital.

"Are you okay with helicopters?" Serafia asked.

Gabriel straightened his tie and nodded. "Helicopters are fine. The weather seems pretty calm today, so it shouldn't be a bumpy ride."

"Good." She sighed with relief. That was one less worry. "The only other option to get out there is to take a boat and get lifted by crane onto the platform while you cling to a rope and metal cage called a Billy Pugh. I wasn't looking forward to that at all."

Gabriel smiled. "That actually sounds pretty cool."

"You're the rebellious one," she said. "I'm interested in staying alive."

"Fair enough. How far out is the oil platform?"

Serafia looked down at her tablet as their car approached the heliport. "The one we're going to is about twelve kilometers off the coast. It's the newest one they've constructed and Patrick is very eager to show off his new toy."

Gabriel frowned. "I'm sure he is."

"What's that face about?"

"I'm not sure how I feel about the Rowlings yet. At least Patrick. He seems a little showy, a little too cocky for my taste. His sons seem nice enough, although I can't wait to see the look on Bella's face when she's introduced to the guy Dad wants her to marry. If there aren't instant fireworks between them, she just might kill our father in his sleep. We might need her to stay at the beach house when she gets here."

"I wouldn't worry too much about Patrick or Bella today. I'm sure the trip will be fine and you'll be off the hook for a while until the coronation. Today, we'll be flying over with Prime Minister Rivera. He asked to join us on the tour."

"What about Hector?"

"Apparently he doesn't do helicopters, but he's briefed everyone and he'll be meeting with you afterward to go over how it went with Rivera."

"That's fine. I've only had one short meeting with the prime minister, so it's probably a good idea to have some more face time. I don't think we'll get much talking done in the helicopter, though. Aren't they loud?"

Serafia had never been in one, but she'd heard they were. "Yes. I'm pretty sure you won't be conducting any business in the helicopter."

He nodded and relaxed back into the seat. "Good. I'm not sure I'm ready for any hard-core discussions. Is the helicopter large enough for the royal guard, as well? That's quite a few of us to fit into one."

Serafia shook her head. "They've already got a crew of guards there at the rig. They cleared the platform this morning and are standing by for your arrival. All the details have been taken care of," she assured him. Turning to glance out the window, she realized they were at their destination. "And here we are."

They climbed from the car at the heliport and made their way over to the helicopter waiting for them. The prime minister was already there, rushing over to shake Gabriel's hand. Then as a group, they climbed into the helicopter and headed out to sea.

Serafia was glad Gabriel was okay with helicopters. She wasn't exactly thrilled with the idea, so it was good that at least one of them wasn't freaking out. When the engine started, she put on the ear protec-

tion and closed her eyes. The liftoff sent her stomach
into her throat, but after a few minutes the movement
was steady. Thankfully it wouldn't take long to get out
there, so she took some deep breaths and tried not to
think about where she was.

A thump startled her, and she opened her eyes in
panic only to realize they'd already landed on the oil
platform. Thank goodness. Everyone climbed out and
Patrick came to greet them. With him, he had the lead
rig operator, his son William and a few members of
Patrick's management team who always seemed to be
following him around. This, in addition to a large con-
tingent of press, as always. They'd come out earlier
on the boat. Once everyone was fitted with hard hats,
the tour began.

With all the cameras so near today, Serafia decided
to take a step back from Gabriel. There was no need
to stir any more rumors or give any of them a reason
to write another scathing article about her family or
their romance. He didn't seem to notice she was gone.
With everything going on, he surged ahead, carried by
the crowd with Rivera and Patrick Rowling at his side.

Serafia trailed the group as they walked around the
open decks of the platform, admiring the massive drill
and other equipment. She couldn't hear what Patrick
and the others were saying, but she didn't mind. She
wasn't really that interested.

After that, they went inside to tour the employee
quarters and cafeteria, the offices and the control room.
It was a tight fit for the men who lived on the rig up to
two weeks at a stretch.

The day was going fairly well, so far. She'd begun
to think she'd been anxious for no reason.

It wasn't until they went back outside and started climbing down a set of metal stairs that went below the platform that Serafia started to feel the niggling of worry in the back of her mind. The only thing below the platform were the emergency evacuation boats, some maintenance equipment and the underwater exploration pod they used for maintenance.

Oh God. Her heart very nearly leaped out of her chest and into her throat when she realized what was about to happen.

The submarine.

She'd forgotten all about it. It had always been a part of the plan. They were to tour the oil rig, and then their exploration pod, which was essentially a small, four-man submarine, would take Gabriel under the surface to see the rig at work. It was a harmless photo op, and when she was given the original itinerary, she hadn't thought a thing about it. Gabriel certainly hadn't mentioned having a problem with it when they discussed the agenda back in Miami.

Since then, she'd learned about Gabriel's issues with small, dark spaces, but so much had happened that the submarine had slipped her mind.

That had to be where they were going. Unfortunately there were twenty people between Gabriel and her on the narrow deck and staircase. He was below the platform and she was stuck above it at the very back of the pack. She was unable to get close enough to warn him before it was too late.

She rushed to the metal railing, peering over the side at the party below. They were still walking around while Patrick pointed out one thing or another, but she could see the open hatch of the exploration pod a few yards in front of them.

"Gabriel!" she shouted, but no one but a few of the reporters and crew members turned to look at her. The sounds of the ocean and the operating rig easily drowned out everything. Everything but the expression on his face.

Serafia knew the instant that he realized where they were going. He stiffened, his jaw tightening. His hands curled into fists at his side. Everyone around him continued to talk and laugh, but he wasn't participating in the discussion. He was loosening his tie, looking around for another option to escape, short of leaping into the ocean and swimming back to the mainland.

Patrick Rowling and the prime minister were the first to crawl inside the exploration pod. Gabriel stood there at the entrance for several moments, looking into the small space. He was white as a sheet and he gripped the railing with white-knuckled intensity. She could tell the others were trying to encourage him, but he likely couldn't hear anything they said if he was having a full-blown panic attack.

Then he shook his head. Backing up, he nearly ran into someone else, then turned and pushed his way through the crowd back to the stairs. Serafia could barely make out the sounds of shouts and words of concern. Patrick climbed back out of the submarine, calling toward Gabriel, but he didn't stop. He leaped up the stairs, finally colliding with Serafia as he reached the top.

He looked at her, but his eyes were wild with panic. It seemed almost as if he didn't really see her at all.

"I'm so sorry, Gabriel. I forgot all about the submarine. I would've warned you if I remembered."

He looked at her, his expression hardening. There was venom in his gaze, a place where she'd only ever seen attraction and humor. She reached out for his arm, but he shoved it aside and took a step back.

"It's not a big deal," she reassured him. "They can go on ahead without you. I'm sure you're not the only person who doesn't fancy the idea of a ride in that thing."

The look on his face made it clear that he didn't agree. It was a big deal, at least to him. Without saying a word, he turned and took off down the metal-grated walkway toward the helipad.

"Gabriel, stop! Wait!" she shouted as she pursued him, but he kept on going. She finally gave up just as she was overtaken by the press. They pushed her aside as they chased Gabriel, but before they could reach him, she spied the helicopter rising over the top of the rig.

With nothing else she could do, Serafia stood and watched the helicopter disappear into the horizon. Once it was gone, all she could see, all she could think of, was the look of utter betrayal on his face. He blamed her for this. And maybe he should. She'd made a very big error today.

"What happened?" The prime minister stopped beside her, his brow pinched in confusion. "Is the prince okay? He looked quite ill."

"I don't know," Serafia said. She wasn't going to be the one to tell him, and any of the surrounding reporters, that Gabriel was claustrophobic. That would make it seem as if she was deliberately trying to undermine him. He should've been the one to say it. All it would've taken was a polite pass and he could've avoided it. Instead, he'd run like he'd been ambushed.

A sinking feeling settled into Serafia's stomach at the thought. Was that what Gabriel believed she was doing? This was just one oversight, but when added to the string of other problems they'd had over the last week, did it add up to the appearance of sabotage? He couldn't possibly believe she'd do that to him. He hadn't given that newspaper article a second thought.

Or had he?

Serafia feared he'd begun to suspect her. That look had said everything. Serafia had ruined it. She hadn't meant to, but she'd ruined her relationship with Gabriel before it ever started.

Even though Gabriel had his driver take him back to Playa del Onda right away, he was discouraged to find Hector already waiting for him there. Judging by his press secretary's dour expression, the news of the incident on the oil rig had beaten Gabriel home. He just wanted to take off his tie, pour a glass of scotch and relax, but Hector was the hitch in that plan.

"Where's Serafia?" he asked as Gabriel blew past him.

"I don't know. I left her at the oil platform."

Hector made a thoughtful noise and followed him into the den. Gabriel poured a drink and ripped off his tie before collapsing onto the couch. "Why?"

"Well, I wanted to speak to you privately about those rumors. I'm concerned that the Espinas may be trying to undermine your coronation."

Gabriel was tired of hearing about this. "We've discussed this already."

"Yes, but that was before the prime minister called and briefed me about what happened today. He was concerned about you. He'd heard about the incident at the winery, as well."

Great. Now they were talking about him and his issues behind his back. "I don't do well in small spaces," Gabriel explained. "When I start having a panic attack, I have a very aggressive flight response. I overreact, I'm aware of that, but in the moment, I just have to get away from the situation. All the pressure I'm under to be poised and perfect every moment is just making it that much worse because I try to fight my way through it and it doesn't work. Then I feel like a fool."

Hector listened carefully. "I'll make certain we don't have these issues in the future. In exchange, I ask that you speak up when you're uncomfortable so we don't make a bigger scene out of it. Does Serafia know about your claustrophobia?"

"Yes." She didn't know until after the winery incident, but she knew today.

"I see. Your Majesty, my concern is about why these situations keep popping up. Rivera said he asked Patrick Rowling about the submarine and said that it had been Serafia's idea. I understand that you two are… whatever you are. But you really need to put your feelings for her aside and consider the possibility that all these unfortunate incidents are actually carefully orchestrated by the Espina family."

Gabriel dropped his face into his hand. He'd had a horrible day and he didn't really want to face this right now. "I'll take care of it," he said.

"Your Majesty, I—"

"I said, I'll take care of it!" Gabriel shouted. Suddenly his overwhelming apprehension had morphed into anger. He knew he shouldn't direct it at Hector, but he didn't care. He would kill the messenger because he didn't know what else to do.

"Very good, Your Grace. Thank you for your time." Hector gave a curt bow and left the room.

Gabriel watched Hector leave, the questions and anxiety spinning in his mind. Unable to sit still, he headed out to the veranda to await Serafia's return to the compound. The longer he waited, the more his blood began to heat in his veins. He had been upset at the oil platform, but after his discussion with Hector, every minute that ticked by tipped his emotions over into pure anger.

If he was right, this was the ultimate betrayal. Serafia would've known exactly what she was doing. She knew he couldn't stand small, confined spaces. How could she schedule him for what amounted to a miniature submarine ride under an oil platform? Even people who hadn't been through the kind of experience he'd had would balk at that. And yet, he felt this pressure as the future king to do it. He had to be strong; he couldn't show weakness. His father expected it. His country expected it. And all it did was backfire on him and make him look like more of a coward when he fled.

The situation had snuck up on him. They were walking around the lower level and the next thing he knew, he was confronted with his personal nightmare. As he'd looked down into the small round hatch at the metal ladder that would take him into a space too cramped for more than four full-grown men, he felt himself launch into a full-blown panic attack.

This wasn't like the incident at the vineyard. There, the room was dark and underground, but he could escape any time he chose, and did. The minute Gabriel climbed down that ladder, and the hatch was sealed, he would be trapped. His lungs had seized up as if a vise was crushing his rib cage. His heart had been racing so quickly he could barely tell the rhythm of one beat from the next. He'd been sweating, wheezing and damn near on the verge of crying while Patrick Rowling and the prime minister tried to coax him on board.

No way. He didn't care if he offended the richest man in Alma. He wasn't about to have that image on him on television, blasted around the internet and on the front page of every paper. New King of Alma Cries Like a Baby When Forced Into a Submarine! They might as well send a stamped invitation for the Tantaberra family to come back and take over again. It was better to leave before it got worse.

It was bad enough everyone had witnessed his behavior. The Rowlings, the press and even the prime minister were all standing by as he'd completely flipped out, shoved people aside to escape and run across the platform to the helicopter pad as if he were on fire. It must have been a sight to see…his guards chasing after him, people shouting at him to come back, the press recording every moment of it… *The Runaway King.* Now, there was a nickname for his upcoming illustrious reign.

He hadn't registered much in the moment. Gabriel had only been motivated by a driving need to get away from that submarine, off the platform and onto dry land with sunshine on his face as soon as possible. But he could hear Serafia as she'd tried to comfort him. He'd registered the panic and worry on her face as she rushed toward him, but he wasn't slowing down for her or anyone else. Besides, it had been too late. The damage was already done.

Of course, that might have been part of her plan, right? The article had insinuated that the Espina family was determined to gain the throne back one way or another. If not through seduction, perhaps through scandal and humiliation. Serafia had been throwing grenades at him since he arrived. The watch, the debacle at the airport, the vineyard and now the oil platform... Even the supposedly successful party at Rowling's house had proven controversial when he snubbed the Gomez girl at Serafia's suggestion.

He'd paid her to help this week go smoothly, to prepare him for any eventuality as king, and it had started to seem more as if she was deliberately setting him up to fail.

He heard the sound of his bedroom door open. After taking a large sip of his scotch, he set the mostly empty glass down. The amber liquid burned in his stomach, just as his anger shot hot through his veins.

Finally Serafia stepped through the open doorway, looking as worn and ragged as if she'd jogged all the way back from the oil platform. Her shirt was untucked and wrinkled. There was a run in her stocking, and her heels were scuffed. Her hair had been up in a bun, but now it was half up, half down in a silky black mess. She was flushed, with bloodshot eyes and dried tear tracks down her cheeks. It made him wonder how long it had taken her to put together this look and assume the role of the innocent in all this. Maybe that was why it took forever for her to get here.

"I'm so sorry, Gabriel. I didn't—"

"Just stop!" he shouted more forcefully than he intended. The anger that had simmered inside him was approaching a full boil now that he was face-to-face with her again. "Don't tell me you didn't know about this, because I know that's a lie." He gestured to the white sheet of paper on the table in front of him. "I found the schedule you gave me back in Miami for this week. This event was on there. Patrick Rowling said you actually suggested it. You knew all this time what we were building up to."

Serafia crossed her arms over her chest in a defensive posture. "In Miami, I didn't know anything about your abduction. Yes, it was my suggestion because I thought it would be an interesting activity for you. When we reviewed your schedule for the visit, I mentioned it and you said nothing. You just tuned me out half the time. I'm surprised you even had the schedule anymore."

"And after you knew about what happened to me in Venezuela? After the incident at the vineyard? Did it not occur to you then that these plans for the visit to the oil platform might be a bad idea?"

"I'd forgotten," she said, tears forming in her eyes again. "With everything that has happened over the past week, I forgot all about the submarine. It slipped my mind and by the time I remembered, it was too late. We were separated by the crowd and I couldn't warn you without making a scene. I was trying to warn you before they got to that part of the tour."

Gabriel stood up, his dark gaze searching her face

for signs of the treachery he knew was there. Hector had helped him cast her under a shadow of suspicion he couldn't shake. She'd been hiding her secret agenda beneath a disguise of coy smiles and stiff, respectable suits, but it was there nonetheless. And he'd fallen for it.

"And you showed up to warn me at the perfect time," he replied with bitterness in his voice. "Late enough for me to embarrass myself and undermine my future as king, but not so late as to convince me that it was deliberate just in case the ploy didn't work and you might still end up queen."

A strange combination of emotions danced across Serafia's face, ending in a look of exasperation. "I don't want to be queen. I never have and you know why!"

If she really didn't want to be queen, that only left one option. "Just wanting to stay close enough to ruin me and my family, then?"

Serafia threw her arms up, spinning in a circle before facing him with her index finger held up. "One incident. *One.* And suddenly those newspaper accusations you dismissed are gospel? Do you have no faith in me at all?"

"I did. For some stupid reason, I pushed aside all my suspicions and allowed myself to trust you more than I've trusted anyone in years. Even when that article came out, I dismissed it as nasty gossip or old news from another time and place. I couldn't believe that you could be using me to get to the throne."

"Because I'm not," she insisted.

Gabriel just shook his head sadly. "You're just as bad as the Gomez family. You know what? You're even worse. At least they're transparent about their ambitions. You and your family just sidle up to us like friends, then pervert the entire relationship to suit your own purposes."

"Gabriel, you said yourself that that story was nonsense. I didn't get planted with you. You hired me."

That was the detail that had bothered him, but the longer he sat on the patio, the more he'd begun to wonder if that was really true. "What *were* you doing in Miami, Serafia? I hadn't seen you in years, and then all of a sudden, you fly all the way to Miami from Barcelona for my going-away party? You could've just waited to see me in Alma if you were that interested in congratulating me, and saved yourself a fortune in time and money."

Serafia stiffened, her eyebrows drawing together into a frown. "I was in the States for another project and my father asked me to attend on behalf of the family."

"What project?" he pressed. "Who were you working for?"

Serafia started to stutter over her words, as though she was failing to come up with an adequate lie when she was put on the spot. "I—it w-was for a confidential client. I can't tell you who it was."

"A confidential client? Of course it was." Gabriel tried not to take it personally that she thought he was so stupid. "You may not have been a plant, but you were a tempting little worm dangling on a hook right in front of me. I snatched you up just as surely as you'd weaseled your way into my inner circle on your own. You pretended to help me be a better king, building up my confidence in and out of bed, while slowly undermining every inch of progress I've made along the way."

Serafia looked at him with hurt reflecting in her

dark eyes. "Is that all you think of the two of us? Of what we have together?"

"I didn't at first, but now I see how wrong I was. I can see it must have been really difficult for you."

She narrowed her gaze at him, her tears fading. "What must be?"

Gabriel swallowed hard and spat out the words he'd been holding in all day. "Trying to screw me in two different ways at once."

Serafia gasped and raised her hand to cover her mouth. She stumbled back on her heels until her back collided with the doorframe. "You're a bastard, Gabriel."

"Maybe," he said thoughtfully. "But it's people like you who made me this way."

"I quit!" she shouted, disappearing into the house.

"Fine. Quit!" he yelled back at her. "I was just going to fire you, anyway."

He heard her bedroom door slam shut down the hallway. With her gone, the anger that had boiled over suddenly drained out of him. He slumped back into his chair and dropped his head into his hands.

It didn't matter whether she quit or he fired her. In the end, the damage was done and she would soon be gone.

Eleven

Harder. Faster. Keep pushing.

It didn't matter if Serafia's lungs were burning or that her leg muscles felt as if they could rip from her bones at any second. She had to keep going.

Just when she hit the point where she couldn't take any more, she reached out for the console and dropped the speed on the treadmill by half a mile. Giving herself only a minute or two to recover, she then increased it by a whole mile. Her sneakers pounded hard against the rotating belt, which was reaching speeds she could barely maintain in the past.

But she had to now. She had to keep running or everything would catch up with her. It wasn't until she could feel her heart pounding like Thor's hammer against her breast that she realized she'd taken this too far. She reached out and pounded the emergency stop button, slamming into the console and draping her broken body over it. The air rushing from her lungs blazed like fire, her heart feeling as if it was about to burst. She'd run for miles today. Hours. Longer and harder than her doctor-appointed forty-five-minute daily limit.

And yet the moment she looked up, the world around her was just the same. The same heartache. The same confusion. The same anger at herself and at Gabriel. All she'd managed to do was pull a hamstring and sweat through her clothes.

She gripped her bottle of water and stepped down onto the tile floor with gelatinous, quivering legs. Unable to go much farther, she opened the door to her garden courtyard. The cold water and ocean breeze weren't enough to soothe her overheated body, so she set down her bottle and approached her swimming pool. Without stopping to take off her shoes, she stepped off the edge, plunging herself into the cool turquoise depths.

Rising to the surface, she pushed her hair out of her face and took a deep breath. She felt a million times better. Her heart slowed and her body temperature was jerked back from the point of disaster.

And yet she was still at a loss over what to do with herself. She had returned home to Barcelona in disgrace. Her last-minute flight had delivered her home late in the night; she hadn't even told her family or staff that she was returning. All she knew was that she had to get out of Alma that instant. She would work the rest out later.

Once she'd escaped…she didn't know what to do. She had no jobs lined up for several weeks. She'd cleared her calendar when she took the Montoro job because she wasn't sure how long it would truly take. The first few days in Miami had been excruciating and she'd wondered if two weeks would be enough.

Two weeks were more than enough, at least for her. And while she was relieved to be home, returned to the sanctuary she'd built for herself here, something felt off. She'd wandered through the empty halls, sat on the balcony overlooking the sea, lay in bed staring at the ceiling…the thought of Gabriel crept into everything she did.

Serafia swam to the edge of the pool and crossed her arms along the stone, lifting her torso up out of the water. She dropped her head onto her forearms and fought the tears that had taunted her the last few days. As hard as she'd resisted falling for the rebellious prince, it had happened, anyway. Even with the threat of returning to the spotlight, the potential for becoming queen and all the responsibilities that held, she couldn't help herself.

And then he turned on her. How could he think she would do something like that on purpose? The minute she realized where they were headed, the panic had been nearly overwhelming. And then when he'd looked at her with the betrayal reflecting in his eyes, she felt her heart break. He was so used to people using and abusing his trust that he refused to see that wasn't what she was doing.

Perhaps she should have stayed in Alma and fought to clear her name. Running away made her look guilty, but she just couldn't stay there. Her family might have been from Alma decades ago, but she was born and raised in Spain and that was where she needed to be.

She just needed to get her life back on track. The

dramas of Alma would fade, Gabriel would choose his queen and she would go on with her life, such as it was.

At least that was what she told herself.

The French doors to the courtyard opened behind her, and Serafia's housekeeper stepped out with a tray. "I have your lunch ready, señorita."

Serafia swam back to the shallow end of the pool to greet her. She wasn't remotely interested in food with the way she felt, but it would hurt her housekeeper's feelings if she didn't pretend otherwise. "Thank you, Esperanza. Please leave it on the patio table."

Esperanza did as she asked, hesitating a moment by the edge of the pool with a towel in her hands. She seemed worried, her wrinkled face pinched into an expression of concern. "Are you going to eat it?"

Serafia frowned and climbed up the steps. "What do you mean?"

"You barely touched your breakfast, just picking at the fruit. I found most of last night's dinner plate scraped into the trash so I wouldn't see it. I have all your favorite snacks and drinks in the house since your return and I haven't had to restock a single thing."

Serafia snatched the towel from the housekeeper's hands, the past anxiety of being caught in the act rushing back to her. "That's none of your business. I pay you to cook my meals, not monitor them like my mother."

The hurt expression on the older woman's face made her feel instantly guilty for snapping at her. Esperanza was the sweetest woman she knew and she didn't deserve that kind of treatment. "I'm sorry. I shouldn't have said that. Forgive me." Serafia slipped down into the patio chair and buried her face in her towel.

"It's nothing. When I don't eat, I get grumpy, too," Esperanza offered with a small smile. She was a plump older woman with a perpetually pleasant disposition. Probably because she got to eat and wasn't eternally stressing out about how she looked. "But I worry about you, señorita, and so do your parents."

Serafia's head snapped up. "They've called?"

"*Sí*, but you were out walking on the beach. They asked me not to tell you. They seemed very interested in your eating habits, which is why I noticed the change. They said if you started visibly losing weight, I should call them straightaway."

Great. Her parents were having her own employee spy on her. They must really be concerned. Serafia sighed and sat back in her chair. They probably were right to be. In the last few days since returning from Alma, she'd already lost five pounds that she shouldn't have. She was at the low end of the range her doctors had provided her. If she got back into the red zone, she risked another round of inpatient treatment, and she didn't want to do that.

Damn it.

"Thank you for caring about me, Esperanza." Serafia eyed the tray of food she brought her. There was a large green salad with diced chicken, a platter with a hard-boiled egg, slices of cheese and bread and a carafe of vinaigrette. Ever hopeful, Esperanza had even included two of her famous cinnamon-sugar cookies. All in all, it was a healthy, balanced lunch with plenty of vegetables, proteins and whole grains. The kind Serafia asked her to make most days.

And yet she had a hard time stopping her brain from mentally obsessing over how many calories were sitting there. If she only ate the greens and the chicken with no dressing, it wouldn't be too bad. Maybe one piece of cheese, but definitely no bread. They were the same compulsive thoughts that she'd once allowed to take over her life. She'd battled this demon for a long time. A part of her had hoped that she'd beaten it for good, but one emotional blow had sent her spiraling back into her old bad habits.

Habits that had almost killed her.

"It looks wonderful," she said. "I promise to eat every bite. Are there any more cookies?"

"There are!" Esperanza said, her face brightening.

"I'll take some of those this afternoon after my siesta."

"Muy bien!" Esperanza shuffled back into the house, leaving Serafia alone on the patio.

She knew she should change out of her wet workout clothes, but she didn't care. She knew that she needed to eat. Now. Voices in her head be damned.

She started with one of the cookies for good measure. It dropped into her empty stomach like lead, reminding her to take it slow. Her doctors had warned her about starving herself, then binging. That was another, all new, dangerous path she was determined not to take.

Nibbling on the cheese and bread, she started to feel better. She knew that her body paid a high toll for her anorexia. As she was driven to exercise and ignore all the food she could, it made her feel terrible. Even this small amount of food made the difference. Picking up her fork and pouring some of the vinaigrette over the salad, she speared a bite and chewed it thoughtfully.

All this was in marked contrast to the way she'd felt in Alma. For some reason, her past worries had slipped away as she focused on preparing Gabriel to be king. Perhaps it was because he thought she was so beautiful, even with the extra pounds she resented. He worshipped every inch of her body in bed, never once stopping to criticize or comment on her flaws. That made her feel beautiful. When they ate together, it was a fun, enjoyable experience. She was too distracted by the good food and even better company to worry about the calories. There were a few days in Alma where she'd even forgotten to exercise. Before that, she hadn't missed a day of exercise in years. When she was with Gabriel, she'd been able to stop fighting with her disease and simply *live*.

She had been doing so well, and the minute it was yanked away from her, the negative thoughts came rushing back in. She couldn't do this. If there was one thing she'd learned in the years since her heart attack, it was that she loved herself too much to keep hurting herself.

Reaching for a slice of bread with cheese, she took a large bite, then another, and another, until her lunch was very nearly gone.

She couldn't allow loving Gabriel to undo all the progress she'd made.

The report on Gabriel's lap told him what he already knew in his heart, but somehow, seeing the words in black-and-white made him feel that much more like the ass he was.

Hector had done as he'd asked. His people in the press office had reached out to the author of the scathing article on the Espinas. It hadn't taken much pressure for him to reveal that he'd been approached by Felicia Gomez. He admitted that while the historical portions of the article were researched and fact-checked, the insinuations of Serafia's nefarious intentions were purely speculation based on Felicia's suggestions. It didn't mean that her family didn't help overthrow the Montoros, but in the end, that really didn't matter anymore. All that mattered was that Serafia was innocent of all those charges.

He knew it. He knew it when he'd read the article the first time and he knew it when he'd thrown accusations at Serafia and watched her heart break right before his eyes. He'd been humiliated. Angry. He'd lashed out at her because he'd allowed his own fears to rule his life and publically embarrass him. It was easier to blame her in the moment than face the fact that he'd done this to himself.

Gabriel felt awful about the whole thing. Serafia had been the only person in his life he thought he could trust, and yet he'd turned around and abused her trust of him at the first provocation. It made him feel sick.

He needed to do something to fix this. Right now.

Looking up from his report, he spied Luca walking down the hallway past his office. "Luca, can you find out if the Montoro jet is still in Alma?"

Luca nodded and disappeared down the hallway.

Gabriel took a deep breath and resolved himself to his sudden decision. He didn't entirely have his plan together, but he knew he needed to get out of Alma to make this happen. That meant getting on a plane. Serafia had returned to Barcelona. He was certain she wouldn't answer his calls if he tried, and anyway, he knew in his heart that they needed to have a conversation in person. The only catch would be whether or not the jet was here. His father had sent for Bella to come to Alma. Gabriel wasn't sure what day that was happening, but if the jet was with her in Miami, he'd have to find another way to get to Serafia. Could a prince fly coach?

He didn't care if he was crammed in a middle seat at the back of the plane, he had to get to her. Saying he was sorry wasn't enough. He needed to follow that up with how he felt about her. It had taken losing her for him to get in touch with how he truly felt. There was nothing quite like waking up and realizing he was in love and he'd just ruined everything.

But maybe, just maybe, apologizing and confessing his love for her would be enough for Serafia to forgive his snap judgments.

Luca appeared in the doorway, an odd expression on his face.

"Where's the jet?" Gabriel asked.

"It's still at the airport in Del Sol, Your Grace."

He breathed a sigh of relief. "Good. Tell them I want to go to Barcelona as soon as possible. I need a car to meet me at the airport and I need someone to track down Serafia's home address. I have no idea where she lives."

"Yes, Your Grace. I will see to all that. But first, you have…a visitor."

Gabriel could feel his own face taking on Luca's pinched, confused expression. "A visitor?" Could people just stroll up to the royal beach compound and knock on the door to join him for tea?

"Yes. It's an old woman from Del Sol. She told the guards at the gate that she took a taxi out here to speak with you. She said it's very important."

Gabriel was certain that everything people wanted to say to the king was very important, but he was at a loss. He wanted to pack his bag and be in Barcelona before dinnertime. Certainly this could wait…

"She says it's about Serafia."

Gabriel stiffened. That changed everything. "Have her escorted into the parlor. Tell Marta to bring some tea and those almond cookies if we have any left. That will give us some time to make the arrangements before I leave."

Luca nodded and went off to fulfill his wishes. Gabriel returned to his closet to pick a suit coat. He'd been dressing himself for the last few days and if he was honest with himself, he wasn't doing a very good job. He knew that Serafia would want him to wear a jacket to greet a guest, especially an elderly one with more conservative ideas about the monarchy. He selected a black suit coat that went with the gray shirt he was already wearing. He knew he should add a tie, but he just couldn't do it. He was in his own home; certainly he could get away with being a little more casual there.

By the time he reached the parlor, all his instructions had been executed beautifully. Marta had placed a tray of lovely treats on the coffee table and was pouring two cups of tea. Seated on the couch was a tiny woman. Perhaps the smallest he'd ever seen, withered and hunched over with age. She was at least eighty, the life shriveling out of her just as the sun had seemed to tan her skin to near leather. Her hair was silver and pulled back into a neat bun. She looked like everyone's *abuela*.

"Presenting His Majesty, Prince Gabriel!" one of

the guards lining the wall announced as he entered the room.

The old woman reached for her cane to stand and curtsey properly, but Gabriel couldn't bear for her to go to that much trouble just for him. "Please, stay seated," he insisted.

The woman relaxed back into her seat with a look of relief on her face. "*Gracias*, Don Gabriel."

He sat down opposite her, offering the woman sugar or cream for her tea. "What can I do for you, señora?"

She took a sip of tea, and then set it down on the china dish with a shaky hand. "Thank you for taking the time to see me today. I know you are very busy. My name is Conchita Ortega. In 1946 when the coup happened, I was just fifteen years old and working as a servant in the Espina household. I have seen what was published in the papers over the last week or so, and now I have heard that Señorita Espina has left Alma."

"Señorita Espina was only working for me for a few weeks. She was always supposed to return home."

The older woman narrowed her gaze at him. "I understand, Your Grace, but I also understand and know *amor* when I see it. I know in my heart you were a couple in love and those vicious lies have ruined it. I had to speak up so you would know the truth."

Gabriel listened carefully, his interest in what the woman had to say growing with each additional word she spoke. Even though he didn't hold the past of her family against Serafia, it would help to know the truth of what really had happened back then. This woman might be one of the only people left alive who knew the whole story. "Please," he replied. "I'd love for you to tell me what you know."

She nodded and relaxed back in her seat with a cookie in her hand. She took a bite and chewed slowly, torturing Gabriel by delaying her story. "By the time everything fell apart," she began, "the hurt feelings about the broken engagement between Rafael the First and Rosa Espina were nearly a decade in the past. Rafael had married Anna Maria, Rosa had married another fine gentleman and the young Prince Rafael the Second, your grandfather, was seven years old. All had turned out for the best. The Espina family would not, and did not, conspire against the Montoros during the coup. In fact, they were your family's closest confidantes."

"How do you know?"

"At fifteen, I was like a little mouse, moving quiet and unseen through the house. I was privy to many discussions with no one giving any thought to my presence. I was serving tea when Queen Anna Maria came to the Espina Estate in secret. She'd come to ask your family to help them. Alma had weathered the Second World War, but they feared the worst was yet to come for them. Tantaberra was growing in power, staging large demonstrations and causing unrest all over Alma. The royal family was worried that they were losing hold of the country.

"The queen asked the Espinas to help them protect Alma's historical treasures by smuggling them out of the country before things got worse. The Montoros had to stay as long as they could to appear strong against their opposition, but they feared that when they did leave, they'd have to leave everything behind. The queen couldn't bear for such important things to be lost, so they arranged for the Espinas to move to Switzerland and take the country's most important historical artifacts with them."

Serafia had mentioned that her family lived in Switzerland before moving to Spain. The article had said the family fled before the coup, which was interpreted as suspicious at the time. "What kind of things?" he asked.

"The royal jewels and stores of gold, an oil portrait of the first king of Alma, handwritten historical records of the royal family...everything that would be considered irreplaceable."

"Were they successful in smuggling everything out?" he asked.

"Yes. I helped load the ship myself. They sailed from Alma with all of their things and a secret cargo of Alman treasure. They traveled down the Rhine River to Switzerland, arriving just weeks before everything fell apart. Your family was not so lucky. They fled to America with nothing, leaving everything else behind for Tantaberra to claim as his own."

"What about you?"

"I had the option to go with the Espinas, but I couldn't leave my family behind. I stayed. But I'm glad I did so I could be here to tell you the truth. The Espinas are not traitors. They're heroes, but no one knows the truth."

"Why doesn't anyone know about this? Not even my father has mentioned it."

"It is likely he does not know. The queen orchestrated everything and may not have told anyone in the family so they could not be tortured for the information. It was a closely guarded secret and everyone was instructed not to speak of it while the Tantaberras were still in power. At the time, they had ties with Franco in Spain and they feared that if anyone knew the truth, their network would seek out the Espinas and retaliate. They were instructed not to breathe a word to anyone until the royal family was restored officially to the throne again."

"Do you think the family still has the treasures after all these years?"

"I have no doubt of it. I ask you to reach out to Señor Espina in Madrid. He can tell you the truth. After all these years, I'm sure he will be happy to return the royal treasure to where it belongs after the coronation."

Gabriel was stunned by the entire conversation. Apparently this information had not been passed down through the generations the way it should've been. But as they finished their tea, a plan started to form in his mind. He arranged for a car to take Señora Ortega home and finalized the preparations for his flight. Instead of going to Barcelona, he decided a visit to Madrid to see Serafia's father was in order. If her family had his country's treasures, they needed to be restored to the people. Once he knew for certain the story was true, he intended for the whole country to know the truth about the Espinas. They deserved a parade in their honor, and all the vicious rumors to be put to bed once and for all.

And while he was there…he wanted to ask Señor Espina for his daughter's hand in marriage.

Twelve

It was a quick flight to Madrid, but still too long in Gabriel's eyes. The car that picked him up at the airport rushed him through the streets of the city to the Espina residence. Now all he had to do was face Serafia's father and accept his punishment for hurting her.

Arturo Espina opened the front door and glared at Gabriel. He had been expecting a less than warm reception. Serafia had no doubt told her family how horribly he'd treated her. He was on a journey to make amends not only with Serafia, but also with her parents. If what Señora Ortega said was true, things needed to be made right with the Espinas. By keeping Queen Anna Maria's secret so diligently, they'd lived in the shadow of suspicion and rumors for too long. And Gabriel had a long path to redemption where Serafia was concerned. The pain would start here, now, but it had to start somewhere.

"Señor Espina," he said, hoping his smile didn't give away how nervous he was. "Hello."

The older man glanced over Gabriel's shoulder at the royal guard hovering nearby. The irritation suddenly faded and was replaced with a respectful bow. "Prince Gabriel. To what do we owe the honor of your presence?"

"Please," Gabriel said. "You bandaged my skinned knee once. Let's drop the formalities. I'm not here as prince. I'm here about Serafia."

Arturo nodded and took a step back to allow him inside. The guard remained outside the door at Gabriel's request. Arturo led him through the large mansion to an inner courtyard landscaped with trees and a sparkling tile fountain. "Please, have a seat," he said. "May I offer you a drink? Something to eat?"

Gabriel shook his head. "No, thank you."

"I'm surprised to see you here, Gabriel. Serafia hasn't mentioned what happened in Alma, but considering how she rushed home, I'm assuming things did not end well. What I've read in the Alma newspapers has been disheartening, to say the least."

"I know, and what I'm really here to do is apologize. And maybe, if my apology is accepted, I'd like some information only you can give me."

Arturo sat down across from him and waited for the questions to come.

"First, I want to apologize for the way I've handled all this. Regardless of the truth, I behaved poorly, lashing out at Serafia, and I'm ashamed of that. Your family, and specifically your daughter, never gave me any reason to doubt your loyalty."

"You are not the first to be suspicious of our family over the years."

"I had never heard any of those stories before," Gabriel explained. "The papers have had some terrible things to say about your family. I grew up in America in a household that very rarely, if ever, discussed Alma and what happened. Our families have always been friends, so I was blindsided by those stories. I feel like a fool, but I allowed those articles to taint my feelings for your family and for your daughter. I shouldn't have let that happen, but I was upset with myself and took it out on her."

"I read about what happened at the oil rig. Am I wrong in thinking that was related to your abduction?"

Gabriel looked Arturo in the eye. "It was. I wasn't sure how many people knew about it. My father wanted to keep it all pretty quiet."

"He called me while it was happening and asked for advice. Rafael was torn up about the whole thing and how it was taking so long to bring you home. Rafael was so frustrated—he felt helpless for the first time in his life. When you showed back up in Miami, I think he was embarrassed about how it was all handled and never wanted to talk about it again. He thought you would blame him for everything, so he wanted to forget about it all."

"I didn't blame him," Gabriel said. "But I've always felt like I was a disappointment to him, somehow. I tried to hide my claustrophobia because I thought he'd see it as another weakness."

"No one—your father included—would hold something like that against you. You went through a terrible experience. He probably thought that putting it behind you would help. We did that with Serafia and I've never been certain it was the right course. But as parents, you do what you can to protect your children."

Gabriel sighed. He'd come here for answers about the Espina family and ended up with more than he'd expected. "Thank you for telling me that. I've never really been able to get past what happened. I don't do well in small spaces since my kidnapping, and I blamed Serafia for not warning me ahead of time about what was in store on the oil rig. It wasn't her fault. I ruined everything with her, and then I find out that all those rumors that poisoned my mind weren't even true."

"Do you mean the rumors about the Espinas helping Tantaberra depose your family?" Arturo asked. His tone was flat, as though he'd had to hear these slanderous charges his whole life.

"Yes. An old woman who worked for your family back then came to the house today and explained the truth about how the Espinas safeguarded the royal treasure. At least, I hope it's the truth."

Arturo nodded. "We've had to keep quiet about our family's role in all this for decades, ignoring the rumors so we didn't risk anyone finding out the truth. I don't think any of them believed the dictatorship would last as long as it has. We feared that the Tantaberras would come after us if they knew what we were hiding, or worse, come after your family if they had any knowledge of it. Even after all this time, we had to deliberately keep it from you and others in your family."

"I can't imagine that burden."

"I think it was worth it. I heard that Tantaberra was furious when he took the palace and all the gold and jewels he'd coveted were gone."

Gabriel had never given much thought to his great-grandmother, Anna Maria, but in that moment, he admired her fire. He wished he could've seen the dictator's face when he realized that the Montoros had outsmarted him. "That means your family still has it?"

Arturo stood. "Wait here. I'll be right back." He disappeared down a hallway and returned a few minutes later with something in his hand. When he sat down again, he placed two small items on the table. One, a gold coin, and the other, a diamond and ruby ring. "This is just a small part of what my family has protected for seventy years."

Gabriel reached out and picked up the coin. It was a coin minted in Alma in the 1800s. "You keep it here?"

"No. I've always kept a few tiny items in my safe for a moment like this, but the rest is in a vault in Switzerland. We were to keep it until the coronation took place, to ensure it was official, and then it can all be restored to the palace. I've always hoped to see this day happen. It's been a weight on my shoulders since my father told me the truth."

Returning the coin, Gabriel examined the ruby ring and felt a touch of sadness come over him. It was so beautiful, with a dark red oval ruby that had to be nearly four carats. It was surrounded by a ring of tiny diamonds and flanked on each side by a pear-shaped diamond. The setting was a mix of platinum and gold filigree. It was more beautiful than any ring had a right to be. He was incredibly grateful the Espinas had hidden it away from the Tantaberras, yet sad that no one had enjoyed the ring for all these years. This ring was meant to be on the hand of a queen—a woman like Serafia.

"I've betrayed the family that I should've trusted above all others. I'm so sorry. I can't apologize enough. I want to see to it that the truth gets out. When the treasure is restored, I want it put on display in Alma's national museum so that everyone will know how the Espinas safeguarded it all these years, and put an end to the rumors once and for all."

"That would be wonderful," Arturo said. "I would like to move back to Alma one day. My father was born there. I grew up in Switzerland, but I've always dreamed of going back to where my people belonged."

Looking down at the ring, Gabriel was reminded of the other reason he'd come here today. The truth was nice, but even if the old woman's story was just a fabrication, his first priority was getting Serafia to forgive—and marry—him. He put the ring back on the table and looked at Arturo.

"I also came here today because I want Serafia in my life," he said. "I…I love her. I want her to be my queen. Do you think she'll ever be able to forgive me for the way I've treated her?"

Arturo sat back in his seat and looked at him with a serious expression. "I don't know. She's taken this very hard. Her mother and I have been worried about her."

Gabriel's gaze met his. "Worried?"

"Did she tell you about her illness?" Arturo asked.

"The anorexia? Yes, but she said that was behind her."

"We'd hoped so," Arturo explained, "but her doctors had warned us that patients are never fully cured of this disease. Stress, especially emotional upheaval, can send her spiraling back into her bad habits. Her housekeeper has told us that she is hardly eating. That she does nothing but exercise and sleep since she returned to Barcelona. There have been a few times where she's fallen into this slump before, but she's righted herself before it went too far. I'm hoping that you can help pull her out of it."

Gabriel sensed the worry and fear in Arturo's voice and felt even more miserable than he had before. He knew how much Serafia struggled with her image and how hard she'd worked to overcome her illness. She'd done so well when they were together that he never would've known about the anorexia if she hadn't told him the truth. If he'd sent her into such an emotional state that she fell prey to it again—if she got hurt because of it—he'd never forgive himself.

"I'm flying directly to Barcelona from here. I'll do everything I can to make things right, I promise. Even if she doesn't want me, even if she won't forgive me, I won't leave until I'm certain she's safe."

Arturo watched him as he spoke, and then nodded. "You said earlier that you wanted my daughter to be your queen. You're serious about this?"

Gabriel swallowed hard. "Yes, sir. With your permission, I'd like to ask Serafia to be my wife. I know that under the circumstances, the public role will not be an easy one for her, but I love her too much to let her out of my life. I don't think I could choose a better woman to help me make Alma that great country it once was."

Arturo nodded. "You are good for her, I know it. I've watched you two on the news together. She looks happier with you than she has been in years. You make sure she stays that way and you have my blessing."

"Yes. Of course. I only want Serafia to be happy. Thank you, Señor Espina."

Serafia's father finally smiled for the first time since Gabriel had arrived, and he felt a weight lifted from his chest.

"Do you have a ring for her?" the older man asked.

Gabriel was embarrassed to admit that he didn't. "I rushed here to see you without thinking all of it through. I don't have anything for her yet."

Arturo reached out and picked up the ruby ring from the table. "This is the wedding ring of Rafael the First's mother, Queen Josefina. If you truly love my daughter and want her to be queen, this is the ring you should give her."

Gabriel took the ring from the man who might soon be his father-in-law and shook his hand. "Thank you, sir. It's perfect."

"Good job," Esperanza said as she took away Serafia's mostly empty dinner plate.

Serafia chuckled. "Does this mean I get the tiramisu you promised me?"

"Of course."

Esperanza disappeared inside, leaving her alone on her patio, watching the sun set. It seemed like only yesterday that she was doing the same with Gabriel, only overlooking the Atlantic instead of the Mediterranean. The moment had been romantic and full of promise.

And now here she was, alone. What a difference a few days could make.

But she wasn't going to dwell on it. She'd had her moment to mope, and now it was time for her to figure out what she wanted to do with her life. Being with Gabriel had helped her realize that she was hiding here in Barcelona. She got out, she worked, but she hadn't really allowed herself to have the full life she deserved. That was over. She was determined that from this point forward, she was going to live her life to the fullest.

"Señorita?" Esperanza was at the door again.

"Yes?" Serafia said as she turned and froze in place. Standing tall behind her tiny housekeeper was Gabriel. He was looking incredibly handsome in a gray shirt and a black suit coat. Without a tie, of course.

She felt her heart skip a beat in her chest when she saw him. Every nerve awakened as her body realized he was so close. She tightened her hands around the arms of her chair to fight her unwanted reaction to him. He was a bastard. He said terrible things to her. She absolutely should not react to him like this. And yet she couldn't help it. He might be a bastard, but she still loved him. She still hadn't managed to convince her heart differently.

Taking a deep breath, she wished away her attraction and tried to focus on more important things, like what had brought him all the way to her doorstep.

Esperanza looked a little stunned. Serafia imagined that opening the door and finding a prince standing there was not exactly what the older woman had anticipated when the bell rang. "Prince Gabriel is here to see you. He would not wait outside."

"I didn't want to give you the chance to turn me away," he said, with a sheepish smile that seemed to acknowledge he was the guilty party.

"Smart move," Serafia noted in a sharp tone. He *was* the guilty party and she wanted to make sure he got his punishment. "Esperanza, could you please bring out a bottle of merlot and two glasses, please?" She wasn't sure how this conversation was going to go, but drinking certainly wouldn't hurt matters. At the very least it would help her relax. She was drawn tight as a drum.

Esperanza disappeared into the house and Gabriel joined Serafia outside. He took a seat in the chair beside her and looked out at the sea as she had been doing earlier.

"You have a beautiful home," he said.

"Thank you."

He turned back to look at her, his concerned gaze taking in every inch of her, but not in the hungry way she was used to. He seemed to be cataloguing her somehow. "How are you?" he asked.

Not once in the weeks they'd spent together had he asked her that question. Now she knew it was probably her parents' doing. They'd started calling each day, never directly asking if she was eating, but hinting around the subject, not knowing Esperanza had already ratted them out. She frowned at him. "Did my family send you down here to check on me?"

"What?" He looked startled. "No. I came here on my own, but I made a stop in Madrid on the way. Your father mentioned they were concerned about you."

"They usually are," she said. "That's why I opted to move to Barcelona and give myself some breathing room. They're very overprotective of me."

"They just want to make sure you're happy and healthy. As do I."

"Is that why you've come?" she snapped. "To make sure you didn't break my heart too badly?"

"No," he said with a grave seriousness in his voice. "I came to apologize."

"It's not necessary," she said.

"Yes, it is. I lashed out at you and it wasn't your fault. I let my own fears get the best of me, then used the most convenient excuse I could find to push you away. It was the dumbest thing I've ever done, and that's saying a lot after the antics I've gotten into the last few years. I've relived that moment in my head over and over, wishing I'd handled everything differently. I was a fool and it cost me the woman I love."

Serafia gasped at his words, but before she could respond, Esperanza returned with the wine. The interruption allowed Serafia a minute to think about his words and consider what her response should be. He loved her. She wanted to tell him that she loved him, too, but she was wary of giving away too much. He'd hurt her, abused her trust. She wasn't just going to take him back because he decided he was in love and that made everything better.

When Esperanza went back into the house, he picked up where he'd left off. "I never believed those stories about your family, and now that I know the truth, I'm going to see to it that those rumors are put to bed for good. The Espinas are heroes and I want everyone to know it."

"Heroes?" Serafia frowned. What was he talking about?

"Your family protected the royal treasure from the Tantaberras. That's why they left before the coup. Your father and I are going to work to have the treasure restored and put on display after the coronation. Without your family's help, the Tantaberras would've used up and destroyed our country's history."

Serafia had never heard any of this before, but she didn't doubt the truth of it. Her father had made more than a few mysterious trips to Switzerland over the years. At the same time, the truth didn't make everything okay, either. "So now that you know I don't come from a line of traitors, you've decided you can love me?"

"No. Stop jumping to these horrible conclusions. I'm happy I found out the truth, but no, that's got nothing to do with why I'm here. I had one foot out the door to come see you when all this fell into my lap. But in the end, none of it has to do with us. That's all in the past. What I'm interested in is you and me and the future."

Serafia's breath caught in her throat. She reached a shaky hand out for her wine, hoping it would steady her, but all she could do was hold the glass as he continued to speak.

"I love you, Serafia, with all my heart and all my soul. I am a fool and I don't deserve your love in return, but if someday I could earn it back, I would be the happiest man in the world." Gabriel reached out and took her hand and she was too stunned to pull away.

"I don't just love you. I don't just want you to come back to Alma. I went to Madrid because I wanted to ask your father for his blessing to marry you. I want you to be my queen."

Gabriel slipped out of his chair and onto one knee. Serafia sat stunned as she watched him reach into his inner breast pocket. She saw a momentary flash of gold and realized he was wearing the pocket watch she gave him, but then he pulled out a small ring box and her thoughts completely disintegrated into incoherence.

"I don't know if I'm the right man to be king. But fate has put the crown in my hands and because of you, I feel like I'm closer than I could ever be to the kind of man my people deserve. With you by my side as queen, all my doubts are gone. We can restore Alma to its former glory together. I don't think Alma could ask for a better queen and I couldn't ask for a smarter, more beautiful, graceful and caring bride. Would you do me the honor of being my wife?"

Gabriel opened the box and stunned her with an amazing bloodred ruby with diamonds. It was unlike any ring she'd ever seen before. It was the kind of ring that was fit for royalty.

"This ring belonged to my great-great-grandmother, Queen Josefina. It was her wedding ring and part of the treasure entrusted to your family to protect. Your father returned it to me today. He told me that it belonged on your finger and I quite agree."

Serafia let him slip the ring onto her finger. She couldn't take her eyes off it and couldn't stop thinking about everything it represented. He loved her. He wanted to marry her. He wanted her to be his queen. In that moment, all her doubts and hesitations about being in the spotlight disappeared. Before, she had been there alone. If Gabriel was by her side, it would okay. She couldn't believe how quickly everything in her life had changed.

"Serafia?"

She tore her gaze away from the ring to look at Gabriel. He looked a little confused and a little anxious as he watched her. "Yes?"

"I, uh, asked you a question. Would you like to answer it so I can stop freaking out?"

Serafia smiled, feeling quite silly for missing the critical step in the proposal process. "Yes, Gabriel, I will marry you."

He grinned wide, opening his arms to catch her just as she propelled herself at him. Her lips met his with an enthusiasm she couldn't contain. Just an hour ago, she thought she might never be in his arms again. And here she was…his fiancée. There was a sudden lightness in her heart and she felt as though she had to cling to Gabriel so she wouldn't float away.

"I love you, Serafia," he whispered against her lips.

"I love you, too, Gabriel," she answered, happy to finally say those words out loud.

Gabriel stood up, pulling her up with him. "The coronation is over a month away. I don't want to wait that long to marry you."

She knew exactly how he felt. She would happily elope if she thought they would get away with it. Unfortunately the people of Alma would want their royal wedding. As would her mother. There was no avoiding that. "How quickly do you think we can pull off a wedding?"

"Well," Gabriel said thoughtfully, "my brother's wedding is already in the works. He abdicated, but he's still prince, so father insisted he and Emily have their ceremony in Alma. That's only a few weeks away. What would you say to a double wedding?"

"A double wedding?"

"Why not? They've already got the plans in place. All the same people will be coming. Why can't we have one giant celebration and both marry at the same time?"

Serafia looked at her handsome fiancé thoughtfully. He was not a woman. He didn't understand what kinds of expectations went into a wedding. Serafia might not mind a double wedding, but Emily certainly might.

"How about this…?" she proposed. "You talk to Rafe and Emily about it. If they are both fine with it, then I'm okay with it, too."

Gabriel grinned wide. "I'm sure they will be, but I'll check. And then you'll be Mrs. Gabriel Montoro, soon to be *Su Majestad la Reina Serafia de Alma*. Are you ready for that?"

Serafia wrapped her arms around his neck and nodded. "I think so, although I'm sure that being queen will be the easy part."

Gabriel arched one brow curiously at her. "What's going to be the hard part?"

She climbed to her bare toes and planted a kiss on his full lips. "Keeping the king out of trouble."

* * * * *

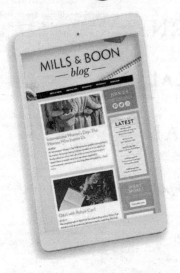

MILLS & BOON

THE HEART OF ROMANCE

A ROMANCE FOR EVERY KIND OF READER

MODERN

Prepare to be swept off your feet by sophisticated, sexy and seductive heroes, in some of the world's most glamourous and romantic locations, where power and passion collide.
8 stories per month.

HISTORICAL

Escape with historical heroes from time gone by. Whether your passion is for wicked Regency Rakes, muscled Vikings or rugged Highlanders, awaken the romance of the past.
6 stories per month.

MEDICAL

Set your pulse racing with dedicated, delectable doctors in the high-pressure world of medicine, where emotions run high and passion, comfort and love are the best medicine.
6 stories per month.

True Love

Celebrate true love with tender stories of heartfelt romance, the rush of falling in love to the joy a new baby can bring, and focus on the emotional heart of a relationship.
8 stories per month.

Desire

Indulge in secrets and scandal, intense drama and plenty of sizzling hot action with powerful and passionate heroes who have it all: wealth, status, good looks…everything but the right woman.
6 stories per month.

HEROES

Experience all the excitement of a gripping thriller, with an intense romance at its heart. Resourceful, true-to-life women and strong fearless men face danger and desire - a killer combination!
8 stories per month.

DARE

Sensual love stories featuring smart, sassy heroines you'd want as a best friend, and compelling intense heroes who are worthy of them.
4 stories per month.

To see which titles are coming soon, please visit

millsandboon.co.uk/nextmonth

JOIN US ON SOCIAL MEDIA!

Stay up to date with our latest releases, author news and gossip, special offers and discounts, and all the behind-the-scenes action from Mills & Boon...

 millsandboon

 millsandboonuk

 millsandboon

might just be true love...

MILLS & BOON
MODERN
Power and Passion

Prepare to be swept off your feet by sophisticated, sexy and seductive heroes, in some of the world's most glamourous and romantic locations, where power and passion collide.

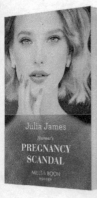
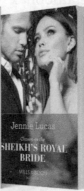
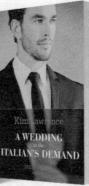
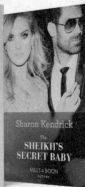